REPRODUCTIVE PRESSURE AND ROYAL COUPLES

BORDERLINES

Further Information and Publications

www.arc-humanities.org/series/book-series/

REPRODUCTIVE PRESSURE AND ROYAL COUPLES

MEDIEVAL ENGLAND AND SCOTLAND, ca. 1200–1400

by

EMMA TRIVETT

ARC HUMANITIES PRESS

British Library Cataloguing in Publication Data
A catalogue record for this book is available from the British Library.

ISBN (Hardback): 9781802702125
e-ISBN (PDF): 9781802704303
e-ISBN (EPUB): 9781802704310

www.arc-humanities.org

Printed and bound in the UK (by CPIGroup [UK] Ltd), USA (by Bookmasters), and elsewhere using print-on-demand technology.

Publisher (manufacturer) details: Arc Humanities Press, 14 Clifton Moor Business Village, James Nicolson Link, York YO30 4XG, United Kingdom.

EU Authorised Representative details (for GPSR purposes): Amsterdam University Press, Nieuwe Prinsengracht 89, 1018 VR Amsterdam, The Netherlands. www.aup.nl

CONTENTS

Acknowledgements and Dedication vi

Abbreviations vii

Royal Introductions 1

The Couples and Their Reproductive Histories 1

Chapter 1. Fertile Ground: Historiographies of Queenship, Kingship, and Infertility 23

Chapter 2. Under Pressure: Contemporary Perceptions of Royal Fertility 43

Chapter 3. Narratives About Royal Childlessness 73

Chapter 4. Cause for Concern: The King's Age, Gender, and Childlessness 97

Chapter 5. Royal Healthcare and Reproductive Medicine 131

Chapter 6. Reproductive Politics: Religious Patronage and Spiritual Support for Royal Fertility 175

Reproductive Outcomes: Conclusions About the Pressure for Royal Fertility 215

Bibliography 221

Index 241

LIST OF TABLES

Table 1. Royal couples from England and Scotland in the thirteenth and fourteenth centuries viii

Table 2. Medicines for Queen Isabella, November 1313 138

ACKNOWLEDGEMENTS AND DEDICATION

THIS BOOK IS based on my PhD from the University of Edinburgh. During my time there, I was supported by a wonderful community of medievalists whose knowledge and insight I am immensely grateful for, none more so than my supervisors, Cordelia Beattie and Zubin Mistry.

I also owe a great debt of gratitude to the History Department at the University of Prince Edward Island, Canada, and particularly Drs. Ed MacDonald, Richard Raiswell, and David Buck, whose encouragement and mentorship led me here; your dedication to your students and your craft still inspires me.

A tremendous, heartfelt thank you to my family, especially my mum and dad. To my parents-in-law, too, who have always made Scotland feel like home. I also had the great pleasure to grow up with grandparents who shared their love and pride for the history of our provinces and families, and nurtured that in me.

Finally, to my own little family: Laing, there are certainly no words that do credit to you and all that you do. Since I finished my PhD, I have become a mother and the struggles and experiences of the royal couples in my research have taken on a more personal meaning. Thank you, Iris and Sorley, for the profound insight that has come from being your mum. I dedicate this to all three of you.

ABBREVIATIONS

CCR	*Calendar of Close Rolls Preserved in the Public Record Office of the Reign of Henry III*. 14 vols. HMSO, 1902–1938.
CDS	*Calendar of Documents Relating to Scotland*. Edited by Joseph Bain. 5 vols. H. M. Public Record Office, 1881–1888.
Chron. Bower	Walter Bower. *Scotichronicon*. Edited by D. E. R. Watt. 9 vols. Aberdeen University Press, 1987–1998.
Chron. Fordun	Johannis de Fordun. *Chronica gentis Scotorum*. Edited by W. F. Skene. Edmonston, 1871.
Chronica majora	Matthew Paris. *Chronica majora*. Edited by Henry R. Luard. 7 vols. Longman, 1872–1883.
CLR	*Calendar of Liberate Rolls Preserved in the Public Record Office of the Reign of Henry III*. 6 vols. HMSO, 1916–1964.
CPL	*Calendar of Papal Letters to Scotland of Benedict XIII of Avignon, 1394–1419*. Edited by F. McGurk. Scottish History Society, 1976.
CPR	*Calendar of Patent Rolls Preserved in the Public Record Office*... HMSO, 1881–.
ER	*Rotuli scaccarii regum Scotorum: The Exchequer Rolls of Scotland*. Edited by John Stuart and George Burnett. 23 vols. H. M. General Register House, 1878–1908.
Flores historiarum	*Flores historiarum*. Edited by Henry R. Luard. 3 vols. HMSO, 1890.
Foedera	Thomas Rymer, ed. *Foedera, conventiones, litterae, et cujuscunque generis acta publica, inter reges Angliae et alios quosvis impeatores, reges, pontifices, principes, vel communitates: Ab ingressu Gulielmi I. in Angliam, A.D. 1066, ad nostra usque tempora habita aut tractate*. 20 vols. 1816.
Historia Anglorum	Matthew Paris. *Historia Anglorum*. Edited by Frederic Madden. 3 vols. Longman, 1866–1868.
HMSO	His/Her Majesty's Stationery Office
ODNB	Oxford Dictionary of National Biography
Rot. Scot.	*Rotuli Scotiae in Turri Londinensi et in Domo Capitulari Westmonasteriensi asservati*. Edited by William Illingworth et al. 2 vols. Eyre, 1814–1819.
RRS	*Regesta regum Scottorum: The Acts of David II, 1329–71*. Edited by Bruce Webster. Edinburgh University Press, 1982.
TNA	The National Archives (Kew)
Wyntoun	Andrew of Wyntoun. *The Orygynale Cronykil of Scotland*. Edited by David Laing. 3 vols. Edmonston, 1872.

Table 1. Royal couples from England and Scotland in the thirteenth and fourteenth centuries

Couples	Marriage date and ages at marriage	Known Births	
Henry III (1207– 1272) Eleanor of Provence (ca. 1223–1291)	1236 Henry (29) Eleanor (12)	1239 Edward 1240 Margaret 1242 Beatrice 1245 Edmund 1253 Katherine	
Edward I (1239–1307) Eleanor of Castile (1241–1290)	1254 Edward (15) Eleanor (13)	1255 daughter ca. 1261/63 Katherine 1265 Joan 1266 John 1268 Henry 1269 Eleanor 1271 daughter 1272 Joan	1273 Alphonso 1275 Margaret 1276 Berengaria 1278 Child (daug 1279 Mary 1280/1? Son 1282 Elizabeth 1284 Edward
Edward II (1284–1327) Isabella of France (ca. 1295–1358)	1308 Edward (24) Isabella (12)	1312 Edward 1316 John 1318 Eleanor 1321 Joan	
Alexander II (1198–1249) Joan Plantagenet (1210–1238)	1221 Alexander (23) Joan (11)		
Alexander III (1241–1286) Margaret of England (1240–1275)	1251 Alexander (10) Margaret (11)	1261 Margaret 1264 Alexander 1272 David	
Alexander III (1241–1286) Yolande de Dreux (1263–1330)	1285 Alexander (44) Yolande (21)		
David II (1324–1371) Joan of the Tower (1321–1362)	1328 David (4) Joan (7)		
David II (1324–1371) Margaret Logie (ca. 1330–ca. 1373)	1363 David (39) Margaret (33)		

Children who died in infancy	Miscarriages/ stillbirths	Illegitimate children and other children
herine d. 1257		
herine d. 1264 a d. 1265 (9 mo) n d. 1271 ry d. 1274 ghter d. 1271 honso d. 1284 engaria d. 1277/78 d (daughter?) d. immediately d. infancy	1255 stillborn daughter 1278 stillborn child?	
	1313 miscarriage or stillbirth?	Adam, illegitimate son of Edward b. before 1305/1306 mother?
		Marjory, illegitimate daughter of Alexander b. before 1221? mother?
	1286 Stillbirth? Fake pregnancy?	
		Margaret had a son from her first marriage

ROYAL INTRODUCTIONS

THE COUPLES AND THEIR REPRODUCTIVE HISTORIES

FOR MANY ROYAL COUPLES in the Middle Ages, concerns about fertility and experiences of reproductive anxiety have gone unstudied. This is because in many cases, such experiences do not fit the limited, medicalized view of "infertility" as the inability to conceive a child.[1] Instead, reproductive difficulties encompassed a broader spectrum of anxieties: delayed conception, pregnancy loss, long intervals between births, and the related experience of high infant mortality that left couples without children. These experiences, scattered across chronicles, administrative records, and devotional practices, reveal that reproductive pressure was a fundamental political reality that shaped royal behaviour, diplomatic relationships, and the performance of medieval kingship and queenship, epitomizing Gayle Davis and Tracy Loughran's observation that "it can seem that infertility is almost everywhere in history, often unrecognized even though it is in full view."[2]

This book focuses on eight royal case studies from thirteenth- and fourteenth-century England and Scotland (Table 1).[3] The indications that these royal couples encountered some kind of reproductive anxiety or difficulty, whether mentioned by their contemporaries or pieced together from other documentary sources for their lives, suggest that pressure for fertility was a significant aspect of medieval monarchy. When examined together, these couples shed light on experiences of infertility. Rather than viewing successful reproduction as evidence of fertility ease, this study demonstrates that even royal couples with fertility "success" navigated complex landscapes of reproductive uncertainty and employed strategies to manage both their bodies and public perceptions of their fertility. This chapter introduces the couples in question and establishes the methodology for including them in this study. It then considers the existing scholarship on these couples, demonstrating how fertility concerns have only been recognized in contexts where couples never produced children—thereby missing the broader story of reproductive anxiety as a feature of medieval royal life.

---

1 Davis and Loughran, "Introduction," 4.

2 Davis and Loughran, "Introduction," 4.

3 Two additional royal marriages will occasionally be considered as well: Alexander II and Marie de Coucy, and Edward I and Margaret of France.

English Royal Case Studies

Henry III (1207–1272) and Eleanor of Provence (ca. 1223–1291)

Henry III became king in 1216 at the age of nine, following the death of his father, King John. He came to the English throne during the crisis of the First Barons' War (1215–1217) and invasion by Prince Louis of France (1216). Hastily crowned at Gloucester, Henry's minority was governed by a regency led by William Marshal and later Hubert de Burgh. The regency government was focused on restoring royal authority after the chaos of civil war and the unpopular reign of John. As part of this, the minority council issued a revised version of Magna Carta in 1216 and again in 1225, helping to re-establish baronial loyalty. After more than a decade as king, Henry declared his majority around 1227, when he was nineteen, and took full control of his government.[4] However, in practice, he continued to rely on the guidance of his mentors, like de Burgh. In 1230, Henry launched a military expedition to reclaim lands in France which had been lost by his father in 1204. Poorly planned and executed, the campaign ended in failure and was widely criticized in England.

Henry married Eleanor of Provence in 1236, but she was not the first woman considered to become his queen. Several other potential brides were proposed, including Margaret, sister of Alexander II of Scotland, and Jeanne de Ponthieu. In 1234–1235, negotiations for marriage to Jeanne progressed to the stage that Henry sought formal papal dispensation because the couple was too closely related, but the match was ultimately abandoned. Shortly after, negotiations began with the House of Savoy and Henry married Eleanor in 1236. Eleanor's arrival in England brought an influx of her foreign Savoyard relatives and Henry granted them lands, offices, and English marriages. The growing influence of the Savoyards provoked resentment among the English barons and sowed seeds of political tension that deepened in the following decades and eventually erupted in the 1250s–1260s.

During their reign, Henry and Eleanor faced mounting opposition over their favouritism, extravagant spending, and failed foreign ventures, particularly Henry's attempt to secure the Sicilian crown for their second son, Edmund. These tensions alienated the king from his nobles and led to the Second Barons' War (1264–1267), during which Henry was briefly captured by the baronial leader, Simon de Montfort's forces. Eleanor went to France to raise funds and political support for the royalist cause, and their

4 Carpenter, *Henry III*, 44.

son, Edward (later Edward I), restored royal authority after defeating Montfort in battle in 1265. After the war, Henry's authority was re-established, but power increasingly shifted toward Edward. After Henry's death in 1272, Eleanor retired to Amesbury Priory, where she lived until her death in 1291.

Henry III and Eleanor of Provence have not previously been considered in studies of infertility and they did ultimately have children together, but contemporary comments about Eleanor's fertility make them an important case for consideration in this book. When they were married, Eleanor was twelve and Henry was twenty-eight.[5] They seem to have consummated their marriage relatively soon after their wedding: there are surviving instructions for their chambers to be connected by passageways in 1237 and they were certainly sharing the same bedchamber by 1238, when Henry survived an assassination attempt in his own chamber because he was sleeping in the queen's.[6] Henry and Eleanor had a close relationship and were frequently together in the early years of their marriage, so there were no lengthy periods of separation that would have initially prevented a pregnancy.[7]

Their first child, Edward, was born in 1239 but not before contemporary chronicler Matthew Paris claimed, in 1238, that "it was greatly feared that the queen was barren."[8] Henry and Eleanor had three more children between 1240 and 1245—Margaret (b. 1240), Beatrice (b. 1242), and Edmund (b. 1245)—followed by no births or evidence of further pregnancies for nearly a decade until their last child, Katherine, was born in 1253.[9] The starting point for my research was Paris's comment about Eleanor's fertility in 1238 because of the ostensible association of infertility exclusively with the very young queen (she was just fourteen), and the fact that this contemporary concern about fertility has gone unexplained by scholars. The lack of historiographical interest demonstrates how concerns about a royal couple's fertility have been overshadowed by our knowledge that they ultimately went on to have children. This approach has influenced how (and

5 Howell, *Eleanor of Provence*, 14–15.

6 *Chronica majora*, ed. Luard, 3:497; *CLR*, 1:305; Carpenter, *Henry III*, 181–82.

7 Carpenter, *Henry III*, 180–81. Henry and Eleanor did have a period when they were not on good terms, in 1251/2, when they were on opposing sides in a dispute between their respective relations, the Savoyards and Lusignans: Howell, *Eleanor of Provence*, 64–70. This period immediately preceded the conception and birth of their final child, Katherine, in 1253.

8 *Chronica majora*, ed. Luard, 3:518: "Timebatur enim vehementer, quod regina sterilis fuisset." English translations are my own unless otherwise stated.

9 Howell, *Eleanor of Provence*, 70.

whose) fertility has been studied—existing scholarship on all eight of the royal couples offers very little sense of when, why and to what extent contemporaries were interested in royal fertility.

Edward I of England (1239–1307) and Eleanor of Castile (ca. 1241–1290)

Edward and Eleanor of Castile were married in 1254 as part of a diplomatic alliance to secure English interests in Gascony and strengthen ties with Castile.[10] Edward was the eldest son of Henry III and Eleanor of Provence, and he became a key political figure in his father's later reign. Eleanor, the daughter of Ferdinand III of Castile and Jeanne of Ponthieu, brought valuable continental claims, including the county of Ponthieu, to her marital family. The couple's marriage seems to have evolved into a strong political and emotional partnership and Eleanor accompanied Edward on the Ninth Crusade (1270–1272). While they were on crusade in 1272, Henry III died, and Edward and Eleanor returned home for their coronation in 1274. Unique amongst the other royal couples in this book, Edward and Eleanor were married for almost two decades before they became king and queen.

As king, Edward I pursued an ambitious agenda of military expansion, legal reform, and centralized governance. His campaigns in Wales resulted in its conquest and annexation in 1284, and he launched prolonged efforts to bring Scotland under English overlordship, beginning the Wars of Scottish Independence in 1296. Eleanor played an important role in royal administration and shrewdly managed her extensive estates, helping to bolster the crown's resources.

Edward deeply mourned Eleanor after her death in 1290, and memorialized her with the Eleanor Crosses, a series of lavish monuments along the route of her funeral procession from Lincoln to London. In 1299, he married Margaret of France, half-sister of the French King Philip IV, to secure peace with France. Though Edward was forty years older than his second queen, they had three children together, Thomas (b. 1300–d. 1338), Edmund (b. 1301–d. 1330), and Eleanor (b. 1305–d. 1311). Margaret is considered in Chapter 5, in discussion about queens and medical care, but her marriage to Edward I is not one of the eight primary case studies of this investigation because there is no indication that they experienced any version of infertility together. It is, however, important to mention their union because it was part of the broader context of Edward I's reproductive life.

---

10 Parsons, *Eleanor of Castile*, 15–17.

Edward I and Eleanor of Castile are a primary case study in this book because they experienced high rates of birth combined with very high infant mortality. When they were married, Edward was fifteen and Eleanor was about thirteen.[11] Within months of their wedding, Eleanor gave birth in May 1255—only about six or seven months into the pregnancy—to a daughter who was likely stillborn.[12] After this, they were perhaps separated to prevent further pregnancies until they were older; at least, there is no evidence that they conceived again until the early 1260s.[13] Six children were born between the early 1260s and 1272, when Edward and Eleanor became king and queen, but only two of those children survived infancy and early childhood.[14] After becoming king and queen, Edward and Eleanor had nine or ten more children together, but their experiences of loss are starkly highlighted by the fact that Edward I was succeeded in 1307 by the couple's youngest child and only surviving son, Edward II.[15]

A key premise of this book is to study the reproductive pressure and experiences of royal couples who do not fit the conventional, medicalized definition of "infertility" as the inability to conceive. Certainly, Edward I and Eleanor did not struggle to conceive. They had a total of fifteen or sixteen pregnancies together, but their experiences of stillbirth, possibly being kept apart for birth control, and prolific, recurrent and unusually high rates of infant and child mortality are an important inclusion in this study of the pressure on royal couples to produce an heir.[16]

11 There is uncertainty about the year of Eleanor's birth: Parsons, "Year of Eleanor of Castile's Birth," 245–49, reasons that she was born ca. 1240–1241.

12 Parsons, "Year of Eleanor of Castile's Birth," 257.

13 Parsons, "Year of Eleanor of Castile's Birth," 257–58.

14 Parsons, *Eleanor of Castile*, 24: Katherine (b. ca. 1261), Joan (b. 1264)—both died by 1265—John (b. 1266), Henry (b. 1268), Eleanor (b. 1269), and a daughter (b. 1271). Only Henry and Eleanor survived after 1272, but Henry died in 1274. See *The Chronicle of Bury St. Edmunds*, ed. Gransden, 49, for John's death in 1272 (under 1271 in the chronicle).

15 Edward and Eleanor probably had a total of fifteen or sixteen children together: Parsons, *Eleanor of Castile*, 33.

16 Parsons, "The Year of Eleanor of Castile's Birth," 257–65. Howell, "Royal Women," 169, for a comparison of Eleanor and Edward's family size with that of other medieval English and French royal couples, who had between three and seven children. Howell suggests that Edward and Eleanor's high birthrate was a response to the high mortality rate of their children. See Orme, *Medieval Children*, 113 for discussion of medieval child and infant mortality rates.

Eleanor and Edward's reproductive history also typifies a broader challenge in the history of (in)fertility, and medieval women more generally: despite Eleanor's many pregnancies, it is frustratingly difficult to determine precise details of the births and even the number and outcome of some of her pregnancies are unclear, despite her position as queen. This confusion reflects a wider issue in the contemporary sources and the approach in historiography, where reproductive lives are not recorded in full and attention is focused on only the surviving births, particularly of heirs, without concern or consideration for the mother's experience.

Edward II of England (1284–1327) and Isabella of France (ca. 1295–1358)

Edward II and Isabella of France were married in 1308 to solidify a diplomatic alliance between England and France. Edward had succeeded his father, Edward I, the year before and his marriage to Isabella, daughter of Philip IV of France, was intended to resolve tensions over the English holdings in Gascony. The union was politically significant but increasingly personally strained because Edward had emotionally close and possibly sexual relationships with male favourites, first with Piers Gaveston and later Hugh Despenser the Younger. The nature of these relationships is debated in scholarship but certainly the king's reliance on his favourites ultimately sidelined Isabella and alienated the nobility by the end of his reign.[17]

Despite scholarly interest in Edward II's sexuality, the primary sources for Edward's reign describe his preference for his favourites, but they do not characterize those relationships as sexual.[18] My focus is on the contemporary perceptions of Edward and Isabella's wait for an heir and reproductive difficulties so the following chapters will consider how contemporary sources mentioned the king's attention to his favourites as it related to royal fertility, but Edward II's sexual identity—if we can even retrospectively assign such a label—and the nature of his relationships are beyond the scope of this book.[19] Contemporaries criticized Edward II's unmanliness, but not on the grounds of his sexuality or the sexual nature of his relationships with

17 Edward II's sexuality has received much scholarly attention. For example, see Dodd and Musson, eds., *The Reign of Edward II*, particularly, Ormrod, "The Sexualities of Edward II," 22–47. For earlier work, see Chaplais, *Piers Gaveston*. Recently, Warner, *Edward II,* claims that Edward II was bisexual.

18 Fletcher, *Richard II*, 136–37.

19 It is important to note that defined categories, such as "homosexual" did not necessarily exist in the Middle Ages, and medieval authors tended to describe acts, such as "sodomy" instead: Arnold, "Gender and Sexuality," 174.

favourites. Labels such as "homosexual" or "bisexual" are products of later interpretation rather than contemporary description.[20]

Another feature of his rule, Edward's reign was marked by ongoing war with Scotland, and ultimately, his military defeat by the Scots at the Battle of Bannockburn in 1314. Peace was not officially agreed until 1328 but Robert the Bruce's position as King of Scots was significantly strengthened after his success at Bannockburn. Edward also failed to decisively defend or support his northern counties against recurrent raids from the Scots. Nobles like Thomas of Lancaster became increasingly resentful of the king's inaction in the north and Edward's weak response to defending this region was a key factor in the wider breakdown of support for his rule and eventual collapse of his authority in the mid-1320s.

By 1325, relations between Isabella and Edward were deeply strained by Edward's promotion of his favourite, Hugh Despenser the Younger. Isabella went to France on a diplomatic mission at the court of her brother, Charles IV, joined by her eldest son, Prince Edward. While in France, she allied with the exiled nobleman Roger Mortimer and, leveraging her powerful position of possessing Edward II's heir, refused the king's request to return to England with their son. She and Mortimer raised a mercenary army and invaded England in 1326.[21] Edward II was deposed, and Isabella had their fourteen-year-old son, Edward, installed as king in 1327. Edward II was imprisoned and died later that year under suspicious circumstances.[22]

Isabella acted as regent during the minority of her son, Edward III, until he seized power in 1330 and ended her and Mortimer's control. Mortimer was executed and Isabella lost much of her political authority, but Edward III treated her with respect as his mother and a dowager queen and allowed her to retain her titles and estates. Isabella withdrew from active court life but continued to engage in religious patronage and some ceremonial duties as the king's mother until her death in 1358.

Like the other two English queens in this study, Isabella was twelve when she married Edward in 1308; Edward was twenty-three.[23] Their first child, Edward, was born four years later, in 1312. Edward and Isabella went on to

---

20 See Seymour Phillip's discussion of Edward's reputation in the centuries following his death: Phillips, *Edward II*, 5–32.

21 Phillips, *Edward II*, 455–519.

22 Phillips, *Edward II*, 560–65, 567. Phillips explains that there was not seemingly immediate suspicion around Edward's death but there were subsequent theories, for example that he had escaped and was still alive in 1330.

23 Phillips, *Edward II*, 132.

have three more children, John (b. 1316), Eleanor (b. 1318), and Joan (b. 1321–future wife of David II).[24] There was a four-year gap between Edward's birth in 1312 and John's in 1316, and there is a surviving list from Isabella's apothecary which suggests she suffered a miscarriage or stillbirth between these births.[25]

Edward and Isabella were not childless for particularly long, and they ultimately had multiple children, yet the delays between pregnancies and the evidence that Isabella received medicines from her apothecary for a miscarriage or stillbirth in 1313 suggests that they experienced some reproductive difficulty and loss. Such experiences of miscarriage and stillbirth are key to studying reproductive difficulty as more than struggling to conceive a child. Furthermore, the similarities between the couples Edward II and Isabella of France, and Henry III and Eleanor of Provence, particularly the queens' age at marriage and the delay before their first pregnancies make these couples interesting comparative cases for investigating the conditions that sparked contemporary attention to a couple's fertility and the problematization of childlessness.

Introducing Isabella and Edward II's case raises a point about terminology: the modern medical distinctions between miscarriage and stillbirth are based on gestational age but I use both terms here because it is impossible to determine the gestation of Isabella's pregnancy in 1313. Modern medicine describes "miscarriage" as loss before twenty-four weeks gestation, and "stillbirth" as loss later in pregnancy, at least after twenty-four weeks gestation.[26] Medieval medical usage was less precise, and medical texts describe birth of a dead fetus, without reference to gestational age.[27] I continue to describe Isabella's loss as "miscarriage or stillbirth" to leave space for two very different experiences: a loss at seven weeks would have been a significantly different experience from one at thirty-six weeks, for instance.

---

24 Phillips, *Edward II*, 102.

25 It is difficult to distinguish a miscarriage from stillbirth using the apothecary list because many of the ingredients in medicinal remedies for miscarriage and stillbirth were similar. This is discussed in Chapter 5.

26 See the *Oxford Concise Medical Dictionary*.

27 For instance, *Trotula*, 97 (miscarriage), 101 (death of fetus during labour), 103 (dead fetus), 123 (dead fetus).

Scottish Royal Case Studies

The remaining royal case studies come from Scotland. The five couples under consideration in the following chapters are Alexander II and Joan Plantagenet, Alexander III and his two queens, Margaret of England and Yolande de Dreux, and David II and his two queens, Joan of the Tower and Margaret Logie. Concern about the royal succession defines late thirteenth- and fourteenth-century Scottish history. Succession became the most pressing issue of the political realm at the end of Alexander III's reign, when he died unexpectedly in 1286, at the age of forty-four. He was predeceased by his three adult children from his first marriage and he and his new queen, Yolande, had not yet produced a child. As a result, the only surviving direct heir to the Scottish throne was Alexander's three-year-old granddaughter, Margaret, daughter of the king of Norway. In 1290, on her way to claim her throne, six-year-old Margaret died, and Scotland was left with no clear heir. Following Alexander's death in 1286, a group of leading nobles, clergy, and royal officials formed a provisional guardianship to maintain stability, safeguard the independence of the kingdom, and oversee the selection of the next ruler.[28] Faced with multiple claimants to the throne from leading Scottish noble families, most notably John Balliol and Robert Bruce, 5th Lord of Annandale (grandfather to King Robert I, "Robert the Bruce"), the guardians invited Edward I of England to arbitrate in 1291. Edward exploited the situation and used his role to assert his overlordship in Scotland. This ultimately led to the Wars of Independence between England and Scotland, which dominated the reigns of Robert I and his son, David II, in the fourteenth century.

This is important context for understanding the reproductive pressure experienced by Scottish royal couples because the succession crisis of the late thirteenth century left a lasting imprint on Scottish political consciousness and profoundly shaped attitudes toward royal succession in the fourteenth century. Alexander III's death without a direct, mature heir, and the succession chaos that followed, reinforced the view that Scotland's sovereignty depended on firm, undisputed royal succession. It also fostered a lasting vigilance amongst the Scottish elite to resist foreign impute and a desire to safeguard national sovereignty. The idea of a community of the realm, or collective responsibility for the rule of the realm, was a defining part of the Scottish political context, and the role of the guardians in the wake of the events of 1286–1290 showed that political authority

28 Duncan, *Kingship of the Scots*, 175–76.

in Scotland could be exercised collectively, especially when the monarchy was weakened or in dispute.[29]

By the time of the succession crisis, the idea that the kingdom's leading magnates and clergy had a collective role and responsibility for the kingdom's governance, particularly during periods when the monarchy was weak or unsettled was not new.[30] Earlier in the thirteenth century, during Alexander II's reign, royal councils and assemblies composed of leading nobility and clergy met with increasing regularity.[31] Although by no means well-defined or fully established by this point, these bodies acted as traditional advisors to the king and they began to see themselves as guardians of the kingdom's laws and interests.[32] During the minority of Alexander III, a group of guardians chosen from the kingdom's elite governed on behalf of the child king.[33] This period reinforced the principle that the realm could be governed by its community when the monarch was unable to rule directly.[34] Therefore, when Alexander III died in 1286, there was already some precedent for electing a group of guardians to defend the kingdom's laws, independence and ensure continuity of governance.

The concept of the community of the realm and governance by guardians also shaped attitudes towards a female heir in Scotland. Like in 1286 when Alexander III's granddaughter, Margaret, Maid of Norway, was accepted as heir to the throne, there were other points when the Scottish political community were accepting of a female heir, or the possibility of a female heir. For instance, in 1261, when Alexander III's first child, Margaret, was born, she was acknowledged as his heir. Willingness to have a female heir must not be interpreted as evidence of a less misogynistic culture in medieval Scotland or a readiness for female rule; a male heir and ruler was still far preferable.[35]

---

29 Reid, *Alexander III*, 5–41; Reid and Penman, "Guardian–Lieutenant–Governor," 191–218; Reid, "The Kingless Kingdom," 105–29; McQueen, "Parliament, the Guardians and John Balliol," 29–49.

30 Reid, *Alexander III*, 36–37; Taylor, *Shape of the State*, 444–55; Oram, *Alexander II*, 27; Stringer, "Kingship, Conflict and State-making," 107.

31 Reid, *Alexander III*, 59; Brown and Tanner, eds., *Parliament and Politics in Scotland*, 1–29; Stringer, "The Scottish 'Political Community,'" 53–84.

32 Reid, *Alexander III*, 59.

33 Reid, *Alexander III*, 75–90.

34 Reid, *Alexander III*, 35–40, 87–90. For more on minorities, see: Ward, *Royal Childhood and Child Kingship*; Dean, "Crowing the Child," 254–80.

35 For a nuanced interpretation of female inheritance in medieval Scotland, see Davis, "Elite Women and Power," 43–51.

Rather, the Scottish elite were open to a female heir because of the collective approach to rulership that had become necessary during previous royal minorities in the twelfth and thirteenth centuries, including Alexander III's own.[36] The political community's support for Margaret in 1261 and the Maid of Norway in 1286 reflected a pragmatic political attitude focused on avoiding civil war and external interference in Scottish affairs.

Alexander II (1198–1249) and Joan Plantagenet (1210–1238)

Alexander II became king in 1216, at the age of sixteen. He had three sisters, but he was his father, William the Lion's only legitimate male heir. From the beginning of his reign, Alexander was focused on consolidating royal authority in Scotland and centralizing Scottish kingship.[37] Despite his youth, Alexander proved himself to be an effective and actively involved warrior king. Relations with England were tense from 1215, when Alexander sided with English barons in their dispute with the English king, John, and he invaded England with his Scottish forces. A peace was agreed in 1217 between Alexander and John's son, the new king, Henry III; as a further act of diplomacy between the two kingdoms, Alexander married Joan Plantagenet, Henry's sister, in 1221.[38]

Queen Joan was active in Anglo-Scottish relations and continued to support diplomacy between her husband and her brother, Henry III.[39] In September 1237, she and Alexander joined Henry III and Eleanor of Provence at York, where they agreed the Treaty of York, which resolved the territorial dispute over border lands between the two kingdoms.[40] When Alexander II returned home, Joan remained in England to go on pilgrimage; she died the following spring, in 1238, at the age of twenty-eight and was buried at Tarrant Crawford Abbey in Dorset.[41] Less than a year later, in 1239, Alexander married Marie de Coucy (ca. 1218–1285), a French noblewoman. Alexander and Marie had one child together in 1241, the future Alexander III.[42] Alexan-

36 Reid, *Alexander III*, 157–58; Reid, "The Kingless Kingdom," 105–29; Ward, *Royal Childhood*, 225–28.

37 Oram, *Alexander II*, 149–91.

38 Oram, *Alexander II*, 108–9.

39 Oram, *Alexander II*, 138.

40 Oram, *Alexander II*, 144–45.

41 Oram, *Alexander II*, 147–48.

42 Oram, *Alexander II*, 156–57. Marie de Coucy and Alexander II's marriage is not one of the primary marriages considered in this study because they had a child together without much delay, so it is difficult to justify this as a case of infertility.

der II's reign was marked by his efforts to extend royal authority both within Scotland and beyond its traditional borders, particularly through campaigns in Argyll and attempts to take control of the Hebrides which were under Norwegian rule. He died suddenly in 1249 on the Isle of Kerrera, while preparing for a military campaign against Norway, and his seven-year-old son became king.

Alexander II and Joan Plantagenet are one of the few couples included in this book whose story is marked by infertility as conventionally—and narrowly—understood by earlier historians as the inability to conceive.[43] When they married in 1221, Joan was eleven and Alexander was twenty-three.[44] They were married for almost two decades until Joan's death in 1238, but they never had any children together and there is no evidence that Joan was ever pregnant. Alexander II did have an illegitimate daughter, Marjory, who was probably born before his marriage to Joan.[45] Alexander and his second queen, Marie, are not a primary consideration in this study, but Alexander's subsequent fertility in his second marriage is important comparative context for considering the perceptions of his first queen, who remained childless.

Alexander III of Scotland (1241–1286) and Margaret of England (1240–1275); Yolande de Dreux (1263–1330)

Following the premature death of his father, Alexander III became king in 1249, at the age of seven. His majority reign was a period often considered a golden age in medieval Scotland, marked by internal stability and economic prosperity. He was focused on securing Scottish independence, strengthening royal authority, and maintaining peaceful relations, particularly with England. One of Alexander's most significant achievements was the assertion of Scottish sovereignty over the western seaboard. Carrying on from the efforts of his father and the conflict with Norway over control of the Hebrides, Alexander successfully concluded the Treaty of Perth in 1266, which transferred the Hebrides and the Isle of Man to Scottish control.[46] This consolidated and extended royal authority further in Scotland than ever before.

---

43 See Davis and Loughran, "Introduction," 8.

44 Oram, *Alexander II*, 68–69.

45 Oram, *Alexander II*, 134, 155, claims that the king's illegitimate daughter affected perceptions of the couple's infertility by serving as proof of Alexander's fertility. See Chapter 4.

46 Reid, *Alexander III*, 189–97.

Alexander III and Margaret of England, daughter of Henry III and Eleanor of Provence, were married in 1251.[47] The marriage, celebrated during Alexander's minority, reinforced peace between Scotland and England and signalled a period of good relations between the kingdoms. Alexander's ability to maintain autonomy while keeping diplomatically close ties with Queen Margaret's natal family was a hallmark of their marriage and his kingship.

The couple had three children together, before Margaret's death in 1275. However, by 1284, Alexander was predeceased by all three of their adult children, creating a dynastic crisis and leaving him with only his infant granddaughter as his heir.[48] This situation was intensified by the fact that Alexander was his father's only legitimate child and, therefore, there were no siblings or their children who could supplement the royal line of succession. In 1285, to produce a new heir, Alexander married a French noblewoman, Yolande of Dreux. Unluckily, in 1286, Alexander died unexpectedly after he fell from his horse during a late-night journey in Fife. Yolande later claimed to be pregnant, but there is no evidence that a living heir was born.[49]

Alexander III was only ten and Margaret was eleven when they were married in 1251. Unsurprisingly, given their age, they did not have a child for some time. Their first child, named Margaret, was born in 1261, a decade after their wedding. Their second child, Alexander, was born in 1264. In an interesting parallel with Margaret's parents, who also had their final child after a long period without conceiving, Margaret and Alexander had nine years without any other (known) pregnancies before the birth of their third and final child, David, in 1273.[50]

Despite the wait for an heir, there are no explicit expressions of concern from contemporaries about Alexander and Margaret's fertility in the 1250s. However, the Scottish magnates prepared in 1260 to accept the couple's first child as Alexander's heir, regardless of sex. When Margaret was born in 1261, she was acknowledged as her father's heir.[51] If not outright concern about fertility, specifically, this response reflects the contemporary attention to the

---

47 Reid, *Alexander III*, 139; Staniland, "The Nuptials of Alexander III of Scotland and Margaret Plantagenet," 22.

48 Reid, *Alexander III*, 340–41.

49 Reid, *Alexander III*, 273–74. Reid cites *Chron. Bower*, ed. Watt, 6:10–11, who claims that Yolande was pregnant, but the birth either failed to take place or ended with a stillbirth. Reid concludes that there is no other surviving evidence for a pregnancy and moves on in his analysis.

50 Reid, *Alexander III*, 215, 264, 290.

51 See discussion in Chapter 2.

fact that there were no other clear heirs to the Scottish throne if Alexander was to die unexpectedly. Margaret and Alexander are a key inclusion in this study of the pressure for royal fertility. The long wait for their first child, coupled with their youth at the time of their wedding offers the chance to consider how concerns about childlessness were related to age and number of childless years.

Alexander III and his second queen, Yolande de Dreux are also one of the primary case studies in this book. Although they were only married for less than a year before the king's premature death, the immense pressure to secure the succession after the deaths of Alexander's adult children makes their marriage a valuable inclusion in this study. Notably, the suggestion that Yolande claimed she was pregnant after Alexander's death but never produced a child requires focused consideration.

David II (1324–1371) and Joan of the Tower (1321–1362); Margaret Logie (ca. 1330–ca. 1373)

David II and Joan of the Tower, and David and his second wife Margaret Logie are the final two case studies under scrutiny. David was the only surviving son of Robert I ("Robert the Bruce"), and he became king in 1329 at the age of five.[52] The year before his accession, David was married to seven-year-old Joan of the Tower, the youngest daughter of Edward II and Isabella of France.[53] David's minority reign was filled with considerable political instability in Scotland and continued war with England. Following the usurpation of the Scottish throne by Edward Balliol in 1332 (supported by Edward III), David and Joan were forced into exile. In 1334, they fled to France for safety, where they were received by Philip VI. They spent seven years in exile at Château Gaillard in Normandy, under the protection of the French crown, strengthening the alliance between Scotland and France.[54]

After returning to Scotland in 1341, aged seventeen, David worked to establish a power base of support in his kingdom. Despite a strong start, he was wounded and captured by Edward III's forces during the Battle of Neville's Cross in 1346 and spent the next eleven years as a prisoner in England (1346–1357).[55] Terms for David's release were debated throughout his

---

52 Penman, *David II*, 34–37.

53 Penman, *David II*, 18.

54 Penman, *David II*, 52–53, 72.

55 Penman, *David II*, 181. He was captured at the Battle of Neville's Cross in October 1346.

imprisonment and one of the key proposals centred on a succession-peace deal: Edward III proposed that if David died without a biological heir, the Scottish crown would pass to one of Edward's sons, likely John of Gaunt, and the ransom owed for David's release would be settled. David promoted the proposal, but the Scottish political community strongly resisted the plan and wholeheartedly rejected it. An agreement for David's release was finally reached in 1357 with the Treaty of Berwick and he returned home to Scotland, owing a huge annual ransom to Edward III for his freedom.

By the time David was released, he and Joan had still not produced any children together and there is no evidence that they had ever conceived. This was not simply because the couple was apart for more than a decade: Joan was granted leave by Edward III, her brother, to visit David in England during his imprisonment.[56] However, when David returned to Scotland, Joan stayed in England with her natal family and died there in 1362.[57]

In spring 1363, David married Margaret Logie, who had probably already been his mistress since the beginning of the decade.[58] Margaret was a Scottish noblewoman who had been previously married and produced a son.[59] David and Margaret had no children together and by 1369 the king seems to have been working on casting aside his second wife in order to marry Agnes Dunbar, another (younger) Scottish noblewoman.[60] David died in 1371, unexpectedly but seemingly of natural causes at the age of forty-six, before he was able to remarry, and without ever producing any biological children.[61]

The absence of a biological heir looms particularly large in the sources for David II's reign: continued childlessness became a precondition for his creative attempt to settle the crippling ransom that was owed to Edward III. To absolve the debt in the 1360s, David pushed his council to accept the succession-peace deal and admit an English prince into the Scottish succession, if he died without producing an heir. David's willingness to take an English prince as his heir was also motivated by his strained relationship with his nephew and heir-presumptive, Robert the Steward (future Robert

56 *Rot. Scot.*, ed. Illingworth et al., 1:729 (1349, for her valet to travel to England), 760 (1352, safe conduct for Joan to travel to England), 822 (1358, safe conduct for Joan to go to England).

57 Penman, *David II*, 204.

58 Penman, *David II*, 269.

59 Penman, *David II*, 247–48.

60 Penman, *David II*, 373–74.

61 Penman, *David II*, 412.

II).[62] Their relationship affected much of David's adult reign and politics, and the power dynamic would have been significantly shifted in David's favour if he had produced his own child to disinherit his nephew, or if his English succession-peace deal with Edward III had been accepted by the Scottish magnates and displaced the Steward in the line of succession.

David II and his two queens are key case studies in this book. Not only was royal childlessness central to the policies that David pursued in the 1360s, as the absence of his own biological heir made it possible to negotiate with Edward III using the dynastic succession as leverage, but David's childlessness in his second marriage, with Margaret Logie offers the chance to investigate the assignment of blame for infertility; how did contemporaries view the couple's fertility given Margaret's fertility in her first marriage but David's childlessness in his?

Historiography of the Couples

The historiographical approach to the eight royal couples and their fertility has been varied. All six kings have received attention from scholars, predominantly in political histories.[63] The three queens of England, Eleanor of Provence, Eleanor of Castile, and Isabella of France, have also interested scholars since the growth of queenship studies in the 1990s.[64] Comparatively, there is a lack of gendered analysis of Scottish medieval queenship and there are still no full-length studies of any of the five Scottish queens; they have been considered only incidentally in the scholarship on their husbands.[65]

---

62 For David's relationship with his nephew and a nuanced reading of the Scottish support for David's proposed succession deal, see Boardman, *The Early Stewart Kings*, 1–38, esp. 19–21 for the succession deal.

63 Carpenter, *Henry III*, 1; Phillips, *Edward II*; Prestwich, *Edward I, King of England*; Oram, *Alexander II*; Reid, *Alexander III*; Reid, *Scotland in the Reign of Alexander III 1249–1286*; Penman, *David II*.

64 Howell, *Eleanor of Provence*; Parsons, *Eleanor of Castile*; Benz St. John, *Three Medieval Queens*.

65 Jessica Nelson's PhD thesis on thirteenth-century Scottish queenship is somewhat of an exception, discussed in more detail in Chapter 1. Otherwise, relatively recent histories of the kings and queens of Scotland continue to discuss the queens in relation to the value of their marital alliance and their contribution/impact on the succession. For example, Duncan, *The Kingship of the Scots*, 65, 123; Oram, ed. *The Kings and Queens of Scotland*, 59, 61, 64. A representative example of the dynamic in scholarship is Fiona Downie's chapter, "Queenship in Late Medieval Scotland," 232–54. Consideration of late medieval Scottish queenship and its part in rulership is limited in this volume to Downie's chapter, which is treated quite separately from the rest of the volume.

The Scottish kings have been studied differently from their English counterparts too, in the sense that they have not received gendered analysis. As this book demonstrates, there is no reason why Scottish kings and queens cannot be studied in this way. With respect to fertility, there is an all-or-nothing quality in the historiographical approach, and it is only discussed when a marriage ended up childless, but never examined otherwise. When these couples' fertility *has* been considered by historians, there is a tendency to fixate on queens and to investigate reproductive difficulties in relation to queenship. A new methodological move in this present study is to consider fertility as a quality and experience of the royal couple.

Historiography for the eight couples approaches their fertility significantly differently depending on whether they had children or not. Scholars only mention the fertility of the kings when their marriages remained childless. The main studies of both Alexander II and David II do acknowledge that childlessness had some effect on the reigns, but infertility is ultimately treated as a side issue—more of a personal disappointment than significant political matter—for both kings. Richard Oram states that Alexander II and Joan Plantagenet were infertile and he suggests that Alexander's desire to produce an heir motivated several of his actions in the 1230s.[66] In his study of David II, Michael Penman acknowledges that childlessness influenced some of David's political actions in the 1350s and 1360s.[67] However, he tends to approach childlessness as a fixed condition, rather than something which was unpredictable and actively negotiated by the royal couples, and which might have significantly contributed to perceptions of David II's masculinity and kingship.[68] Oram and Penman both acknowledge that not having a bio-

66 Oram, *Alexander II*, 216–23.

67 For instance, Penman, *David II*, 156, 165.

68 Penman does not approach infertility with precision: for instance, he says that David's political standing could have been improved by producing an heir in 1345 (when he was twenty-one), but he "was childless and likely to stay that way, for he may already have become estranged from Queen Joan or have shown himself to be incapable of fatherhood, even with mistresses," *David II*, 113. Penman later states that David and Joan's relationship might have improved, and the king had "only turned-twenty-five years old in March 1349—attaining his official majority—and he must have been confident in his ability to have children"; *David II*, 156. Penman does not signal why having turned twenty-five in March would have necessarily made David particularly confident in his fertility, especially after claiming that the twenty-one-year-old king was thought to be incapable of reproducing. Ultimately, Penman's approach to David's childlessness seems framed by the knowledge that the king had a known successor in his nephew, Robert the Steward, who would become king after David died without producing his own biological heir. This knowledge seems

logical heir affected the political dynamics and circumstances of Alexander II and David II's reigns, respectively, but their works are not gendered analyses of medieval kingship nor royal infertility.

Conversely, fertility and the importance of their reproductive duty is at the centre of the historical analysis of Alexander and David's queens. There are no full-length studies of Joan of the Tower or Margaret Logie, but they appear intermittently in work on David II. Penman mentions Joan when the details of her life impacted David's, primarily the possible breakdown of the royal marriage and separation after 1357–1358, and the impact that living apart had (and was perceived to have had by contemporaries) on the couple's ability to produce an heir.[69] He describes Margaret Logie mainly in relation to her reproductive value, stating that when David and Margaret married in 1363, she was in her mid-thirties, "a little old for a royal bride" but "undoubtedly fertile" because she had produced a son in a previous marriage.[70] Penman's discussion of the queens appears mostly in the context of mentioning David's childlessness, reflecting the assumption that a queen's most significant role was to produce an heir.[71] He acknowledges that David felt pressure to produce an heir and frequently describes it as *his* infertility, while also ultimately relying on unchallenged assumptions about the importance of fertility for queens.[72] This approach implies the misleading presumption that David's queens were insignificant because they never produced heirs.

Scholarship on Joan Plantagenet is also fixated on her childlessness. Jessica Nelson argues that Joan's failure to produce a child in sixteen years of marriage with Alexander II prevented the queen from being fully accepted in her marital land and role as queen of Scotland. On the basis of Joan's limited political influence and posthumous commemoration in Scotland, Nelson claims that this queen's liminal position was because she was childless.[73] This interpretation relies too heavily on an assumption about the automatically marginalizing consequences of infertility for queens and the retrospective knowledge that Joan would never have a child; instead, we must analyze

---

to have affected Penman's interpretation of David and his queens' experience of and perspective on their own infertility.

69 Penman, *David II*, 204–41.

70 Penman, *David II*, 271.

71 Penman, *David II*, 327.

72 Penman, *David II*, 113, for instance.

73 Nelson, "Queens and Queenship," 164–89.

the pressure on Joan *and* Alexander for fertility before Joan's premature death when she was only twenty-seven.

Fixating on childlessness in connection with queens can generate misleading pictures. For example, Matthew Hammond argued that the foundation and dedication of Balmerino Abbey in Fife was in response to Joan Plantagenet's childlessness in the mid to late 1220s.[74] Alexander II and his mother, Ermengarde, founded the new royal abbey and dedicated it to St. Edward the Confessor, an unusual choice in early thirteenth-century Scotland.[75] Hammond interpreted this dedication to be an effort by the dowager Queen Ermengarde to enlist St. Edward's support for Joan and Alexander's production of an heir because Joan had just turned sixteen but remained childless.[76] Hammond's analysis hinges on the fact that Joan never produced a child with Alexander II, rather than on any evidence of contemporary concern about her fertility in the 1220s. Hammond contrasted Ermengarde, who produced an heir and lived a long life, with Joan, who, he claimed, was sickly, never had a child and died "at the relatively young age of 27."[77] This gives the impression that these circumstances informed the planning of Balmerino in 1226, when in reality such a perspective on both women's lives would have been impossible at that point, more than a decade before Joan's death in 1238. Just because *we* know that Joan—or any other queen—would never have children, her life should not be framed artificially by that retrospective knowledge. This misleading interpretation of the dedication of St. Edward as an aid for Joan's fertility epitomizes a broader problem in current scholarship on queens who died childless. One of the aims of this book is *not* to automatically place the burden of childlessness entirely on the queens, or to explain their queenship solely in terms of their ultimate reproductive success or failure.

Scholars have approached the couples who *did* ultimately produce children very differently from those who did not: reproductive anxieties are barely, if at all, part of the story. The indications that Henry III and Eleanor

---

74 Hammond, "Queen Ermengarde and the Abbey of St. Edward, Balmerino," 1–27.

75 Hammond, "Queen Ermengarde," 4; Carpenter, "King Henry III and Saint Edward the Confessor: The Origin of the Cult," 867–68.

76 The argument based on sixteen as a "coming of age" point is discussed in more detail in Chapter 4.

77 Hammond, "Queen Ermengarde," 3, cites *Chronica majora*, ed. Luard, 3:479, for Joan's sickliness. This is a misrepresentation of the source material: Paris does mention Joan's death in England in 1238 in the cited passage, but he does not say that Joan was sickly, just that she had a fatal illness.

of Provence, and Edward II and Isabella of France encountered reproductive problems or felt concerned about their fertility have been overlooked by historians because of the knowledge that they went on to have children. Henry III and Eleanor of Provence's family life is described as particularly harmonious and their approach to raising their children has been noted as especially caring.[78] Scholarship on Eleanor of Provence, and medieval queenship more broadly, regularly cites Matthew Paris's report of concern about the fourteen-year-old queen's fertility, but there has been no attempt to explain why there was anxiety about such a young queen's reproductive ability.[79] Noticeably, studies of Henry III do not even mention Paris's comments about Eleanor's fertility.[80] It seems that the fact that they went on to have five children proved the contemporary concerns about fertility to be unfounded and thus they have been overlooked in scholarship. Isabella of France and Edward II have both received attention from scholars of medieval queenship and kingship.[81] However, despite indications that chroniclers were worried about the couple's delay conceiving early in their marriage, and evidence that Isabella received medical treatment for a reproductive issue, they also had four children and their fertility has gone unstudied.[82]

Two of the couples—Edward I and Eleanor of Castile, and Alexander III and Margaret of England—were married as young adolescents and their youth has likely discouraged historians' interest in the delayed fertility of both couples. The chief political history of Edward I concentrated on his and

78 For instance, see Earenfight, *Queenship in Medieval Europe*, 143–45; Carpenter, *Henry III*, 205–11; Howell, *Eleanor of Provence*, 44–45, 99–103.

79 Laynesmith, *The Last Medieval Queens*, 134; Benz St. John, *Three Medieval Queens*, 100; Parsons, *Eleanor of Castile*, 20. On the other hand, Earenfight, *Queenship in Medieval Europe*, 143–45, does not mention Paris's comments and presents Eleanor as an exemplary royal mother who gained an influential role at court partly because of her maternity.

80 For instance, David Carpenter, *Henry III*.

81 For example: Benz St. John, *Three Medieval Queens*; Ormrod, "Monarchy, Martyrdom"; Slater, "Rumour and Reputation," 257–92; Fletcher, "Manhood, Kingship and the Public in Late Medieval England," 123–42.

82 Scholars have noted the four-year delay between the couple's marriage in 1308 and the birth of their first child in 1312. Roy Haines argues that early pubescent twelve-year-old Isabella was "unlikely to have provided much sexual interest" for Edward II, who was in his mid-twenties: Haines, *King Edward II*, 61. Parsons, "Mothers, Daughters, Marriage," 66–68 states that Edward might have postponed consummating his marriage with Isabella until she could safely endure pregnancy and childbirth. This does not align with the contemporary chronicle relief when Edward was born, though, and needs some focused consideration.

Eleanor's fecundity and perpetuated the assumption that Eleanor's "main activity [was] the production of children."[83] Edward has similarly been characterized as particularly fertile; when Edward was on crusade and told that his father (Henry III) and his young son had both died, he allegedly said that it was easy to have sons, "but the loss of a father was irredeemable."[84] This tale—whether authentic or not—has left a mark on historiographical impressions of Edward's fatherhood, suggesting that he viewed children as easily replaceable and fertility as unproblematic. This not only diminishes the potential impact of child loss on the king but also obscures any reproductive anxieties he may have experienced. Parsons's foundational study of Eleanor's queenship began to remedy the historiographical approach to this couple's reproductive lives, and nuanced understanding about Eleanor's activities as queen by moving beyond focus on her motherhood and fecundity. He also drew attention to "the apparent lack of concern for [Eleanor's] fertility" in the first two decades of the couple's marriage.[85] Parsons described the contemporary silence as "puzzling," but, in the three decades since his work, scholars have yet to examine Eleanor and Edward's fertility in any depth.

Alexander III and Margaret of England's youth in the 1250s, followed by fertility in the 1260s–1270s, has prevented scholars from asking questions about their reproductive experiences too. Nelson included Margaret in her doctoral thesis on thirteenth-century Scottish queenship but she focused on the diplomatic nature of Alexander and Margaret's marriage, Margaret's management of her own household and access to resources, and the evolution of her status from the precarious early years when she was caught between her natal and marital lands, to her place at the centre of the Scottish royal family in the 1260s.[86] Nelson argued that a turning point for Margaret's integration into the Scottish royal family and her position as queen was the birth of her first child in 1261 and her willingness to "sacrifice a high profile political role" in order to escape the criticism and suspicion that this engendered.[87] Nelson contended that motherhood was pivotal for Margaret's queenship, but she did not consider whether Margaret experienced

83 Prestwich, *Edward I*, 121.

84 Mentioned by Prestwich, *Edward I*, 82, who cites Rishanger's chronicle: William Rishanger, *Chronica et annales*, ed. Riley, 78.

85 Parsons, *Eleanor of Castile*, 20.

86 Nelson, "Queens and Queenship," 213–38, at 233.

87 Nelson, "Queens and Queenship," 251.

pressure to produce an heir in the decade before 1261, or how she might have negotiated such pressure in her role as queen.

The existing scholarship on all eight royal couples, indeed, for medieval kings and queens more generally, has a tendency to think about fertility only when a royal couple never produced a child, to relate successful queenship to a queen's maternity and to forget about kings when considering royal fertility. The following analysis remedies these gaps in the study of royal infertility because couples struggled with fertility and pressure to produce children beyond complete and permanent childlessness, there was more to the queen's role than producing an heir, and ultimately, fertility involved the king too.

Chapter 1

FERTILE GROUND

HISTORIOGRAPHIES OF QUEENSHIP, KINGSHIP, AND INFERTILITY

EQUATING INFERTILITY WITH childlessness has resulted in a limited approach to the study of infertility in history; other concerns about fertility have been missed by scholars because "infertility" has been narrowly understood as the inability to conceive and studies have therefore ignored the experiences of couples who ultimately did have children.[1]

Adopting a more expansive approach to the study of infertility and distinguishing between the overlapping but distinct concepts of *childlessness, infertility*, *sub-fertility*, and *secondary infertility*, this book applies these terms in ways that avoid anachronistic assumptions about medieval royal reproductive lives.

Before turning to the existing scholarship on medieval queenship, kingship, and the history of infertility, it is essential to clarify the key terms that frame this study. *Childlessness* refers to a state—the absence of living children at a given moment—rather than a permanent condition. It is, by nature, transient: a royal couple might have been childless early in their marriage but later had children, or lost children and returned to a state of childlessness. Scholars often use the term retrospectively to only describe kings and queens who died without ever producing children, but this is misleading. This collapses the lived experience of uncertainty into a foregone conclusion. For the couples themselves, childlessness was not a fixed identity but a temporary, and potentially reversible, circumstance. In this study, couples who ultimately had children, such as Henry III and Eleanor of Provence, are described as childless when discussing specific periods before the birth of their first surviving child.

In contrast, *infertility* is the persistent biological inability to conceive (for males or females) or carry a pregnancy to term.[2] While infertility might be suspected in cases of prolonged childlessness, it can never be diagnosed with certainty in the Middle Ages, and even in modern medicine it is defined

1 See Davis and Loughran, "Introduction," 8, for a discussion of how the conventional and "medicalized" definition of infertility as the inability to conceive has shaped the study of infertility in history.

2 *Oxford Concise Medical Dictionary*.

probabilistically rather than absolutely. Applying the label retrospectively to medieval couples risks imposing a retrospective medical framework and obscuring the fact that, in their own time, the outcome of their fertility was still unknown. Ultimately, this book is concerned with the contemporary perceptions of royal couples' fertility at precisely this stage, when their reproductive future was still uncertain. The term "infertility" is used in the following chapters when referring to the field of study known as "the history of infertility" or when discussing specific understandings of "infertility" in medieval medicine, for instance.

Finally, *sub-fertility* and *secondary infertility* are important concepts in this book. *Sub-fertility* describes a reduced capacity to conceive that does not rule out eventual pregnancy. This could result in a long wait for conception or irregular reproductive success over a couple's lifetime. In a medieval context, sub-fertility is often an appropriate description for couples whose reproductive histories included long intervals between births, repeated pregnancy loss, or delayed first pregnancies, even when they ultimately produced heirs. *Secondary infertility* refers to trouble conceiving more than one child, or difficulty reaching a desired family size or number of children.[3]

Kings, Queens, and Infertility in History

Approaching royal fertility and reproductive difficulty from this broader perspective, the purpose of this study is not to determine the value of motherhood for queenship or explore how royals navigated childlessness in the absence of biological parenthood. Instead, it examines the full spectrum of fertility problems experienced by medieval royal couples. This includes not only what we conventionally label as infertility, but also the often-overlooked experiences of sub-fertility and secondary infertility in royal couples who did have children. Such couples have attracted little scholarly attention precisely because their eventual parenthood obscures earlier or ongoing struggles to conceive. By considering kings and queens together and treating fertility as a shared issue, this book reconsiders the pressure endured by royal couples to produce children and how those pressures were understood in relation to the male and female life course. The following chapters ask several questions: when and why was royal childlessness problematized in some cases but not others? What made a couple seek remedies or support for their fertility? What did they do? How was the management of fertility

3 Davis, "Oral History and Women's Accounts of Infertility," 135.

gendered? By thinking about how and why couples experienced pressure to be fertile and produce children, the following investigation considers when and why the wait for a child received contemporary attention and treats fertility as a shared, relational issue rather than an attribute of either spouse in isolation.

This book developed from the intersection of three distinct but overlapping fields of study. Queenship scholarship has long acknowledged the centrality of maternity in shaping perceptions of a queen's success or failure, while kingship studies have rarely treated fertility as a significant factor in a king's reign. Even though the importance of producing heirs is widely recognized in studies of medieval masculinity, fertility, and fatherhood are not regularly included in analyses of kingship, nor examined with the same precision as maternity in queenship studies. As a result, discussions of royal fertility have largely focused on queens alone. At the same time, the emerging history of infertility has encouraged historians to move beyond an exclusive focus on the inability to conceive and instead to consider a spectrum of reproductive experiences, including delay, loss, and uncertainty. Bringing these strands together, this chapter situates the book within the historiographies of queenship and motherhood, kingship, masculinity and fatherhood, and infertility studies, and argues that integrating them offers a fuller understanding of the pressures placed on royal couples to reproduce. In doing so, it extends existing work that has examined how monarchs such as Richard II and Anne of Bohemia navigated their roles without children, by also considering couples who did have heirs but nonetheless faced reproductive challenges.

Queenship and Motherhood

Interest in queenship as an office and societal role, distinct from biographical approaches to individual queens' lives, emerged in the wake of second-wave feminism with Marion Facinger's article on Capetian queenship from 1968.[4] Facinger studied Capetian queens in the tenth to thirteenth centuries and argued that in the twelfth century there was a shift in the nature of queenship, as royal power was consolidated and bureaucratized. The king's and queen's households became more distinct from each other and the queen's

4 Facinger, "A Study of Medieval Queenship," 1–48. Generally, scholarship on medieval women emerged in the 1970s and 1980s, in the UK and the US, following the second wave of feminism: see Rubin, "A Decade of Studying Medieval Women," 213–39; Mosher Stuard, ed. *Women in Medieval History and Historiography.*

political position was diminished and marginalized as a result.[5] Facinger argued that the queen's personal relationship with the king became her chief way to achieve political influence.[6] In the early 1980s, Pauline Stafford reassessed the marginalization of early medieval queens from medieval politics.[7] Her initial work emphasized the importance of the female life course for the queen's exercise of official power, and she argued that the gendered roles of wife, mother and widow were fundamental to the queen's ability to access influence and power.

There was a growth and shift in scholarship on queenship in the 1990s, epitomized by John Carmi Parsons's work on English medieval queens. He reasoned that, far from being marginalized, queens exercised power through their gendered roles in "informal, unofficial spheres," particularly childbearing and rearing, and their family networks and connections.[8] Parsons argued that "the familial context" was the arena in which queens operated.[9] This was similar to medieval women generally, but queens had unique access to wealth, the international stage, and the king, the official political leader of the realm.[10] Parsons also highlighted that queens were active in raising their children, particularly daughters, and that a queen's influence as a mother was critical for her power. Her motherly instinct to protect children was an acknowledged and acceptable justification for a queen's political involvement during her husband's reign.[11] Studies of the ritual aspects of medieval queenship have maintained that maternity was especially emphasized in ritual displays of the queen's role, particularly in coronations.[12]

---

5 Facinger's argument about queenship was in line with wider arguments in historiography at this time about the decline of women's positions. See McNamara and Wemple, "The Power of Women Through the Family," 126–41. For an outline of the state of the field since the 1960s, see Tanner, Gathagan, and Huneycutt, "Introduction," 1–18.

6 Facinger, "Medieval Queenship," 35–40.

7 Stafford, *Queens, Concubines and Dowagers*, xvii. Stafford went on to update her conclusions about this in the early 2000s: see Stafford, "Powerful Women," 409–10.

8 Parsons, *Eleanor of Castile*, 249.

9 Parsons, "Family, Sex and Power," 2.

10 Parsons, *Eleanor of Castile*, 249.

11 Parsons, "Mothers, Daughters, Marriage, Power," 63–78.

12 Parsons, "Ritual and Symbol in the English Medieval Queenship," 60–77; Stafford, *Queens, Concubines and Dowagers*, 87, 89, 130–31, 191–92; Stafford, "The King's Wife in Wessex 800–1066," 16–17. Scholars have since examined the coronation ritual for queens and shown that it also emphasized the queen's duty to support good works and justice. See Nelson, "Early Medieval Rites of Queen-Making," 301–15; Smith,

The foundational work of the 1990s emphasized the importance of maternity for queenship.[13] After Parsons's pioneering work on Eleanor of Castile and thirteenth-century queenship, Margaret Howell examined the queenship of Eleanor of Provence and argued that while a queen faced gendered expectations in her role, her success was ultimately determined by her personal agency.[14] Eleanor successfully wielded political influence through management of her household and her children, but Howell noted that Eleanor's power as queen was ultimately because Henry III "allowed room" for her to apply her ability and skill.[15] Howell scrutinized how Eleanor of Provence's lived experience of queenship reflected the gendered ideals of queenship and argued that Eleanor's maternity was fundamental for her access to authority as queen.[16]

Examining later medieval English queenship, Joanna Laynesmith reassessed major arguments about the queen's role that had been established in queenship scholarship in the 1990s; notably, the importance of the queen's income and household, her role as the king's counsellor, and the significance

---

"The Earliest Queen-Making Rites," 18–35; Mistry, "Ermentrude's Consecration (866)," 567–88.

13 Distinct strands of queenship studies have emerged since the 1990s, organized around the core functions of medieval queenship that had been identified in the earlier foundational work. Motherhood is one of these strands. They also include the queen as intercessor and counsellor, her piety and activity as religious and cultural patron, as well as her influence through gift-giving and the management of her household and access to income as part of her ability to exercise political power. Recently, there has been interest in queens' formations of identities and reputations. For some historiography on medieval queenship, see: Parsons, "Intercessionary Patronage of Queen Margaret and Isabella of France," 191; Huneycutt, "Intercession and the High-Medieval Queen," 126–46; Webb, "Queen and Patron," 205–21; Huneycutt, "'Proclaiming her Dignity Abroad,'" 155–74; Garcia Herrero and Munoz Fernandez, "Queenship and Monastic Foundations," 16–48; Geaman, "Beyond Good Queen Anne," 67–89; Earenfight, ed. *Royal and Elite Households in Medieval and Early Modern Europe*; Adams, "Anne de France and Gift-Giving," 65–84; Mielke, "Doubly Crowned," 1–23; Earenfight, "Without the Persona of the Prince," 1–21; Dunn and Carney, eds., *Royal Women and Dynastic Loyalty*; Comba, "Methods of Queenship in Matrimonial Diplomacy," 1–9; Woodacre, "Cousins & Queens," 30–45; Brown, "Family Female Networking," 209–40. Rohr and Benz, eds., *Queenship, Gender, and Reputation*; Fleiner and Woodacre, eds., *Virtuous or Villainess?*; Evans, *Inventing Eleanor*; Harrill, "Politics and Sainthood."

14 Howell, *Eleanor of Provence*, 286.

15 Howell, *Eleanor of Provence*, 286.

16 Howell, *Eleanor of Provence*, 46–48. See also, Howell, "Royal Women of England and France," 169–71.

of motherhood and family.[17] Laynesmith approached maternity as a useful category of analysis for understanding late medieval queenship; she argued that the role of mother was empowering for queens, while also a uniquely political and public role because of the significance that producing an heir had for the wider political community. Laynesmith nuanced Parsons's earlier argument by questioning the centrality of maternity in the ritual displays of queenship. She posited a more complex interpretation of queen-making rites, in which marriage to the king was the defining role of queenship, not motherhood.[18] The expectation of motherhood was not unique to queens but shared by all married medieval women. Producing children only helped the queen to affirm her marital role as the king's wife.[19] Laynesmith suggested that it was not specifically the queen's potential to produce heirs that was emphasized in rituals like the coronation rite, but rather the queen's role as a fundamental component of the king's public body.[20] Motherhood did not make a queen, but it was the "most public aspect of the queenly function of complementing kingship in a hereditary monarchy."[21] Related to this, Lisa Benz St. John reasoned that the queen's position was exceptional in fourteenth-century English society because of her status as the king's wife, and that status was enabled by her gender and the biological roles associated with it.[22] More recently, historians have explored the idealized images and models of queenly motherhood, and studied how individual queens employed and navigated their maternal identity in relation to their political role.[23] Queenship scholars have moved beyond examining queens' agency and influence as a derivative of motherhood, but motherhood continues to be seen as a fundamental aspect of successful queenship.

In her survey of medieval queenship in western Europe, Theresa Earenfight suggested that the importance of motherhood for queenship should be re-examined.[24] She drew attention to the fact that many medieval queens who were childless were still able to maintain influence and authority as

---

17 Laynesmith, *The Last Medieval Queens.*

18 Laynesmith, *The Last Medieval Queens*, 180.

19 Laynesmith, *The Last Medieval Queens*, 180.

20 Laynesmith, "Fertility Rite or Authority Ritual?," 52–68.

21 Laynesmith, *The Last Medieval Queens*, 179–80.

22 Benz St. John, *Three Medieval Queens*, 164.

23 Fleiner and Woodacre, eds., *Virtuous or Villainess?*; Aram, "Authority and Maternity," 121–29. For the early modern period: Strohman, "'A More Natural Mother.'"

24 Earenfight, *Queenship in Medieval Europe.*

the wife of the king and were not repudiated by their husbands.[25] Kristen Geaman also questioned the importance of motherhood for late medieval English queens in her doctoral thesis on Anne of Bohemia and Richard II, and Margaret of Anjou and Henry VI.[26] She examined perceptions of Anne of Bohemia as a good queen despite the fact that she never produced children, while Margaret of Anjou was harshly judged for her childlessness in the eight-year-long wait for an heir and motherhood did not sufficiently redeem her political standing even once she had produced a son. Geaman concluded that biological motherhood was not as crucial for successful queenship as we have previously supposed, and that Anne of Bohemia was successful because she ably executed other feminine and key roles of monarchy, complimenting Richard II's kingship with queenly intercession and patronage. Following her death, Richard II emphasized Anne's career as intercessor to reconstruct her image as a nurturing, maternal queen despite her childlessness.[27] The queens considered in this book were not condemned as harshly as Margaret of Anjou was for the eight-year wait for her first child, nor did any of the royal couples investigated in the following chapters repackage their childlessness like Richard and Anne. Rather, couples with less conspicuous experiences of fertility problems are the focus of this study. How did queens navigate the pressures of their gendered role and deal with the realities, and uncertainties, of reproduction in more typical examples of medieval rulership than the turbulent reigns of Richard II or Henry VI?

Scottish kings and queens make up more than half of the case studies in this book. There has been much less consideration of medieval Scottish queens than their husbands or their English counterparts.[28] The most sys-

25 Earenfight, *Queenship in Medieval Europe*, 180. Earenfight also muses on this point on her blog, theresaearenfight.com (posted September 6, 2013).

26 Geaman, "Childless Queens and Child-like Kings."

27 Geaman, "Childless Queens and Child-like Kings," 181–227.

28 This gap may owe, in part, to how infrequently Scottish queens appear in the contemporary sources. Interest in Scottish queens has focused predominantly on the later medieval queens of the Stewart dynasty, see: Hayes, "The Late Medieval Scottish Queen"; Downie, *She is But a Women*; Fitch, "Maternal Mediators," 1–35. Work on earlier Scottish queens is limited to St./Queen Margaret and her daughter, Matilda, queen of England: Huneycutt, "Public Lives, Private Ties," 295–309; Huneycutt, *Matilda of Scotland*; Huneycutt, "The Idea of the Perfect Princess," 81–98; Lee, "The Miracles and Cult of St. Margaret of Scotland," 1–11. Generally, work on Scottish gender and women's history has been slower compared to the English context (for example) and continues to be left out of mainstream political and social histories. See Ewan, "A History of Women in Scotland"; Ewan, "A New Trumpet?"; Ewan and

tematic investigation of high medieval Scottish queenship is Jessica Nelson's unpublished doctoral dissertation.[29] Noting the continuities between queens, Nelson claimed that queens served as powerful signs of good faith between Scotland and their natal lands (usually in England), and the increasing preference for patrilinear succession put the queen's motherhood, particularly production of sons, "firmly in the public sphere."[30] Nelson concluded that successful maternity placed the queen at "the centre of the royal family...but a queen who was not a mother was at best a disappointment, and at worst a target for gossip and scapegoating."[31] This book challenges this interpretation by arguing that there is not such a discernible difference in contemporaries' comments about queens who were childless compared to queens who were mothers.

Nelson drew attention to the fact that between 1221 and 1286, only four Scottish royal children were born, and only one—Alexander III—survived his father.[32] She describes it as ironic, because "just as the kings were becoming firmly committed to linear succession, their queens were losing the ability to produce healthy children."[33] If motherhood was a queen's critical role for determining her success or failure, and queenly fertility diminished in thirteenth-century Scotland, we must ask if there are any signs of increasing anxiety or criticism on these grounds in contemporary sources. Additionally, Nelson's comment highlights the flawed approach to royal fertility in historiography: the ability to produce healthy heirs depended on the king as well as the queen.

Queens as mothers is an enduring category of analysis in queenship studies, and considering problems with fertility and reproductive anxieties is a new way to assess the significance of maternity for queens. However, the primary focus of the following chapters is not to determine the importance of motherhood for a queen's success, or how royals negotiated their role in the *absence* of fertility, as Geaman has done. Rather, this is a broader study of experiences of reproductive anxiety and difficulty, including not only what

Meikle, eds., *Women in Scotland*; Ewan, "Women's history in Scotland," 155–64; Meikle, "The World of Women," 71–77; Barclay, Cheadle, and Gordon, "The State of Scottish History," 83–107.

29 Nelson, "Queens and Queenship."

30 Nelson, "Queens and Queenship," 271.

31 Nelson, "Queens and Queenship," 272.

32 Nelson, "Queens and Queenship," 273.

33 Nelson, "Queens and Queenship," 273.

we conventionally think of as infertility but also the often-overlooked experiences of sub-fertility and secondary infertility of royal couples who did have children.[34]

Ultimately, this study does not dismiss the importance of motherhood for queens. However, we do need to consider the realities of queens' experiences, including the uncertainties of pregnancy and fertility problems beyond childlessness, to be able to understand the pressure felt by a queen to produce an heir, and indeed, other children. When and why did a queen's fertility receive contemporary scrutiny, and what was at stake as a result? The historiographical focus on queens' successful maternity has resulted in a lack of nuance in our understanding of both childless queens and the significance of royal fertility for queens; ultimately, this book studies royal fertility not only as the queen's ability to produce healthy children, but the king's too. The following chapters consider how royal couples shouldered the pressure and divided the labour of managing reproduction.

Kingship and Fatherhood

There is a distinct divide between kingship and queenship studies when it comes to considering fertility. While motherhood is a pillar of queenship studies, scholars of kingship rarely consider the reproductive life or fatherhood of kings with any precision or gendered analysis. The gendered analysis of medieval kingship developed out of the scholarly interest in the history of masculinity, which itself developed from the history of women and gender studies. The history of masculinity has expanded in several distinct directions since the 1990s, based on the concept that masculinity is not innate, but formed through behaviours and expressed to varying degrees by different men. Vern Bullough argued in the early 1990s that men demonstrated that they were men by "impregnating women, protecting dependents and serving as provider to one's family."[35] The work of sociologist R. W. Connell was also influential; she suggested that there are multiple masculine ways of life in a society, but a particular set of behaviours, core values and functions become idealized by the dominant socio-political group. Connell described

---

34 Davis, "Oral History and Women's Accounts of Infertility," 135.

35 Bullough, "On Being a Male in the Middle Ages," 34. Subsequent work on medieval masculinities includes Karras, *From Boys to Men*; Neal, *The Masculine Self*; McLaughlin, "Secular and Spiritual Fatherhood in the Eleventh Century," 25–43. Fletcher, "The Whig Interpretation of Masculinity?" 57–75. Davis, *Writing Masculinity*; Bruso, "Bodies Hardened for War," 255–77. Hodgson, "Normans and Competing Masculinities on Crusade," 195–213.

this as "hegemonic masculinity"; the masculinity perpetuated by a society's most powerful men and aspired to by other men lower down the social strata.[36] While slower than the attention to medieval men more generally, interest has extended to medieval kingship, too, due to the king's position at the top of the medieval social structure.

Specifically, scholars have questioned how expectations of normative masculinity informed the ideals of medieval kingship and influenced perceptions of the conduct of individual kings.[37] Mark Ormrod contended that the medieval ruler was meant to encompass both masculine and feminine qualities, and there was an informal division of these gendered attributes between the roles of king and queen.[38] Ormrod, in his analysis of Richard II's kingship, argued that the king had an unusual understanding of his role as ruler and increasingly diminished and overshadowed the queen's position as an active and essential part of monarchy.[39] Christopher Fletcher also demonstrated how using contemporary ideals of manhood and masculinity to understand Richard II's reign shows that it was not just rhetoric used to critique and control his problematic rule, but that "ideas of how a "man" should act" underwrote the practice of medieval politics.[40] In her study of late medieval English kingship, Katherine Lewis argued that medieval kings Henry V and Henry VI were judged on their ability to embody the ideal qualities of medieval masculinity, but the essential traits of manhood were not static, and a king's gender identity was formed through "the balance of these [traits] within the wider configuration of qualities which together made up the social presence of their manhood and kingship."[41]

Following the argument that "impregnating women" was fundamental to manhood, gender scholars have explored the social implications of infertility for the formation of medieval masculinity more generally. Rachel Middlemass and Theresa Tyers investigated medieval medical theory about

36 Connell, *Masculinities*, 76–81. See also Connell's subsequent thought on this: Connell and Messerschmidt, "Hegemonic Masculinity," 829–59.

37 An example of this from the early modern context: Doran, "Monarchy and Masculinity," 201–23.

38 Ormrod, "Monarchy, Martyrdom and Masculinity," 175.

39 Ormrod, "Monarchy, Martyrdom and Masculinity," 181–82. For Richard II's unusual approach to another aspect of his role, producing an heir in this case, see Lewis, "Becoming a Virgin King," 86–100.

40 Fletcher, *Richard II*, 276–78.

41 Lewis, *Kingship and Masculinity*, 257. Also see Lewis, "Edmund of East Anglia, Henry VI and Ideals of Kingly Masculinity," 158–73.

sexual dysfunction and masculinity and argued that the threat to manhood posed by impotence and infertility was mitigated in contexts where masculine identity was associated with the role of father rather than reproduction. The responsibilities and self-control of parenting could still be displayed in alternatives to biological reproduction such as fostering children and taking on the responsibility of parents despite not having produced offspring.[42] However, Middlemass and Tyers concluded that more commonly, the ability to reproduce was critical for manhood because of the association of masculinity with physical perfection and "any form of physical weakness or defect, whether arising from disability or disease, [was] a serious threat to men's capacity to meet the most highly prized masculine ideals."[43] Meanwhile, Rachel Moss argued that fatherhood, not just the ability to reproduce, was the defining behaviour for distinguishing mature masculine adulthood because it showed that along with the functions of providing for and leading a household, a man had contributed to the future of his dynasty.[44] She reasoned that infertility was a barrier to a man's ability to achieve socially recognized maturity because biological fatherhood, as opposed to just impregnating a woman, demonstrated the self-restraint, leadership and assumption of responsibility required to hold the socio-political positions of power associated with manhood.[45]

Yet, despite the interest in kings, fatherhood, and medieval masculinity, and the focus on maternity in queenship studies, the significance of fatherhood for medieval kingship is still neglected in scholarship.[46] Kristen Gea-

---

42 Middlemass and Tyers, "Disabling Masculinity," 53.

43 Middlemass and Tyers, "Disabling Masculinity," 54. On male impotence, see: Kane, *Impotence and Virginity*; Rider, "'A Defect of the Mind or Body,'" 193–210.

44 Moss, *Fatherhood and its Representations*, 71.

45 Moss, *Fatherhood and its Representations*, 60–63.

46 Additionally, there is a distinct lack of gendered analysis of Scottish medieval kings, compared to their English counterparts. Other scholars have highlighted and discussed this deficit: Smith, "Assessing Gender in the Construction of Scottish Identity"; Barclay, Cheadle, and Gordon, "The State of Scottish History," 98–99. Some exceptions are Melissa Hollander's consideration of fatherhood in early modern Scotland, and Katie Barclay's examination of early modern marriages in which she considers how both husbands and wives negotiated of their roles and identities. See Hollander, "'The Name of the Father,'" 63–72; Barclay, *Love, Intimacy and Power*; Abrams and Ewan, eds., *Nine Centuries of Man*, 2, 5. From the same volume, see Neville, "Making a Manly Impression," 101–21. Most recently, Lucy Dean's chapter on age and medieval Scottish kings has taken a step towards filling this historiographical gap: Dean, "Negotiating Youth, Old Age and Manhood," 192–208.

man suggested that this is because the king (usually) inherited his position and did not have to negotiate his political role and status in the same way that the queen did, so there has been no intrinsic link made between being a king and being a father.[47] That said, the importance of kings' fatherhood has been shown in certain individual cases. Edward III's fatherhood helped confirm his maturity in the 1330s and demonstrate his right to rule, while later in his reign, his many children were an indication of the future stability of his dynasty[48] In her work on Richard II and Henry VI, Geaman argued that fatherhood was crucial for marking a king's adulthood and being childless had negative consequences for a medieval king's masculine identity.[49] Geaman's argument is based on two kings who had unusual reigns and expressions of kingly, mature masculinity though; Richard II's youth was used as justification to control his power during his adolescence, and opposition to his authority as an adult king continued to be couched in terms of his tyrannical youthfulness and immaturity.[50] Henry VI failed to display most important qualities of hegemonic masculinity, not helped by the fact that his manhood was always doomed to comparison with the legendary manliness of his father, Henry V.[51] Any conclusions about kingship, masculinity and fatherhood need to be tested in less exceptional reigns. Accusations of immaturity or effeminacy were prevalent in contemporary criticism of Richard II and Henry VI and political opposition to both kings' reigns was based on more than their childlessness. Therefore, it is difficult to extricate concerns about fertility, specifically, from the criticisms of their behaviour more generally.

This present study investigates the relationship between masculinity, kingship, and fertility in cases where the king's behaviour did not rouse such anxiety and public controversy as reigns like Richard II and Henry VI. It examines the significance of reproduction and fatherhood for kingship by considering how royal couples managed fertility and felt pressure to produce children and considers the importance of reproduction in relation to perceptions of the male life course. This will include investigation of how

---

47 Geaman, "Childless Queens and Child-like Kings," 31.

48 Ormrod, "Personal Religion of Edward III," 849–77; Binski, *Westminster Abbey and the Plantagenets*, 92, 198–99; Shenton, "Philippa of Hainault's Churchings," 105–21; Geaman, "Childless Queens and Child-like Kings," 32–33.

49 Geaman, "Childless Queens and Child-like Kings," 32.

50 Fletcher, *Richard II*, 276–78.

51 Lewis, *Kingship and Masculinity*, 257.

kings experienced pressure for fertility, as scholars have done for queens.[52] Building on Geaman's interpretation about the implications of fatherhood for a king's social maturity, this study finds that the king's age and life stage were crucial for determining if and when a royal couple felt pressure to produce a child.

The History of Infertility

Within the last decade there has been a marked shift towards studying the history of infertility. Previously it was included as a sub-topic in broader studies of family, women, gender, sex, and medicine.[53] For instance, Joan Cadden's foundational study of medieval natural philosophical conceptualizations of sex difference, first published in 1993, has a chapter titled "sterility" in which she showed that medical understandings of and treatment for infertility were based on contemporary ideas about the innate differences between male and female bodies.[54] In her study of men's role in women's healthcare in the Middle Ages, Monica Green argued that male physicians claimed authority on treating and diagnosing infertility by the fourteenth century.[55] Both Cadden and Green's work uncovered medieval medical understandings about the causes of sterility and revealed therapeutic approaches to infertility. However, it was not until 2016, with a special issue of the journal *Social History of Medicine*, that there was focused attention dedicated to infertility in medieval and early modern medicine. The articles in this issue went beyond examining theoretical medical explanations to investigate various social dimensions of infertility and the applications and intersections of theory and practice.[56]

---

52 For example, Pauline Stafford pioneered this connection between queenship and the female life course: Stafford, *Queens, Concubines and Dowagers.*

53 Cadden, *Meanings of Sex Difference*, 228–58; Green, *Making Women's Medicine Masculine*, 71–111; Lindgren, "The Wandering Womb"; Tyers, "The Rebirth of Fertility." For the early modern context: Evans, *Aphrodisiacs, Fertility and Medicine*, 51–86; Berry and Foyster, "Childless Men," 158–83. An early exception which does focus on infertility is Bologne, *La naissance interdite.*

54 Cadden, *Meaning of Sex Difference*, 249–58. Cadden's chapter is titled "sterility," and her focus is specifically on medieval medical understandings of the condition, causes and treatments for infertility. I use the term here to discuss her work but acknowledge that we cannot retrospectively diagnose the medical condition.

55 Green, *Making Women's Medicine Masculine*, 86–111.

56 Oren-Magidor and Rider, "Introduction," 221.

The special issue focused on the gendered experience of infertility, particularly in relation to seeking and receiving treatment. While medieval writers recognized that men could theoretically be infertile, the authors in the special issue investigated the extent to which infertility was considered to be the woman's fault and her problem to solve: Catherine Rider showed that, although Latin medical texts discussed male infertility and a range of reproductive disorders as theoretical possibility, the practical texts used by physicians placed greater emphasis on treating infertility in women (even though there are still remedies included for men).[57] Sarah Toulalan considered early modern medical writers' ideas about old age and fertility; she argued that fertility was thought to decrease for both men and women in old age but reproductive ability featured more prominently in discussions of aging women and the decline in fertility was thought to be quicker and more dramatic for women than for men.[58] Geaman's article demonstrated that remedying infertility fell to Anne of Bohemia, not Richard II, as it was the queen who purchased the medicines for herself. However, none of the articles suggested that infertility was approached solely as the woman's problem, and Rider and Daphna Oren-Magidor urged in the introduction that "more work is needed on how ideas about who was responsible for infertility shifted depending on context and circumstance."[59] This book intervenes precisely on that point by showing that infertility was significant for kings as well as queens, and the behaviour of the king shaped how contemporaries perceived a royal couple's fertility.

Scholars have also started asking questions about the gendering of control and access to medical knowledge in relation to infertility. Monica Green's work laid the foundations for this, as she showed that male practitioners were able to exert increasing authority over the practice of women's (reproductive) medicine from the thirteenth to fourteenth century, by controlling the teaching of medical knowledge in universities and production of texts.[60] Daphna Oren-Magidor showed that, in practice, early modern women collected remedies for reproductive disorders from male physicians as well as other women and implemented them in their own self-treatment

57 Rider, "Men and Infertility," 245–66. See also Rider, "Men's Responses to Infertility," 273–90.

58 Toulalan, "'Elderly Years Cause a Total Dispaire of Conception,'" 333–59. For more recent work on old age and infertility, see Rider, "Gender, Old Age, and the Infertile Body," 267–88.

59 Oren-Magidor and Rider, "Introduction," 222.

60 Green, *Making Medicine Masculine*, especially at 71–111, in relation to infertility.

and existing knowledge of reproduction.[61] Tyers argued that an aristocratic female manuscript owner possessed and administered medical knowledge for herself and for her household.[62] More recently, Sara Verskin examined women's experience of infertility in medieval Islamic society, and focused on approaches to infertility in Islamic law, Arabo-Galenic medical theory and practice, and the treatment options available to medieval Muslim women.[63] While focused on a different medieval context, Verskin considers important questions about gendered medical care and challenges assumptions about women's roles. Verskin showed that there was societal trust in women to monitor and interpret the signs of their own reproductive bodies. These studies have nuanced our understanding of the gendered practice and control of medieval reproductive medicine, particularly highlighting female agency. The following chapters contribute to this point by examining the agency of queens in royal healthcare, while also uncovering the active role taken by kings to encourage royal fertility and seek remedies when the couple were concerned about fertility and reproduction.

Gayle Davis and Tracy Loughran took a big step towards establishing themes and inspiring further research on historical infertility.[64] Their volume gave attention to women's gendered experiences of infertility, reproductive labour, technologies and "stratified reproduction" (the inequalities and differences in access to care and treatment between socio-economic groups) across time and space.[65] This volume raised the question of how to usefully define infertility for research. A basic premise of the volume was the multidimensional nature of the experience of infertility, and Davis and Loughran argued that using "a medical model of infertility" hides from researchers the broader gamut of involuntary childlessness experienced by those who did not seek medicalized treatment or did not see their condition in medicalized terms.[66] Davis and Loughran observed that pathologized infertility is often the most visible to historians, and so "infertility" has been written about in terms of the medicalized problem of conceiving and being

61 Oren-Magidor, "Literate Laywomen," 290–310.

62 Tyers, '"In the Merry Month of May,'" 267–89. Also see Toulalan, "'Elderly Years Cause a Total Dispaire of Conception,'" 339.

63 Verskin, *Barren Women*.

64 For recent works that explore questions about infertility in history: Toepfer, *Negotiating Childlessness*; Toepfer, *Infertility in Medieval and Early Modern Europe*; Rider, "Gender, Old Age, and the Infertile Body," 267–90; Oren-Magidor, *Infertility*.

65 Davis and Loughran, "Introduction," 5–7.

66 Davis and Loughran, "Introduction," 5–7.

childless, "even though scholars are aware that this constitutes at best only one aspect of the experience of infertility."[67] Davis and Loughran urged historians of infertility to abandon such a limited "definitional certainty" and instead embrace "complexity, ambiguity, and questions about intentionality" to study infertility in history.[68]

A core purpose of this book is to investigate fertility concerns beyond the conventional and limited concept of infertility as the inability to conceive, the approach highlighted by Davis and Loughran. In the process of researching an oral history of motherhood in twentieth-century Britain, Angela Davis found that the women of her study did not describe their experiences as "infertility," yet many of them faced secondary infertility, meaning they had a child but experienced subsequent fertility problems, or sub-fertility, with delays and trouble conceiving. These struggles have been masked by the women's adoption of fatalistic attitudes towards their fertility and downplaying or remaining silent about their experiences because they did not fit the conventional idea of "infertility."[69] Sub-fertility and secondary infertility widely affected the women in Davis's study, and had a significant and powerful effect on their lives, but this had been missed because all of the women were biological mothers.[70] Indeed, Davis had not even been looking for stories of fertility problems when she uncovered these stories. Medieval royal couples experienced sub-fertility and secondary infertility too. Yet the experiences of fertility problems and low fertility for kings and queens as opposed to conventional cases of "infertility" have been neglected.[71] The following investigation asks why, and under what conditions childlessness became problematized for a royal couple and it brings to light royal couples' reproductive anxieties which have previously been overlooked because many of them became biological parents.

67 Davis and Loughran, "Introduction," 8.

68 Davis and Loughran, "Introduction," 7. Davis and Loughran noted how "infertility" can be variously construed in different contexts. They mentioned how having no sons, taking "too long" to conceive a child, and having one or two children when seven or eight was the norm might be perceived as infertility or taken as evidence of some "reproductive abnormality" in some contexts.

69 Davis, "Oral History," 123–40.

70 Davis, "Oral History," 135.

71 Davis, "Oral History," 135: Davis references Elizabeth Roberts, who uses "low fertility." See Roberts, *Women and Families*, 81–82.

Royal Infertility

Scholars of both infertility and monarchy flag up the value of examining infertility in a royal context: Oren-Magidor and Rider claimed that studying infertility is a particularly useful lens for understanding the behaviours of those for whom producing an heir was crucial.[72] Russell Martin wrote that the most precarious moment "in the life of the political system" was "the transfer of power from one ruler to the next";[73] therefore, royal childlessness jeopardized the future of a dynasty and the stability of the political system when it came to the power-transfer moment after a king's death.

Scholarly interest in royal couples and infertility has so far centred on how couples navigated the absence of biological heirs and explored the strategies they employed to compensate for childlessness.[74] Geaman's unpublished PhD dissertation on Anne of Bohemia and Richard II and Henry VI and Margaret of Anjou is the first focused study of royal infertility in medieval England.[75] She argued that these royal couples compensated for their reproductive failures by substituting alternatives to biological reproduction (fostering children), and supplying explanatory narratives about marital chastity to account for their continued childlessness.[76] Subsequently, Geaman and Earenfight argued that in the absence of biological motherhood, queens "nurture[d] their subjects" through non-biological roles like intercession with the king and religious and cultural patronage, and they were still able to exert significant political influence and power without producing an heir.[77] Lewis has also demonstrated how Richard II aligned himself with an alternative model of kingship and masculinity which did not require producing an heir through his public devotion to the childless king and saint, Edward the Confessor.[78]

Advancing the existing approaches to medieval royal infertility, this book considers the fertility of royal couples in cases where, unlike Richard II/Anne of Bohemia and Henry VI/Margaret of Anjou, the behaviour of the king and queen was not transgressive of gendered roles, nor did the king's

---

72 Oren-Magidor and Rider, "Introduction," 216. For the dynastic significance of producing heirs: Bartlett, *Royal Blood*.

73 Martin, "Introduction Part III: Dynasty and Succession," 418.

74 For early modern France, see: Roberts, "Sterility and Sovereignty," 151–69.

75 Geaman, "Childless Queens and Child-life Kings."

76 Geaman, "Childless Queens and Child-life Kings," 143–80.

77 Earenfight and Geaman, "Neither Heir Nor Spare," 528.

78 Lewis, "Becoming a Virgin King," 86–100, esp. 91–93.

masculinity become the focal point in contemporary opposition to turbulent reigns. Laynesmith has shown that a queen's ability to fulfil her gendered role was as much determined by perceptions of her husband's masculinity as by her own behaviour, so Anne of Bohemia and Margaret of Anjou faced different conditions and gendered pressures than other medieval queens. Neither Richard II and Anne nor Henry VI and Margaret demonstrated the "normative" gendered roles of medieval kingship and queenship.[79] Assessing the significance of their childlessness and how they negotiated infertility does not reveal widely applicable results relevant to medieval royal couples who demonstrated more conventionally gendered roles and approaches to rulership.

There is a distinct divide between kingship and queenship studies when it comes to considering (in)fertility, and this book addresses this by focusing on how royal couples negotiated pressure for, and problems with, fertility. Parsons, Ormrod, and Earenfight have all suggested that medieval rulership contained a balance of masculine and feminine qualities in the relational pairing of kingship and queenship.[80] Earenfight encourages us to conceptualize medieval monarchy as a dynamic relationship within which gender and people worked together in the exercise of power.[81] The relational nature of men's and women's experiences is also highlighted by historians of infertility. Studies such as Oren-Magidor's monograph on early modern infertility, and articles in the *Social History of Medicine* special issue show how men's and women's roles in reproduction were interwoven with the sense that infertility impinged on both partners' ability to execute prescribed social roles.[82] Yet there is still a tendency by historians to think about infertility in relation to queenship rather than to approach reproduction as a function of monarchy. The *Routledge History of Monarchy* volume is an example of this one-sided approach: Geaman and Earenfight's chapter considered only how queens managed and succeeded in the absence of biological motherhood and there is no comparable chapter dedicated to the negotiation of childlessness by their husbands or any other kings. If we should think about

79 Laynesmith, *Late Medieval Queens*, 72–130. See also Herrup, "The King's Two Genders," 493–510, for her argument about the necessary use and demonstration of both masculine and feminine qualities in individual rulers.

80 Parsons, "Intercessionary Patronage"; Ormrod, "Monarchy, Martyrdom," 175; Earenfight, "Without the Persona," 1–21.

81 Earenfight, "Without the Persona," 10.

82 Oren-Magidor, *Infertility*; Oren-Magidor and Rider, "Infertility in Medieval and Early Modern Medicine," special issue *Social History of Medicine* 29, no. 2 (2016).

kingship and queenship as a relational pair in concepts of medieval rulership, we must certainly consider them as a pair in respect to reproduction and the social consequences of infertility.

Book Structure

This study examines the pressure for fertility experienced by conventionally infertile couples and offers a reconsideration of the overlooked reproductive concerns and experiences of couples who also had fertility success stories. The following chapters ask: what raised contemporary concerns about a royal couple's fertility? When and why did they experience pressure to be fertile? Did this pressure change after the birth of an heir? How did couples react to the pressure and concerns about their fertility? How were the practices for managing reproduction gendered?

Chapter 2 considers what contemporary narrative sources recorded about the royal couples' fertility and analyses comments and concern about childlessness. It investigates how royal fertility was written about by chroniclers and uncovers attention to couples' fertility which has been missed by scholarship because many of the couples ultimately had children. It highlights chroniclers' association of reproduction with queens but argues that perceptions of the kings shaped what chronicles wrote about royal fertility. Chapter 3 focuses on how chroniclers wove royal fertility into their narratives. It analyses accounts of David II's childlessness and the allegations that two Scottish queens faked pregnancies, arguing that these comments reflected the authors' broader perceptions of the reign, and thus reveal the importance of fertility for good queenship and kingship. Chapter 4 identifies a pattern of behaviour in the devotional practices of three childless kings, and exposes a connection between the king's behaviours, chronological age, and concerns about childlessness. This chapter suggests that royal couples experienced scrutiny of their fertility when the king reached the age associated with physical perfection and maturity in the male life course. Chapter 5 traces evidence of royal medical care and asks how we might identify reproductive medicine in payments to physicians and connections to medical practitioners and texts. The chapter illustrates key patterns in royal healthcare to illuminate how royal couples medically managed fertility. It argues that royal healthcare was gendered, and reproductive medicine was focused on the queen, but queens had an influential role in the transmission and control of the medical care accessed by the royal couple. Chapter 6 examines how royal couples used spiritual practices to manage reproduction and address fertility problems. It argues that these practices served dual purposes: they were strategic communications to control perceptions of the couple's fertility, while also allowing couples to convey broader political messages about their power and legitimacy.

Ultimately, this book considers the pressure for fertility experienced by royal couples, and how they navigated this using medical and spiritual support. The analysis moves on from questioning how queens and kings negotiated their gendered roles in the absence of reproduction and uncovers the significance of fertility for contemporary perceptions of kingship and queenship. It shows how the uncertainties of reproduction affected and were managed by kings and queens, but in different and gendered ways. Ultimately, the following chapters demonstrate that a more open analysis of infertility is necessary for understanding with greater precision the experience of childlessness, and the importance of fertility for both gendered roles of kingship and queenship.

Chapter 2

UNDER PRESSURE

CONTEMPORARY PERCEPTIONS OF ROYAL FERTILITY

THE HISTORY OF reproduction and infertility is inherently private, making it challenging to access the experiences of individual couples. This chapter turns to medieval chronicles to explore how royal fertility and reproduction were perceived and recorded by the couples' contemporaries. Chronicles are not balanced accounts of events, nor systematic records of royal reproduction; instead, they highlight moments of delay, abundance, or loss that carried political or providential significance. Their value in this chapter lies precisely in this selectivity: their perspectives and agendas provide insight into contemporary perceptions of royal fertility and childlessness. This chapter focuses on what chroniclers actually recorded about royal reproduction, treating royal fertility as an ongoing concern rather than a retrospective outcome. In doing so, it uncovers anxieties that modern scholarship has often overlooked. To understand these contemporary perspectives, it is important to briefly explain the intellectual framework of medical knowledge within which medieval observers operated.

Medieval medical writers offered a range of explanations for conception. Drawing on Aristotelian and Galenic traditions, they debated the respective roles of men and women in generation: Aristotle's "one-seed" model conceptualized the male seed as the active principle which shaped and animated the female material, while Galen's "two-seed" model theorized that both sexes produced seeds which were vital in the right proportion and quality for conception.[1] Conception was understood as a cooperative process, dependent on the health, balance, and proper functioning of both partners. Writers also discussed factors such as age, humoral balance, menstrual health, and sexual pleasure in shaping the likelihood of conception. These ideas framed the intellectual landscape of the thirteenth and fourteenth centuries and circulated in learned medicine.[2]

---

1 Cadden, *Meaning of Sex Difference*, 15–26; 108–9.

2 In the thirteenth century were Avicenna's *Canon*, an Arabic text that combined and analyzed the Hippocratic, Galenic, and Aristotelian thought on medicine and

In theory, these medical models allowed for the possibility that infertility could originate with either the man or the woman, or with both. Medical treatises acknowledged male infertility, often attributing it to defective seed caused by imbalance in the humours, blockages in the seminal passages, or weakness in the generative organs.[3] Female infertility was explained through humoral imbalance, obstructions in the womb, failure of menstruation, or insufficient sexual pleasure to produce seed. Remedies for both sexes ranged from dietary adjustments to purgatives, fumigations, and more invasive procedures, and many medical authors described diagnostic tests aimed at determining which partner was at fault.[4] However, while the learned medical tradition formally assigned reproductive responsibility to men and women, in practice, women were more likely to bear the brunt of suspicion when a couple failed to produce children, and receive the medical treatment for reproductive problems.[5]

While medical explanations and remedies for reproductive problems existed in theory and practice, the royal couples themselves and their political communities were not medical practitioners, nor necessarily versed in contemporary medicine, and perceptions of their fertility cannot be reconstructed from medical texts alone. This chapter therefore moves from medical theory to narrative evidence, asking what contemporaries noticed and recorded about royal fertility. At times chroniclers drew on medical tropes, such as the significance of age or a tendency to focus on women in relation to fertility, but they applied them selectively and when

---

natural philosophy. Together with a core collection of Graeco-Roman texts usually bound together from the twelfth century and known as the *Ars medicinae* or *Articella*, Avicenna's *Canon* formed the foundation of medicine education in the medical faculties at the universities of Salerno, Paris, and Bologna (among many others). Indeed, by the thirteenth century, Avicenna's *Canon* likely superseded the *Ars medicinae* as the foundation of medicine in universities. The universities in Paris, Bologna, and Salerno were particularly known for medicine in the Middle Ages: Green, "Articella: Earlies Copies," 1; O'Boyle, *Art of Medicine*, 83, 95, 102–4; Cadden, *Meaning of Sex Difference*, 67; Jacquart, "Aristotelian Thought in Salerno," 407–28.

3 Hippocratic *Aphorisms*, bk. 5, chap. 62, discusses male and female fertility. Avicenna covers male and female seed and conception in bk. 3 of the *Canon*. *Trotula*, 95, 113, 115 and acknowledges male factor infertility. See also Rider, "Men and Infertility"; Lindgren, "Wandering Womb."

4 *Tractatus de sterilitate mulierum*, ed. Cartelle, 130–59; Pseudo-Arnald, *Tractatus de sterilitate*, ed. Cartelle, 25; Green, *Making Women's Medicine Masculine*.

5 *Tractatus de conceptu*, 48; Rider, "Men and Infertility," 257–61.

it served their narrative purposes.[6] Crucially, chroniclers were not physicians, but usually monastic men who had minimal contact with women, and it is important to acknowledge the gendered nature of these accounts.[7] Their ability (and inclination) to know about matters of pregnancy and reproduction was inevitably limited. Nonetheless, what chroniclers chose to record, and how they framed issues of succession and reproduction, captures attitudes about a couple's fertility that would otherwise be lost to us. This chapter argues that by tracing what was emphasized or omitted in these accounts, we can uncover some contemporary perceptions of a royal couple's fertility—perceptions shaped less by medical theory than by chroniclers' narrative choices and the cultural importance of royal reproduction and the succession.[8]

The following discussion first focuses on what contemporary sources explicitly documented about royal fertility, in particular, what chroniclers knew and wrote about royal births. Next, it investigates when and why chronicles problematized royal fertility. To understand why royal childlessness was concerning in some cases and not others, we might consider what they wrote about the fertility of pubescent kings and queens. Is there any correlation between the onset of concern about royal fertility and the couple's age? Did a certain age or number of childless years trigger concerns about fertility, or was there always pressure to produce an heir from the moment a couple was married and able to consummate their marriage? Finally, this chapter investigates when and why narrative sources problematized royal fertility by analyzing comments about the wait for an heir and assessments of couples who never had children together.

---

6 For the construction of chronicles, see Weiler, "Matthew Paris and the Writing of History," 277; Galloway, "Writing History in England," 255; Given-Wilson, *Chronicles: The Writing of History in Medieval England*, 65–78.

7 However, some chroniclers, like Matthew Paris were very well-connected to the secular world and royal court. For instance, marginal notes in his *Book of St. Albans*, a beautifully decorated text on the life of the saint, indicate that he loaned it to Sanchia of Provence, Eleanor of Provence's sister who was married to Henry III's brother, Richard. See Dublin, Trinity College, MS 177, fol. 2r for the note. Binksi, "Reflections," 336–37.

8 For some discussion of the effects of gender on chronicle narratives, see the edited volume, Dresvina and Sparks, eds, *Authority and Gender in Medieval and Renaissance Chronicles*; particularly, Nelson, "Hussies, Matrons and Others in Carolingian Chronicles," 5–31.

Royal Births

Royal births—a visible sign of fertility—are the most commonly recorded aspect of royal reproduction in chronicles. How chroniclers recorded births, including the inaccuracies and discrepancies in their accounts, is revealing of what they considered most important about royal reproduction. This evidence suggests that the birth of a royal heir was most significant because it was most accurately and consistently recorded in chronicles.

Henry III and Eleanor of Provence had five children together: Edward (b. 1239–d. 1307), Margaret (b. 1240–d. 1275), Beatrice (b. 1242–d. 1275), Edmund (b. 1245–d. 1296), and Katherine (b. 1253–d. 1257). Contemporary chronicler from St. Albans, Matthew Paris recorded the births of all five children in his chronicles, *Chronica majora*, *Historia Anglorum*, and *Flores historiarum*.[9] The *Chronicle of Bury St. Edmunds*, produced by the monks of St. Edmund of East Anglia, who were well-connected to the royal court, also recorded all five royal births.[10] Seven other thirteenth-century chronicles for Henry's reign give a more varied numbering of Eleanor and Henry's children.[11] The heir Edward's birth is consistently mentioned in all eleven chronicle accounts, while only Matthew Paris, the Bury St. Edmunds chronicler, and the *Annals of Winchester*—notably, accounts by authors who had close connections to the royal family and court—record the birth of the couple's youngest child, Katherine, in 1253.[12] This suggests that Edward's birth, as the heir, was most important to the chroniclers and their audience.

9 *Chronica majora*, ed. Luard, 3:539–40 (Edward); 4:48 (Margaret), 223 (Beatrice), 406 (Edmund), 415 (Katherine). *Historia Anglorum*, ed. Madden, 2:422 (Edward), 438 (Margaret), 464 (Beatrice), 499 (Edmund); 3:148 (Katherine). The *Flores historiarum* was an institutional history produced at St. Albans Abbey, first by Roger Wendover, a monk from St. Albans, and continued by generations of monks after his death, including Matthew Paris. *Flores historiarum*, ed. Luard, 2:231 (Edward), 239 (Margaret), 255 (Beatrice), 286 (Edmund), 393 (Katherine).

10 *The Chronicle of Bury St. Edmunds*, ed. Gransden, 10 (Edward), 11 (Margaret; recorded under 1241, rather than 1240), 12 (Beatrice; under 1243, not 1242), 13 (Edmund), 19 (Katherine).

11 Six of the seven chronicles are the chronicles of Winchester, Burton, Osney and Wykes, Tewkesbury, Dunstable, and Waverly. They are printed in Luard, ed. *Annales monastici*, ed. Luard, vols. 1–4. The seventh chronicle is the continuation of Gervase of Canterbury's *Gesta regum*: *The Historical Works of Gervase of Canterbury*, ed. Stubbs, vol. 2.

12 "Annales Monasterii de Wintonia," *Annales monastici*, ed. Luard, 2:94; *Chronicle of Bury St. Edmunds*, ed. Gransden, 19; *Historia Anglorum*, ed. Madden, 2:148; *Chronica majora*, ed. Luard, 4:415.

At the other end of the spectrum of recording royal births, a manuscript version of the *Flores historiarum*—the St. Albans institutional history by Roger of Wendover and continued by Matthew Paris—attributes four additional sons to Henry and Eleanor, all supposedly born between 1247–1256.[13] The births and names of Richard, John, William, and Henry are inserted in the margins of the manuscript by an early fourteenth-century hand.[14] The additional sons in the *Flores* manuscript are not easily dismissed. The manuscript with the insertions was the copy written at St. Albans during Matthew Paris's lifetime and then passed to Westminster ca. 1265, shortly after Paris's death in 1259.[15] St. Albans was well-connected to the royal family and court and Henry III was a regular visitor to Westminster Abbey, so both institutions were particularly close to the royal family and many of the events described in chronicles.[16]

While there are discrepancies in the recording of the births of Henry and Eleanor's children in the chronicles, there is plenty of evidence for five children in other contemporary sources. The chancery rolls from Henry's reign, particularly the liberate rolls, contain preparations and provisions for the births, baptisms, and early childhoods of Edward, Margaret, Beatrice, Edmund, and Katherine; this can be inferred from payments for things like wax tapers to be burned on altars in thanks for their births, prayers for their health, and orders for new clothing and living expenses.[17] By contrast, there is no evidence for any other children born to Henry and Eleanor in these accounts; certainly not four additional sons. Margaret Howell argues that Henry and Eleanor most likely did not have four otherwise un-recorded sons, but she suggests that perhaps they had two sons who might have died as infants, maybe with some form of disability, or who were stillborn between 1246–1252.[18] However, Howell's assertion seems implausible. Matthew Paris describes the couple's youngest child, Katherine, as "mute and useless," so she perhaps had a congenital condition or degenerative illness.[19] After her

13 Howell, "The Children of King Henry III and Eleanor of Provence," 59–60.

14 Howell, "The Children of King Henry III and Eleanor of Provence," 59–60.

15 Howell, "The Children of King Henry III and Eleanor of Provence," 59–60.

16 Carpenter, *Henry III*, 319–48.

17 *CLR*, 1:388, 393, 395, 398, 401, 404, 406, 418, 435; 2:2, 6, 9–10, 15, 18, 19, 86, 148, 191, 210, 213, 215, 275, 284, 286, 288–89, 292; 3:56, 65, 83, 165, 169, 210, 270, 289, 340, 360; 4:183, 289.

18 Howell, "The Children of King Henry III and Eleanor of Provence," 60–71.

19 *Chronica majora*, ed. Luard, 5:632, "muta et inutilis"; Howell, *Eleanor of Provence*, 101, suggests that Katherine had a degenerative condition.

death in 1257 at the age of three, there are orders for commemorative works, including a bronze image for her tomb, documented in the liberate rolls, and Matthew Paris (explicitly noting the king and queen's grief) recorded her death.[20] Given this response to their young daughter's death, it is unlikely that the four sons mentioned in the *Flores* manuscript ever existed, as Henry and Eleanor would surely have mourned and commemorated them if they had been stillborn or died in infancy. Moreover, Matthew Paris's silence is significant given his attention to recording details about the couple's other five children.

Without the births of four additional sons, there are eight years, between 1245–1253, when there is no evidence that Eleanor of Provence conceived or gave birth.[21] Eleanor was only twenty-one in 1245, so it would be unusual for the couple's stalled fertility to have been due to perimenopause or menopause. The Westminster *Flores*'s inclusion of additional sons reads as near-contemporary confusion over the absence of royal births in the period 1245–1253. It may reflect that the absence of births for eight years was hard to believe or at least it confused the early-fourteenth-century writer and prompted his assumption that other children *must* have been born in those years. Perhaps the insertion of four extra sons was even meant to correct the record or smooth over the absence of royal pregnancies and births.[22]

---

20 *CLR*, 4:376 (Katherine's tomb, and an image in gilt bronze for her tomb); *Chronica majora*, ed. Luard, 4:632, "Regina autem mater ejus dolore concepto infirmitate quasi irremediabiliter occupabatur, nec potuit ei phisica vel humana consolatio suffragari" (The queen mother was overcome with sadness and became ill as if she would never recover, and no medical nor human consolation comforted her). When Prince Edward was ill in 1246, Henry III's orders for offerings at shrines, chaplains to celebrate divine services daily, and electuaries (compound medicines) shows his concern and attention to the health of his children, too: *CLR*, 3:18, 30, 36, 37, 54, 56, 65. A year later, Henry was still so thankful for Edward's recovery that he fed the poor in the Great Hall at Westminster "for the love of him who made the king's son safe and sound": *CLR*, 3:165.

21 There is still some chance that Eleanor was pregnant and miscarried in these years, but I have not found any evidence of it. Howell, *Eleanor of Provence*, 70, notes that we still do not know why Eleanor did not conceive in these eight years. The couple were not apart for long stretches in these years and despite a marital rift in 1252, Eleanor still conceived their final child in early 1253.

22 It is possible that an eight-year gap between royal pregnancies and births reflected badly on the king and queen (in particular, the nature of their relationship in the late 1240s–1250s), and so the fourteenth-century chronicler attributed other royal children to Henry III and Eleanor of Provence.

Chronicle records of Edward and Eleanor of Castile's children born before 1272 make for an interesting comparative example and indicate that chronicler interest in royal births was focused on the children of the king and queen. Contemporaries did not consistently or accurately record the children who were born before Prince Edward and Eleanor of Castile's accession in 1272. The birth of their stillborn daughter in 1255 and Katherine, in 1261 are not mentioned by any chroniclers, nor is the birth of the couple's third child, Joan, in January 1265.[23] A son, John was born in July 1266 and his birth was noted by several chroniclers.[24] The *Flores historiarum* recorded his birth year as 1267 though, and the Bury St. Edmunds chronicle gives his name as "John of Winchester," instead of "John of Windsor," showing some confusion or disinterest about where he was born.[25] Three more children were born before Edward and Eleanor's accession: Henry (b. 1268–d. 1274), Eleanor (b. 1269–d. 1298), and a daughter whose name is unknown (b. 1271–d. 1271?).[26] The Bury St. Edmunds chronicler had accurately recorded the birth of John under 1266, but he noted Eleanor's birth a year late, under 1270 rather than 1269.[27] Of the six children born between 1255–1271, only Henry and Eleanor lived past 1272 and their parents' accession, but by 1274 Henry too had died. Edward and Eleanor of Castile had a total of fifteen or sixteen children altogether, and the chronicles were markedly more interested in mentioning their children and accurately recording births (and deaths) *after* the couple became king and queen.[28]

23 Henry III seems to have paid for medicines at Joan's birth: Trease, "Spicers and Apothecaries of the Royal Household in the Reigns of Henry III, Edward I and Edward II," Document B, at 40. Trease interprets the "domine Alyneore" mentioned in the document as Eleanor of Provence, but it is unlikely that the queen would have been called "Lady Eleanor," so the medicines were probably ordered by Henry III for Eleanor of Castile after Joan's birth. Both Katherine and Joan had died by 1265. See Parsons, "The Year of Eleanor of Castile's Birth," 250.

24 "Annales Londoniensis," ed. Stubbs, 76.1: 71; *Chronicle of Bury St. Edmunds*, ed. Gransden, 49. Worcester chronicle: *Annales monastici*, ed. Luard, 4:457. Winchester chronicle: *Annales Monastici*, ed. Luard, 2:104.

25 Parsons, "The Year of Eleanor of Castile's Birth," 250

26 Parsons, "The Year of Eleanor of Castile's Birth," 250–52: anonymous daughter b. 1271 in Acre when Eleanor and Edward were on crusade, and Joan, b. 1272, also in Acre.

27 *Chronicle of Bury St. Edmunds*, ed. Gransden, 47.

28 Parsons, "The Year of Eleanor of Castile's Birth," 253–65: nine children were probably born between 1272 and 1290, when Eleanor of Castile died. All are mentioned by chroniclers except for a child born in 1278 who died immediately, so

The focus on the birth of the king's heir explains the silence about Prince Edward and Eleanor of Castile's fertility in the 1250s–1260s and the inaccuracies in the contemporary chronicle records of the births and deaths of their children prior to 1272. This concentration on the king and queen's children also explains the Westminster *Flores historiarum*'s attribution of four additional sons to Henry III and Eleanor of Provence. That manuscript came from Westminster Abbey, where the supposed royal children were buried, so the insertion was likely made in good faith and with knowledge of actual tombs.[29] Whoever inserted the names in the early fourteenth century knew that young royals had been buried in the abbey several decades earlier.[30] It is possible that the Westminster *Flores* assumed that four children of Edward and Eleanor of Castile who had died prematurely in the mid-thirteenth century were the children of the king and queen at that time, Henry III and Eleanor of Provence.

This focus on the birth of the king and queen's heir is also reflected in the Scottish chronicle evidence and record of the births of Alexander III and Margaret's children. The birth of the couple's first child, Margaret, in 1261 received considerable contemporary attention.[31] Chronicles also recorded the birth of the couple's son, Alexander, who replaced his older sister as their father's heir, in 1264.[32] However, the birth of David, eight years later, in 1272, receives less attention from the chroniclers than Margaret's birth in 1261 and there is no contemporary comment on the eight-year span between the births of the king and queen's second and third children.[33] The consistent reporting of Margaret's birth compared with the dwindling interest in noting the birth of her youngest brother, David, suggests that contemporary interest was not determined by the sex of the child, or time between births, but whether it was the birth of an heir to the throne or not.

Finally, it is worth noting that the way in which births are mentioned by chroniclers demonstrates the confusion around recording and, indeed,

---

it seems that the chronicles did not record or perhaps know about births when the baby was stillborn or died very soon after birth.

29 Howell, "The Children of Henry III and Eleanor of Provence," 59, 71.

30 Due to building works in the fourteenth century, many tombs were disrupted and reburied at Westminster Abbey, leading to confusion: Howell, "The Children of Henry III and Eleanor of Provence," 67–71.

31 *Chronica de Mailros*, ed. Stevenson, 185; *Flores historiarum*, ed. Luard, 2:460, 461, 463 (an English chronicle from St. Albans); See discussion below, 57–58.

32 *Chron. Fordun*, ed. Skene, 301.

33 Of the Scottish chronicles, only the *Chronicle of Melrose* recorded David's birth.

even knowing about royal fertility. Even if the birth of the king's heir was the most important aspect of royal fertility for chroniclers, the details of royal pregnancies and births—such as location and date of birth—were not necessarily easily known by the writers of these accounts. With the exception of Howell's essay on Henry III and Eleanor of Provence's four additional sons, this confusion is not reflected in historiographical discussions of the royal couples considered here.

Age and Fertility

To understand when pressure for royal fertility began, this section examines what contemporaries wrote about fertility in adolescent royal couples. Did youth delay expectations, or did pressure for fertility begin immediately, once a couple was married and considered sexually mature? The following discussion explores medieval ideas about age of sexual maturity and reproductive readiness and considers how these ideas shaped perceptions of delays between when a couple consummated their marriage and produced children; it questions whether some delay was treated as a normal phase of young marriage or interpreted as evidence of infertility, regardless of age.

In medieval medicine and theory about the life course, twelve and fourteen were important coming-of-age points for girls and boys, respectively. For both boys and girls, the transition from childhood to adolescence was understood to be marked by puberty, signifying the onset of reproductive ability.[34] While puberty was generally considered to be around fourteen for boys, it was anticipated at a slightly younger age for girls, around twelve to fourteen.[35] There was some disagreement about the typical age of menarche, as contemporary medical authors placed it variously between twelve and fifteen, likely reflecting reality.[36] The higher echelons of society had better nutrition which probably enabled earlier puberty, so menarche might have been closer to twelve than fifteen for medieval queens.[37]

34 Phillips, *Medieval Maidens*, 24, 26.

35 These ages are varied in legal sources too: Bracton gives fifteen as the age for female inheritance, *Bracton: On the Laws and Customs of England*, ed. Woodbine, trans. Thorne, 2:251. The *Regiam majestatem* gives fourteen for female inheritance: *Regiam majestatem*, ed. Cooper, 154. For discussion of the variation of age depending on gender and locality, see Youngs, *The Life Cycle in Western Europe*, 127.

36 Phillips, *Medieval Maidens*, 25.

37 Phillips, *Medieval Maidens*, 25. See also Green "Flowers, Poisons and Men: Menstruation in Medieval Western Europe," 51–64. For archaeological work on the age of

These ages of puberty informed ideas about sexual maturity and the ability to marry. The age of sexual maturation concerned medieval canon lawyers because it helped determine the age of consent for marriage. The minimum age for marriage was placed at twelve for girls and fourteen for boys in canon law, based on the understanding that these were the ages when they *first* possessed the intellectual and physiological capacities that were fundamental for marriage.[38] However, legal texts did not always explicitly articulate this connection between reproductive ability and marriageable age. In his monumental effort to codify church law in the twelfth century, Gratian does not mention reproductive ability in his discussion of minimum marriageable age, although he does state that mutual consent and sexual intercourse, together, were one way to contract a marriage, implying the need for both physical and intellectual capacity.

Although age of puberty, reproductive ability, and marriage were related in theory, reproduction was not necessarily expected of twelve-year-old brides. There was awareness and acceptance that age was only a theoretical marker and puberty was ultimately distinguished by signs of physical development rather than chronological age. A twelve-year old queen might have been legally old enough to be married but consummation would have been delayed if she had not physically reached puberty.[39] There was also a belief that there should be some years between menarche and childbearing, for the health of both the mother and child. For instance, Peter of Auvergne—an influential thirteenth-century commentator on Aristotle—reasoned that the canonical ages for marriage for girls and boys were not the *best* time for marriage, but the threshold point from which it was possible.[40] Marriage was allowed at twelve for girls and fourteen for boys because they were capable of consent *if* they had reached puberty, but they were still physically imperfect

---

menarche in the Middle Ages: DeWitte and Lewis, "Medieval menarche"; Lewis et al., "On the Threshold of Adulthood," 48–56; Gilchrist, *Medieval Life*.

38 Phillips, *Medieval Maidens*, 27: Marriages contracted at the age of seven, or earlier, could and did happen in practice and when the underaged partner reached canonical age of consent, it could be annulled. Marriages made "in the cradle" were covered in canon law as "pro bono pacis," which worked to legalize very young royal marriages.

39 Phillips, *Medieval Maidens*, 28; Parsons, "Mothers, Daughters," 67–8; Biller, *Measure of Multitude*, 336, cites Peter of Auvergne, a thirteenth-century commentator on Aristotle.

40 Biller, *Measure of Multitude*, 337–38.

until they finished growing.[41] Ultimately, physical development was the essential determiner of readiness for reproduction, not chronological age.

Medieval medical authorities reinforced these concerns about the timing of reproduction, advocating for delays well beyond the canonical marriage ages. Another well-known thirteenth-century writer and commentator on Aristotle, Giles of Rome, argued that intercourse and childbearing was unhealthy for the growing bodies of *both* young men and women and would cause them to have "feeble" children.[42] Two manuscript copies of the *Trotula* compendium, the most widely-circulated and popular set of medieval texts on women's health, advise women to wait until at least fifteen before having intercourse or they risked barrenness, lasciviousness and a lifetime of bad breath.[43] According to Peter of Auvergne, the best time for reproduction was "when the bodies of [man and woman] have been perfected, at the time determined by the Philosopher, or thereabouts."[44] Aristotle—the "Philosopher" referred to by Peter—placed the perfect age of man between thirty and thirty-five. Giles of Rome was perhaps more realistic than Aristotle, and he advised that men should at least wait until twenty-one and women until eighteen to have intercourse and reproduce, when they were safely fully grown.[45] Overall, it was widely believed that while young married couples *could* produce children, it was better to wait for a few years after puberty.[46]

Indeed, in practice, many medieval noble and royal women did not marry until they reached their later teens and, if they were married earlier, consummation was delayed for a few years.[47] Kim Phillips has also emphasized that the distinguishing features between childhood and adolescence were quite blurry in reality and often happened later than the official

---

41 In Aristotle's view, women were always physically imperfect in relation to men but, in this instance, perfection refers to physical maturation of women. Biller, *Measure of Multitude*, 336–37.

42 Phillips, *Medieval Maidens*, 26.

43 Phillips, *Medieval Maidens*, 26: London, British Library (BL), MS Sloane 421A, fols. 6v–7r, and BL, MS Additional 12195, fol. 163v. This passage is not in Monica Green's edition of the *Trotula*.

44 Biller, *Measure of Multitude*, 336.

45 Phillips, *Medieval Maidens*, 26; Beattie, "The Life Cycle: The Ages of Medieval Women," 19–20.

46 Phillips, *Medieval Maidens*, 26.

47 Parsons, "Mothers, Daughters," 67–68.

canonical age of twelve suggests; there were also differences across social strata.[48] Phillips cautions against interpreting maturation as a "swift or smooth movement from one life-phase to another," determined by any singular age, quality or position.[49] Indeed, while some of the royal brides in question here were not yet twelve when they married and others were twelve or in their early teens, royal marriages appear to have been consummated at various ages that are mostly undocumented—though likely at least some of these very young marriages were left unconsummated for years.

The royal couples in this study illustrate the varying experiences around the timing of consummation. There are some indications that Eleanor of Provence and Henry III consummated their marriage soon after their wedding. By 1238, when Eleanor was thirteen or fourteen, she and Henry (who was thirty-one) were at least sharing the same bedchamber because the king was saved from an assassination attempt in the middle of the night because he was sleeping in the queen's bedchamber.[50] In contrast, Joan Plantagenet was only eleven when she married Alexander II in 1221 (he was twenty-three), but it is impossible to tell when their marriage was consummated. Joan of the Tower was just seven when she and David II married in 1328 (and David was only four), so their marriage was surely unconsummated for many years.

Prince Edward and Eleanor of Castile seem to have consummated their marriage very quickly. When they were married in 1254, Eleanor was thirteen and Edward was fifteen, both a year older than the respective twelve and fourteen cited in canon law.[51] They consummated their marriage without delay because Eleanor gave birth in May 1255, only about seven months after their wedding.[52] John Carmi Parsons has suggested that after this, Edward

48 Phillips, *Medieval Maidens*, 35–36.

49 Phillips, *Medieval Maidens*, 36.

50 Henry III saved from assassination: *Chronica majora*, ed. Luard, 3:497. There are also instructions for a passage to be made between the king's and queen's chambers at Bruhulle in December 1237: *CLR*, 305.

51 Phillips, *Medieval Maidens*, 27. Eleanor's birthdate is not certain, but John Carmi Parsons argues that she was born in 1240 or 1241: Parsons, "The Year of Eleanor of Castile's Birth," 245–49.

52 They were married in November 1254. Parsons, "The Year of Eleanor of Castile's Birth," 257. The evidence for a stillborn daughter comes from accounts of the king's wardrobe: 15 Ed. 1 1286–1287, (the entries are published in Trabut-Cussac, "Itinéraire d'Édouard I en France, 1286–1289," 178n54). It was recorded that the queen gave a gold cloth for the anniversary of her daughter on May 29, and Parsons agrees with Trabut-Cussac that this can only have been a daughter born in

and Eleanor were kept apart from each other for some time, to prevent them from conceiving again for a few years after the trauma of the premature stillbirth.[53] At least, after their first pregnancy in 1255, there is no indication that Eleanor was pregnant again until around 1261, when their second daughter, Katherine, was born.[54]

On the other hand, we know that the consummation of Alexander III and Margaret's marriage was delayed because of their youth. They were only ten and eleven, respectively, when they were married in 1251 and, according to Matthew Paris, their marriage was unconsummated for several years. Paris initially reported that Margaret's father, Henry III, had ordered that the consummation of the marriage be delayed "because of their tender age" in 1251.[55] Then, Paris claimed that four years later, in 1255, Margaret complained to her mother's physician because she was miserable at the Scottish court and kept from her husband.[56] According to Paris, the men tasked by Henry III in 1251 with safeguarding Margaret's wellbeing, Robert de Ros and John Balliol, were promptly removed from their posts because of their unjust handling of the situation, and the young king and queen were "allowed to sleep together in one bed as husband and wife."[57]

1255 because Eleanor and Edward only had two children with them in Gascony in 1286–1287, Alphonso and Joan d'Acre, and neither died in that year, nor is Eleanor known to be pregnant or to have given birth in Gascony in 1286–1287.

53 Parsons, "The Year of Eleanor of Castile's Birth,'" 257–58.

54 Our knowledge of the birth in 1255 comes from Edward's wardrobe accounts, 15 Ed. 1 1286–1287, which records a gift to the Dominican priory in Bordeaux on the anniversary of a daughter's birth. We know about Katherine from the record of expenses for her burial in 1264 (*CLR*, 5:142–43); Parsons, "Year of Eleanor of Castile's Birth," 258. The chroniclers say hardly anything about Eleanor of Castile, or her pregnancies and births before 1272, but the fact that children born after 1261 are mentioned by the chroniclers and the chancery sources does indicate that there were probably no births between 1255–1260.

55 *Historia Anglorum*, ed. Madden, 2:117: "Dictumque illi et praeceptum, ne permitteret regem et reginam Scociae condormire, propter eorum aetatis teneritudinem."

56 *Chronica majora*, ed. Luard, 5:501. Matthew Paris attributes this control to Henry III and Eleanor of Provence, Margaret's parents, but Nelson, "Queens and Queenship," 219, discusses how consummation might have been delayed by the Scots as a tactic to ensure that Margaret's dower would not have to be paid and impoverish the Scottish crown if Alexander died prematurely.

57 *Chronica majora*, ed. Luard, 5:505–6: "Feceruntque eos licenter in uno lecto, regem videlicet et Scotorum reginam, ut sponsum et sponsam, condormire."

Based on Paris's account, there was a point after which the marriage should rightfully have been consummated.[58] The king's age seems critical for determining when this was. The comparative examples of Eleanor of Provence, Eleanor of Castile, and Isabella of France imply that eleven or twelve was not an unusually young age for a queen at marriage, and Margaret had already turned twelve in 1252.[59] The premise of Paris's account is that it was unlawful (thus prompting Henry III's involvement in Scotland) to continue to keep Alexander and Margaret from consummating their marriage by 1255. Notably, the king had only just reached fourteen in 1255—the canonical minimum age for boys that theoretically marked his readiness for marriage. Paris's account relies on (and in doing so, reveals) contemporary understanding that the king's achievement of the canonical age threshold provided legitimate grounds for demanding consummation. The significant difference between Margaret and Alexander's early marriage and other couples was Alexander's particularly young age when first married. It was Alexander's youth that provided the rationale for delaying the consummation of the marriage and therefore fertility until 1255.

Once the political pressure for consummating their marriage was resolved in 1255, Alexander III and Margaret did not have their first child until 1261. There is no comment about the delay in the chronicle sources, even though their daughter, Margaret, was born a decade after their wedding and, if we follow Paris, five or six years after their marriage had been consummated. Jessica Nelson speculates that Margaret might have already "had previous unsuccessful pregnancies" by 1261.[60] It is possible that Margaret had suffered pregnancy loss before 1261, but there is no evidence that she did.

Although there is no explicit anxiety about the young couple's fertility in the 1250s, unease over the unsettled succession is evident in the careful preparations for their first child's birth in 1261. Alexander and Margaret travelled to England in the autumn of 1260, when Margaret was already about four or five months pregnant. At this time, Henry III swore an oath that *if* Margaret was pregnant when she and Alexander came to England (the likelihood being that everyone involved knew she already was), he would only allow her to stay to give birth if Alexander and his Scottish counsellors

58 It is worth noting that Paris's explanation of these events may have served as a convenient justification for Henry III's interference in Scottish governance.

59 See Phillips, *Medieval Maidens*, 38–39.

60 Nelson, "Queens and Queenship in Scotland," 237. Nelson does not cite any evidence for her claim that Margaret had earlier pregnancy losses.

agreed and, afterwards, both queen and child would be promptly sent home to Scotland.[61] When, in November 1260, Margaret arrived in England, Henry III promised that if she died in childbirth, her child would be handed back to Alexander and the Scots.[62] As Nelson has noted, it is clear that the child who was about to be born was to be Alexander's heir, with no distinctions or stipulations made about the sex of the unborn child.[63] The baby, Margaret, is called Alexander's "primogenita" in the *Chronicle of Melrose*'s announcement of her birth instead of the more usual "filia," further emphasizing that the baby was officially recognized as Alexander's heir.[64]

The recognition of the royal infant as Alexander's heir, regardless of sex, indicates growing concern about the succession and the lack of heir by 1261. The need for Henry III to make public promises ensuring that the baby would be returned to Scotland as quickly as possible indicates how politically significant this unborn child was to the Scots. Alexander III was an only child and so there were no close relatives to fall back on if he died unexpectedly and before he produced an heir. His father, Alexander II had three sisters, but they had all died by 1259 and only one had produced a child, a daughter who died in 1237.[65] So Margaret and Alexander III's child would be the only living and legitimate heir from two generations.

Indeed, the concern about the lack of heir is also indicated by the fact that the willingness to welcome a female heir in 1261 was not lasting. Margaret was quickly replaced as her father's heir in 1264, when a baby boy, Alexander, was born and immediately became heir presumptive.[66] Henry III also seems to have valued the birth of a grandson in 1264 over his granddaughter in 1261, as the messenger who brought him the news of Margaret's birth in 1261 was given 10 marks annually for the news, but £10 a year was granted

---

61 *CPR 1258–1266*, 95; *CDS*, ed. Bain, 1:no. 2206; Latin text printed in *Foedera*, ed Rymer, 1.1:402: "Dictam Reginam sponsam suam, cum sua prole, qualem bonorum omnium Dispensator ordinaverit, ad dicti Regis voluntatem & mandatum, ad regnum suum Scotiae, sine dilation qualibet & difficultate, vel cujuscumque contradictionis obstaculo, rehabere; & quod ispa, una cum prole, per nuncios suos, pro ipsis destinandos ad ipsum Regem & regnum." The choice of "prole" to describe the child is significantly ambiguous and inclusive of a male or female baby.

62 *CPR 1258–66*, 128; *CDS*, ed. Bain, 1:no. 2229.

63 Nelson, "Queens and Queenship in Scotland," 238.

64 *Chronica de Mailros*, ed. Stevenson, 185: "Nata est etiam in Anglia primogenital regis Scotiae, nominee Margareta."

65 Oram, *Alexander II*, 152, 216.

66 *Chron. Fordun*, ed. Skene, 301.

to the messenger in 1264 when he announced the birth of Alexander.[67] There is no contemporary comment by chroniclers or even scholarly interest in Alexander and Margaret's wait for an heir, but the willingness of the Scottish political community to accept a female infant as heir in 1261 preserves contemporary anxiety about the couple's childlessness in the 1250s.

The comparative cases of Edward and Eleanor of Castile, and Alexander III and Margaret of England are valuable for understanding when a royal couple's childlessness roused contemporary concern. In both couples, husband and wife were in their teens (or younger) when they married, and the youthfulness of both partners appears to have initially delayed expectations of their fertility. In Edward and Eleanor's case, their youth was acknowledged by delaying marriage until both had passed minimum canonical age, and they may have been kept apart for years after a stillbirth in 1255. In Alexander and Margaret's case, they were initially kept apart, and consummation was deliberately delayed until they both reached the minimum canonical ages for marriage and the anticipated onset of physical maturity.

The silence in chronicles initially gives the impression that there was no concern about these young couples' fertility. There are certainly no explicit expressions of anxiety in the first decade of their marriages. Nevertheless, the birth of Alexander and Margaret's first child in 1261 appears to have been anxiously anticipated. The formal preparations and insistence on the infant's swift return to Scotland underscore the political weight of her arrival. In contrast, there was a distinct lack of interest from contemporaries in the births of Prince Edward and Eleanor of Castile's children, or the couple's experiences of infant loss, before they became king and queen in 1272. The difference in contemporary reactions and attention to these similarly aged couples suggests that it was royal status, as reigning king and queen rather than heirs, that influenced whether their delay in producing a (living) child became concerning.

The Wait for an Heir

Explicit scrutiny of royal fertility is rare in medieval chronicles, but when it does appear, it offers invaluable insight into the significance of royal reproduction for kings and queens. This section examines Matthew Paris's claim that there was concern over Eleanor of Provence's fertility, and chroniclers' expressions of relief at the birth of Edward II and Isabella of France's first child.

67 *CPR 1258–1266*, 5:175, 382; *CPR 1266–1272*, 6:395; Nelson, "Queens and Queenship," 224.

Why did childlessness attract attention in these cases but not in others? Ultimately, Paris's comment is unique, but his statement exposes a fundamental point that typifies a broader dynamic in the chronicle evidence; overt scrutiny of the queen's fertility was rooted in concerns about the king's behaviour. Previous scholarship has missed a crucial point: in the moments when chroniclers seem to be focused on the queen, they were, in fact, also thinking about the king.

The starkest problematization of a royal couple's fertility is by Matthew Paris. Under 1236, the same year that Henry III and Eleanor of Provence were married, Paris wrote that Henry's younger brother, Richard of Cornwall, was not allowed to travel to the court of the Holy Roman Emperor, Frederick II (who was married to Henry and Richard's sister, Isabella), to help the emperor make war with France because Richard was:

> confirmed as the only clear heir to the king and realm, and after the king, everyone's hopes fell on him. For the king, although married, has no children, and it is still unknown whether his wife the queen, because of her youth, will be fertile or barren.[68]

It is not so strange that Paris—and Henry, if he was the one who stopped Richard from leaving—viewed the twelve-year-old queen's fertility like this, but it is odd that Paris felt this was something worth recording. There is some uncertainty about Eleanor's birthdate, but Paris describes Eleanor as being "already twelve" in 1236.[69] Even if she was slightly younger than twelve, Paris's explicit declaration that she *was* twelve, and therefore above the threshold age for marriage, and so consummation, frames his comments about (and expectations of) the young queen's fertility.[70]

By 1238, when Eleanor was fourteen, she and Henry (who was thirty) had still not had a child. Matthew Paris recounts how another sister of Henry III, Eleanor, married Simon de Montfort, earl of Leicester, and within the same

---

68 *Chronica majora*, ed. Luard, 3:340: "Cum unicus et manifestus haeres regis et regni comprobetur, et spes omnium in ejus sinu post regem reponatur. Rex enim, quamvis uxoratur, liberis caret, et uxor ejus regina, utpote juvencula, utrum sit foecunda an sterilis ignoratur." For Henry and Eleanor's wedding in 1236, see: Howell, *Eleanor of Provence*, 1. Matthew Paris describes the wedding: *Historia Anglorum*, ed. Madden, 1189–1245, 2:397; *Flores historiarum*, ed. Luard, 2:217; *Chronica majora*, ed. Luard, 3:340.

69 *Chronica majora*, ed. Luard, 3:335, Paris says Eleanor was "jamque duodennem" (already twelve) when negotiations for the marriage were taking place in late 1235, which is relevant for reading his comment about her fertility in the *Chronica majora*. However, he also says Eleanor was "aetate fere duodennem" (nearly the age of twelve) in 1236 in *Historia Anglorum*, ed. Madden, 2:386.

70 Phillips, *Medieval Maidens*, 27. Biller, *The Measure of Multitude*, 336.

year gave birth to their first child and heir, who was named Henry, "for the strength and solace of the kingdom," because "it was greatly feared that the queen was barren."[71] Paris's comment is ostensibly about the queen, but it seems just as concerned with the king and the context of his succession: the remark about Eleanor is situated in the narrative in a way which demonstrates that the birth of de Montfort's heir drew attention to the fact that the king, unlike the men around him, had still not produced his own heir and the succession was reliant on his brother, Richard, and new infant nephew.

While Paris's explicit concern about the queen's fertility is unique, chroniclers imply concern in their expressions of relief following the birth of Edward II and Isabella of France's first child in 1312. Like Eleanor, Isabella was twelve when she was married. Also, like Eleanor and Henry, Isabella and Edward's first child was not born for four years, although no chronicler doubted Isabella's fertility in the first years of the marriage. However, while Edward and Isabella's wait for a pregnancy is not openly problematized in contemporary sources, the marked relief and joy in the chronicle reports of Prince Edward's birth in 1312 is noticeable.

The *Vita Edwardi secundi* reports under 1312 that, "a handsome and *long-desired* son was born to the king," and claims:

> [This] *longed-for* birth was timely for us, because by God's will it fortunately had two consequences, as it greatly lessened the grief which the king had experienced from [Piers Gaveston's] death and provided a sure heir for the realm. For if the king had died without issue, the crown would certainly have remained in dispute.[72]

This distinct sense of relief is demonstrated by several other chroniclers too. The fourteenth-century annals from St. Albans Abbey similarly state that: "all of England expressed enormous delight [at the birth of Prince Edward], and his father who had been consumed by grief for Piers Gaveston's death, tempered his sorrow and was quite light-hearted."[73] The *Annales Paulini* from St. Paul's Cathedral in London says that "there was great dancing in

---

71 *Historia Anglorum*, ed. Madden, 2:414; *Chronica majora*, ed. Luard, 3:518: "ad robur et solatium regni...Timebatur enim vehementer, quod regina sterilis fuisset."

72 *Vita Edwardi secundi*, eds. Childs and Denholm-Young, 63: "Natus est regi filius formosus et dudum affectatus...Hec adoptata natiuitas tempore accepto nobis aduenit, quia duos effectus Deo disponente feliciter impleuit. Dolorem namque regis quem ex morte Petri conceperat ualde mitigauit, et certum heredem regno prouidit. Nam, si rex decessisset sine prole, pro certo mansisset corona sub lite."

73 "Johannis de Trokelowe Annals," ed. Riley, 79: "Ob cujus ortum tota Angliae ingenti plausu laetata est, et pater ejus tam hilaris efficitur, quod dolorem, quem

the city because of his birth," while the *Annales Londoniensis* goes into much more detail and describes how Prince Edward's birth "brought the greatest joy to all the realm" and:

> when the news of his birth reached the citizens of London, the mayor and aldermen danced through the whole city from day to night, and so did large groups of citizens, no matter who they were, because of their great joy; and the fishmongers arranged a special dance for the queen's arrival at Westminster...and so dancing in the presence of the queen, all of them [the fishmongers] rode through the middle of the aforesaid city before the queen on horse-back, accompanying her to Eltham, and to all onlookers, they showed unheard of relief.[74]

The *Flores historiarum* is less exuberant but prefaces the announcement of Edward's birth by noting that "the great kingdom of England was adorned with noble progeny."[75] Geoffrey le Baker's *Chronicon* reports the birth and then states that, "this year the source of joy [was] the son born of the queen and she was greatly appreciated and most tenderly cherished."[76] The Bridlington chronicler noted Edward's birth, and included a celebratory verse and prayer for the child's safety.[77]

---

pro morte Petri conceperat, temperaret." The author of these annals (spanning 1307–1327) is now thought to be William Rishanger, and Trokelowe his scribe.

74 "Annales Paulini," ed. Stubbs, 76.1:273: "Et maximum tripudium fuit in civitate ob causam illius nativatis," "Annales Londoniensis," ed. Stubbs, 220–1: "Toto regno gaudium conferens permaximum...Cum rumor ejusdem nativitatis civibus Londoniensibus pervenisset, major cum aldermannis per totam civitatem, diebus et noctibus continuis, choream duxerunt, et quaelibet contubernia civium catervatim prae nimio gaudio hoc idem fecerunt: sed et piscenarii, contra adventum dominae reginae Westmonasterio se praeparantes, inaestimabilem ordinaverunt choream... et sic coram regina karolantes, et per medium praedictae civitatis ante reginam equitantes, conducendo ipsam versus Heltham, omnibus intuentibus, inauditum praemonstraverunt solatium."

75 *Flores Historiarum*, ed. Luard, 3:153: "Altissimus regnum Anglorum generosa progenie decorare."

76 Geoffrey Le Baker, *Chronicon*, ed. Thompson, 6: "Hoc anno laeticia nati filii et regine quam nimium dilexit et tenerrime confovit."

77 *Chronicles of the Reigns of Edward I and Edward II*, ed. Stubbs, 76.2:45: "Natus est Edwardus tertius post conquaestum, et sextus post Brutum; unde scribitur versus" (Edward is born, the third after the conquest, and sixth after Brutus; for whom these lines are written):

Hunc natum cura, virgo vincens nocitura, (Care for this child born, virgin conquering harm)
Casta creatura, quae salvasti peritura, (O chaste creature, who saved the doomed)
De puero pura specialis sit tibi cura, (Let you give care to this pure and special child)
Ut permansura sibi semper sint sua jura. (So that his rights will always be lasting)

Chroniclers' accounts of widespread relief at Edward's birth indicate that there was concern about Edward II and Isabella's childlessness before 1312. This concern seems to stem from a contemporary impression that Edward II had neglected his queen and delayed the birth of an heir because of his focus on his favourite, Piers Gaveston.[78] Just before describing the rejoicing at Edward's birth in 1312, the chronicle from St. Albans mentions Isabella's sorrow because of Edward's neglect, when he chose to flee from his nobles with Gaveston instead of staying with his "then pregnant" queen.[79] This episode highlights the perceptions of Edward's unmanly and un-kingly behaviour, juxtaposed in the narrative with Isabella's imminent fulfilment of her maternal and queenly duty. At the close of his account for 1312, the *Vita Edwardi secundi* author summed up Edward's reign to that point, stating that, despite having reigned now for six full years, "he has achieved nothing praiseworthy or memorable, except that he has made a splendid marriage and produced a handsome son and heir to the kingdom."[80] Earlier in the account, the chronicler described how Edward grieved for Piers Gaveston "as a father at any time grieves for his son." The statement cleverly emphasizes Edward's prioritization of his relationship with Gaveston and highlights the neglect of his duty to both Isabella and his kingdom to provide a legitimate biological heir, an *actual* son.[81]

Two other accounts offer insight into contemporary perceptions of Edward II's fondness for Gaveston and his neglect of Isabella. Writing in the later fourteenth century, Thomas Walsingham of St. Albans claimed that in 1308, Isabella wrote to her father, Philip IV of France, complaining that Edward was ignoring her in favour of Piers Gaveston.[82] Similarly, the *Annales Paulini* reported that after Isabella's coronation that same year, "the queen's

---

78 For discussion of Edward's relationship with Gaveston, see Ormrod, "The Sexualities of Edward II," 22–47. Ormrod argues against the retrospective labelling of Edward's sexuality, and interpretation that Edward and Piers had a homosexual relationship. See also: Menache, "Isabella of France: A Postscript," 499–500.

79 "Johannis de Trokelowe," 75, claims that the king decided to go to Newcastle, not thinking of the risk, "nor the weeping queen, then pregnant" (*nec fletibus Reginae, tunc praegnantis*) so that he could be with Piers.

80 *Vita Edwardi secundi*, eds. Childs and Denholm-Young 68–69: "Ecce nunc rex noster Edwardus sex annis complete regnauit, nec aliquid laudabile uel dignum memoria hucusque patrauit, nisi quod regaliter nupsit et prolem elegantem regni heredem sibi suscitauit." English translation is by Childs.

81 *Vita Edwardi secundi*, eds. Childs and Denholm-Young 52–53: "Sicut aliquando dolet pater de filio."

82 Thomas Walsingham, *Historia Anglicana*, ed. Riley, 1:125.

uncles saw that the king used Piers's bed more than the queen's, and they returned to France in anger. As such, a rumour spread throughout the land that the king loved the wicked man more than his wife, the most elegant and beautiful lady."[83] While neither chronicle explicitly links this to the absence of an heir, both suggest that Edward's intimate relationship with Gaveston was seen as interfering with his marital and dynastic duties. The implication is that his sexual preferences—or at least his emotional dependence on Gaveston—were perceived as a reason for the delay in producing a child.

The chroniclers' impression that Edward II had neglected his wife and the legitimate succession may also have been influenced by contemporaries' knowledge that the king was capable of having a child. Edward had at least one illegitimate son, Adam, who is mentioned in the wardrobe accounts from 1322 when the king paid for his son to join the campaign in Scotland in 1322.[84] Nothing else is known about Adam or his mother, but he was likely born before Edward and Isabella married in 1308 because he was old enough to be a soldier in 1322.[85] Chronicler judgements that Edward and Isabella's childlessness was caused by the king's neglect of his queen and his duty might reasonably have been amplified by knowledge of his reproductive ability.

The births of Edward and Isabella's other children were not recorded with as much celebration as Prince Edward's, but Isabella's fertility earned noticeable praise from the chroniclers.[86] John of Eltham was born in 1316, four years after his brother Edward, and the *Flores historiarum* depicts Isabella's success in light of her fertility, commenting "at Eltham in Kent on the 15 August, Lady Isabella the queen was adorned with a twin bloom when

83 "Annales Paulini," ed. Stubbs, 262: "Patrui reginae, cernentes quod rex plus exerceret Petri triclinium quam reginae, cum indignatione ad Franciam remigarunt. In omnem igitur terram exit rumor iste, quod rex plus amaret hominem magnum et maleficium quam sponsam suam elegantissimam dominam et pulcherrimam mulierum."

84 Phillips, *Edward II*, 102, 428–29; Blackley, "Adam, the Bastard Son of Edward II," 76–77, cites BL, Stowe MS 553, fol. 27.

85 Phillips, *Edward II*, 428–29 suggests that he was likely born in 1305 or 1306.

86 The *Vita Edwardi secundi* does not mention John's birth in 1316, but remarks that there were devastating grain shortages, excessive rain, floods and "fruitful land [was] turned into barrenness" that year: *Vita Edwardi secundi*, eds. Childs and Denholm-Young, 120–21. Perhaps recording royal fertility was too uncomfortable a juxtaposition (and too favourable to Edward II) for the *Vita* chronicler to stomach. The silence might be because two leaves covering 1316 are missing from the sole extant manuscript of the chronicle. Mentioned by Childs in her introduction to the edition: *Vita Edwardi secundi*, xv.

she gave birth to the lord king's second son...In light of giving birth to these noble offspring, the said queen was famous for her fertility."[87]

Edward and Isabella had two more children together, Eleanor (b. 1318) and Joan (b. 1321). The *Annales Paulini* mentions Eleanor's birth in 1318 and describes that the queen "was purified with great ceremony and celebrations."[88] The *Vita Edwardi secundi* does not record Eleanor's birth in 1318, but the chronicler states under that year that hope grew because "God has gladdened the king and people with many signs of prosperity," and "England became fruitful with a lavish profusion of all good things."[89] A royal birth would also have been a sign of prosperity for Edward, Isabella and the kingdom. While Edward II and Isabella have not previously been considered to have suffered from infertility, the contemporary evidence shows that there was considerable apprehension about the wait for a royal heir in the first four years of their marriage. Notably, this initial delay is blamed on the king, and there is distinct sympathy for the queen and celebration of her fertility in narrative sources.

Edward II's deposition by his son and queen in 1326 adds another layer to consider when interpreting how chronicles problematized the couple's wait for an heir. Many of the histories that cover the events of Edward II's reign were edited after his deposition in 1326, or compiled in his son Edward III's reign.[90] Mark Ormrod argued that Edward II struggled to display the critical masculine qualities expected in kingship, while Isabella's leading role in the overthrow of her husband and position as regent in the early reign of her son was a significant transgression of her gendered role as both a consort and a mother.[91] Ormrod has suggested that after the removal of Edward III's

---

87 *Flores historiarum*, ed. Luard, 3:176: "Domina Isabella regina, gemino flore decorate, apud Eltham in Cantia, quinto decimo die mensis Augusti, domino regi filium peperit secundum...Ante ortum hujus regalis propaginis, qua dicta regina nobiliter exstitit prole foecunda."

88 "Annales Paulini," ed. Stubbs, 283: "Purificata fuit ibidem cum magna sollempnitate et tripudio."

89 *Vita Edwardi secundi*, eds. Childs and Denholm-Young, 154–57: quotes from 154, "Deus in multis prosperis regem et populum exhillarauit"; "et habundancia omnium bonorum terram Anglorum multipliciter fecundauit."

90 See Childs's introduction to the *Vita Edwardi secundi*, xvii–xx. *Chronicles of the Reigns of Edward I and Edward II*, ed. Stubbs, 76.1:xvi–xlvi.

91 Ormrod, "Monarchy, Martyrdom," 178. Edward III was fourteen in 1327 and Ormrod argues that he did not really need a regent and should have been allowed to rule in his own right, so, as such, Isabella also manipulated her maternal role to secure power for herself.

mother and Roger Mortimer from power in the 1330s, "it was therefore especially important and relevant that his regime should seek to re-establish the gender norms implicit in the theory and practice of monarchy."[92] Edward III worked to rebuild his father's masculinity by imposing a gendered and conventional widowhood on his mother, correcting rather than punishing her transgressions, and controlling the narrative of his father's deposition so that it became the result of an unruly queen rather than an unmanly king.[93] Similarly, the chronicles' knowledge of Edward II's deposition—whether they were written/compiled before or after 1326—ultimately contributed to how they depict his kingship and Isabella's queenship before 1326.

Specifically, comments about the royal couple's delayed pregnancy in the 1310s apply gendered narratives to the king and queen. The chronicles completed before the deposition demonstrate Edward's shortcomings as a king through his neglect of his reproductive duty in the 1310s, while the accounts compiled *after* 1326 help to re-establish the correct gendering of Isabella's role as a queen and a mother by emphasizing and praising her fertility. The portion of the *Vita Edwardi secundi* that covers 1307–1326 seems to have been written by the end of that period, just before Isabella's invasion of England and overthrow of Edward.[94] Highly critical of Edward II, but seemingly without knowledge of how his reign was to end, the *Vita*'s comments about the delayed birth of the couple's heir show sympathy for Isabella as consort and condemn Edward's behaviour as husband/king, a sentiment which we might expect from an account written before Edward was deposed. Compiled after 1326, the *Flores historiarum*, *Annales Paulini*, and *Annales Londoniensis* (the latter two are based on the *Flores historiarum*) also described the relief and joy at the birth of the future Edward III and extolled Isabella's fertility. They present the same narrative about the couple's fertility as the *Vita*, but written after Edward's overthrow, the narrative re-establishes Isabella's role as a good wife and mother. How accurately the chronicles preserve contemporary perceptions of the couple's fertility in the 1310s is difficult to determine, but we are able to see how chronicles scrutinized the wait for a

92 Ormrod, "Monarchy, Martyrdom," 178.

93 Ormrod, "Monarchy, Martyrdom," 178–79.

94 *Vita Edwardi secundi*, eds. Childs and Denholm-Young, xx (introduction to the chronicle). Chris Given-Wilson argues that the *Vita Edwardi secundi* was composed at regular intervals throughout Edward II's reign, up until 1325, because there seems to be no knowledge of the events of 1326: Given-Wilson, "*Vita Edwardi secundi*: Memoir or Journal?" 165–76.

child to criticize the king's behaviour, and how they emphasized successful fertility to redeem the queen's transgressions.

Chronicle comments on delayed royal pregnancies reveal that fertility anxieties were rooted in concern about kingly behaviour and succession fears, rather than queenly inadequacy. Matthew Paris's attention to Eleanor of Provence's fertility when she was still so young has been overlooked by scholars, but his ostensible concern about Eleanor actually reflected fears about Henry III and his succession. Similarly, while Edward II and Isabella have not previously been considered to have suffered from infertility, contemporary chronicles show considerable apprehension about the unsecured succession during their first four years of marriage. Significantly, chroniclers blamed the couple's childlessness on the king while expressing sympathy for Isabella and celebrating her eventual fertility. Later chroniclers, writing after Edward's deposition during Edward III's reign, used gendered narratives about the wait for an heir to demonstrate Edward II's failure and to reconstruct Isabella's correctly gendered role as his wife and queen. These examples demonstrate how the problematization of royal childlessness was consistently related to kingly behaviour and context rather than queenly deficiency.

Royal Couples Who Never Had Children

How did chroniclers treat the royal couples who remained childless? Were queens who died without producing children discussed differently in contemporary sources than those who successfully produced heirs? While chronicles typically focused explicitly on the queen when mentioning fertility, this chapter has demonstrated that the king's status and behaviour significantly influenced attention to a couple's fertility. This pattern raises important questions: did chroniclers assign blame for ongoing childlessness, and if so, to whom? The evidence for Alexander II's first and second queens, Joan Plantagenet and Marie de Coucy, suggests that chroniclers held kings at least as accountable as queens for royal childlessness.

Chronicles mention remarkably little about the childlessness of Alexander II and Joan Plantagenet, given the focus on Joan's fertility in modern scholarship. The *Chronicle of Melrose* does not say much at all about Joan, only noting the royal marriage in 1221 and the queen's pilgrimage to Canterbury in 1237, "for the sake of praying there."[95] The only other mention of Joan

95 *Chronica de Mailros*, ed. Stevenson, 138 (marriage), 148 (pilgrimage). The *Chronicle of Melrose* seems to have been written contemporaneously with the events it describes between 1171 and 1263. For detailed discussion of the physical

is a passage about her death in England, after "protracting a severe illness" following her journey to St. Thomas Becket's shrine in Canterbury.[96] The *Melrose* chronicler explains that in March 1238, the queen, "having received the sacraments of the church, and without children [...died] in the arms of her brothers Henry, king of England, and Richard, duke of Cornwall."[97] The passage about Joan's death is followed a few lines later by an equally brief one on Alexander's marriage to Marie de Coucy in May 1239.[98] The birth of Alexander's heir in 1241 is recorded, but Marie is not named nor actually mentioned in the entry about the royal birth.[99]

The *Chronicle of Lanercost*, like *Melrose*, mentions Joan and Alexander's marriage in 1221, but does not have much else to say about Joan.[100] Under 1238 it states that "Joan, daughter of king John of England, and queen of Scotland died."[101] Unlike *Melrose,* there is no mention of the queen's childlessness. Alexander's marriage to Marie de Coucy in 1239 is described very briefly and, when their son Alexander was born in 1241, the chronicler states simply that "a son was born to Alexander king of Scotland, and his name is Alexander in memory of his father, produced by his fertile wife who he married from overseas,

---

complexities of the manuscripts and contents and composition of the *Chronicle of Melrose*, see: *The Chronicle of Melrose*, eds. Broun and Harrison; Broun, "Creating and Maintaining A Year-by-Year Chronicle: The Evidence Of The Chronicle of Melrose," 141–52; Duncan, "Sources and Uses of the *Chronicle of Melrose*, 1165–1297," 146–85.

96 *Chronica de Mailros*, ed. Stevenson, 148: "Gravi infirmitate detenta."

97 *Chronica de Mailros*, ed. Stevenson, 148–49: "Domina Johanna regina Scocie... perceptis ecclesiasticis sacramentis, absque liberis...inter manus fratrum, H. scilicet regis Anglie et R. ducis Cornubie."

98 *Chronica de Mailros*, ed. Stevenson, 149.

99 *Chronica de Mailros*, ed. Stevenson, 154: "Natus est primogenitus domini Alexandri regis Scocie apud Rokesburch, in die translationis sancti Cuthberti, pridie nonas Septembris, feria iiii[a] dictusque est Alexander; natus est autem anno etatis patris sui xliii[io] incipiente, tunc regni sui xxvii" (The firstborn son of Alexander, King of Scots was born at Roxburgh, on the Translation of St. Cuthbert, 4 September, and he is called Alexander; he was born when his father was aged 44 years, then the 27th year of his reign).

100 *Chronicon de Lanercost*, ed. Stevenson, 29. Despite its English origins, *Lanercost* is a valuable and knowledgeable, if sometimes hostile, source for thirteenth-century Scotland. Herbert Maxwell argues that the chronicle was compiled or composed in Carlisle, despite its association with the neighbouring Lanercost Priory; *Chronicle of Lanercost*, ed. Maxwell, xiii–xx. For more discussion this source, see also Kehnel, "The Narrative Tradition of the Medieval Franciscan Friars on the British Isles," 507–9; Gransden, *Historical Writing in England, c. 550–c. 1307*, 1:494–501; Nelson, "Queens and Queenship," 281.

101 *Chronicon de Lanercost*, ed. Stevenson, 47: "Johanna, filia regis Johannis Angliae, ac regina Scotiae, in fata collapsa est."

known as Marie, from the Coucy family."[102] *Lanercost* was produced in Northern England, so the author's silence about Alexander and Joan's childlessness might reflect a lack of interest or knowledge, or perhaps he did not wish to imply any negative comparison with Alexander's first and English-born queen.

Other Scottish chronicles mention just as little about both Joan and Marie de Coucy. The contemporary thirteenth-century source *Gesta annalia I*, preserved in John of Fordun's fourteenth-century *Chronica gentis Scotorum*, mentions that Joan and Alexander were married in York in 1221, when Joan was a "girl of most tender age," likely an acknowledgement that she was only eleven and officially too young to be married.[103] The couple's almost twenty years of marriage are covered in a few passages, with just a description of a meeting between Alexander II and Joan and Henry III and Eleanor of Provence in York in 1237. Alexander returned home to Scotland after the meeting ended, reports the *Gesta* author, but Joan stayed in England to go on a pilgrimage to Canterbury with Eleanor of Provence.[104] Like the *Chronicle of Melrose*, the *Gesta* notes that Joan died in March of 1238, in the arms of her brothers. Unlike *Melrose*, there is no mention of the queen's childlessness. The only comment about the absence of a royal heir is made in the entry about Alexander's second marriage, which happened very soon after Joan died (and is described in the same passage as Joan's death):

> Therefore, since the king produced no sons or daughters with [Joan], he took to be his wife the daughter of the nobleman Ingram of Coucy, who was named Marie, on Pentecost, the Ides of May at Roxburgh in 1239. And she gave him a son, who was given the name of his father.[105]

---

102 *Chronicon de Lanercost*, ed. Stevenson, 48–49: "MCCXLI. Eodem anno natus est Alexandro regi Scottorum filius, ad memoriam patris Alexander nominatus, ex fecunda uxore quam de partibus transmarinis duxit, Maria scilicet, genere de Curcys."

103 *Chron. Fordun*, ed. Skene, 288: "puellam adhuc tenerrimae aetatis." John of Fordun's *Chronica* is a compilation of older sources rather than his own original work. The narrative from 1153 to early 1285 is an older history known as *Gesta annalia I*, probably written in the thirteenth century, while the account from late 1285 to 1363 is another distinct source, known as the *Gesta annalia II*. See Broun, "A New Look at *Gesta annalia*," 9–30.

104 *Chron. Fordun*, ed. Skene, 291: "Peractis quoque tractatibus rex Scociae prospere repatriavit. Sed regina Scociae cum regina Angliae, causa orationis, Cantuariam adiit, quae juxta Londonias defuncta est anno sequente, videlicet, anno Domini MCCXXXVIII, IIII nonas Martii, inter manus Henrici regis Angliae et Ricardi ducis Cornubiae, fratrum dictae reginae."

105 *Chron. Fordun*, ed. Skene, 291: "Cum igitur rex filios aut filias ex ea minime procreasset, consilio suorum procerum filiam duxit uxorem nobilis viri Ingerami de

The paragraph does not add anything else about Alexander and Marie's marriage and ends with the king's death in 1249. The explanation that Alexander married Marie because "the king produced no sons or daughters [with Joan]" makes Alexander at least as accountable as Joan for the infertility of their marriage.

The *Gesta annalia I*'s comments about Joan and Alexander's marriage and childlessness are repeated in Walter Bower's fifteenth-century *Scotichronicon*. Bower used Fordun's work (Fordun's narrative up until early 1285 is the *Gesta annalia I*) for much of his account, but he also had access to other narratives which the *Gesta annalia I*/Fordun seem not to have known.[106] Bower mentions Joan's death in England in 1238, after the pilgrimage to Canterbury with her sister-in-law, Eleanor of Provence, but he includes nothing about childlessness in the record of her death.[107] Bower echoes the *Gesta annalia I* under 1239, stating that "as King Alexander did not have any offspring with his first wife," he married Marie de Coucy.[108]

Despite never producing an heir, Joan comes off quite well in the *Orygynale Cronykil* by Andrew of Wyntoun.[109] Wyntoun covers Alexander and Joan's life together in just a few lines, stating that after their wedding in 1221 in England, Alexander brought her back to his own country, but "he had no children with that lady. For she died after that."[110] Despite noting that Alexan-

---

Cuchy, Mariam nomine, die Pentecostis Idus Maii apud Roxburgh anno MCCXXXIX, de qua genuit filium, cui nomen patris impositum est."

106 Watt, *Chron. Bower*, ed. Watt, 9:243–51. Broun, "A New Look at *Gesta annalia*," 14–15; Boardman, "Chronicle Propaganda in Fourteenth-Century Scotland," 24–25; *Chron. Bower*, ed. Watt, 9:204–9.

107 *Chron. Bower*, ed. Watt, 5:160. The *Liber Pluscardensis*, the later fifteenth-century account based on Bower's work, repeats Bower's description of Alexander's need to remarry because he and Joan had no children but adds that Joan died in Cupar, Fife, perhaps confusing her with Alexander III's queen, Margaret: *Liber Pluscardensis*, ed. Skene, 1:52.

108 *Chron. Bower*, ed. Watt, 5:166–68: "Cum igitur rex Alexander de prima conjuge sua natos non haberet."

109 Wyntoun had access to a now lost thirteenth-century account, probably from St. Andrews. See Broun, "A New Look at *Gesta annalia*," 14–15; Boardman, "Chronicle Propaganda," 25–26. *Chron. Bower*, ed. Watt, 9:234–51, esp. 244–45. Wyntoun produced three versions of his chronicle. The first edition was written by about 1408 and the third by 1424. The first and third are edited and published in *The Original Chronicle of Andrew of Wyntoun*, ed. Amours. The second edition was edited by Laing, *The Orygynale Cronykil of Scotland by Andrew of Wyntoun*. I use Laing's edition.

110 *Wyntoun*, ed. Laing, 2:238: "On that lady na barne he gate./Fra scho ded wes, efftyre that."

der produced no children with Joan, this does not seem to be an evaluation of the marriage or queen's worth; Wyntoun goes on to describe that their union brought stability to Scotland, as "all was quiet, settled, and peaceful. For [Henry III and Alexander] were two kings of peace."[111] He explicitly acknowledges that Joan was crucial to this: "there was the Queen, this Alexander's wife, this Henry's sister: without her, strife."[112]

Like the other chronicles, Wyntoun also mentions the talks that happened in York in 1237 between Henry and Alexander and their queens, and "afterwards [Joan] bade farewell to her lord, for he rode home to Scotland: for her purpose was to go on pilgrimage to Canterbury. There she died with honour and was buried in holy sepulcher."[113] Wyntoun follows his lines about Joan's death in 1238 with a very similarly structured and brief comment about Alexander II's second wife and the outcome of that marriage: "he married Lady Mary, Sir Ingram de Coucy's daughter. With her he had Alexander the Third, who became king after him."[114] Jessica Nelson claims that Joan's burial in England indicates her failure to be fully accepted in Scotland and her lack of success as Alexander's wife and queen, primarily because she failed to produce an heir.[115] This is clearly not the impression given by Andrew of Wyntoun though, who says more in praise of Joan than Marie de Coucy, even though Marie ultimately gave Alexander II an heir.

On the whole, Joan and Marie are depicted comparably in the Scottish chronicles—both in the frequency of comments and in what was written about them—despite the fact that Joan and Alexander were childless for almost two decades, and Marie produced a son within two years of marriage. There is no special praise for Marie's fertility or expression of relief about Prince Alexander's birth as there was by the English chroniclers after the birth of Edward II's heir in 1312. Comparing the chronicle comments about Joan with those about Marie de Coucy shows that Joan's childlessness

---

111 *Wyntoun*, ed. Laing, 2:239: "wes ay qwyete, rest, and pes./ Kyngis off Pes for-thi thai twa."

112 *Wyntoun*, ed. Laing, 2:243: "Thare wes the Qwene, this Alysandrys wyff/This Henrys systyr: for-thi, but stryff."

113 *Wyntoun*, ed. Laing, 2:243: "Efftyre [Joan's] Lord off Lewe scho bade,/Fra he hame in till Scotland rade:/ In till pilgrimage to pas/Till Cawntyrbery hyr purpos wes./Thare scho deyd with honwre,/ And layd in halowyd sepulture."

114 *Wyntoun*, ed. Laing, 2:238: "To wyff he weddyt Dame Mary,/ Schyr Ingramys dowchtyr De Cowcy./ Alysandyr the thryd on hyr he gat,/ Nest hym that Kyng wes efftyr that."

115 Nelson, "Queens and Queenship," 182–89.

was thought worth mentioning by the *Melrose* chronicler, but the comment seems quite a neutral assessment of Joan as queen. Moreover, the language of the *Gesta annalia I* suggests that Alexander and Joan's infertility might have even been acknowledged as their shared burden. Ultimately, the impression from the contemporary chronicles does not convey the sense that Joan's "failure to bear a child made her, in essence, a failure as queen."[116]

* * *

Contemporary medieval sources reveal far more concern about royal fertility than modern historians have acknowledged. Stripping back historiographical impressions of royal couples and examining what chroniclers actually wrote about fertility revealed significant contemporary concern about reproduction for couples like Henry III and Eleanor of Provence, and Edward II and Isabella of France, despite their eventual success at producing multiple children. Scholarship has overlooked the anxieties about delayed pregnancies and other fertility challenges that existed during these couples' lives by narrowly focusing on ultimate reproductive outcomes rather than contemporary perceptions during these couples' lives. Chroniclers' ostensible association of reproduction with queens has further reinforced a scholarly fixation on the childlessness of queens like Joan Plantagenet, obscuring the important role kings played in contemporary perceptions of fertility.

Despite this association of queens with reproduction, the chronicle evidence also challenges existing assumptions about medieval perceptions of reproductive responsibility. While reproduction was closely associated with queens—like Matthew Paris's comments about Eleanor of Provence's possible sterility and the treatment of Joan Plantagenet and Marie de Coucy by Scottish chroniclers—chronicles did not openly blame queens for the lack of heirs. Joan Plantagenet was not condemned for her childlessness and the chroniclers seemed to view infertility as much the king's issue as the queen's. Similarly, attention to queens who produced heirs, such as Marie de Coucy, does not appear markedly different from that given to those who did not, suggesting that scholarly assumptions about a queen's worth being tied to fertility should be reconsidered. While chroniclers celebrated queens' fertility—Isabella of France's success after bearing sons, for instance—they also recorded concern over reproductive issues in ways that implicate the king and broader contextual factors, like in the cases of Eleanor of Provence and Margaret of England.

---

116 Nelson, "Queens and Queenship," 189.

Furthermore, the chronicle records of the reproductive histories of queens, like Eleanor of Castile, illustrate the broader difficulty of reconstructing women's maternal experiences, even at the highest social levels. Despite Eleanor's numerous pregnancies, details about their timing, outcomes, and maternal experience are incomplete which reflects the broader trend in medieval sources of privileging the birth of heirs over the mother's bodily history. Chronicles often record only surviving children, especially sons, or note reproductive events in passing, underscoring the marginalization of women's, even queens', experiences.

Ultimately, this analysis has revealed the previously overlooked importance of kings in contemporary perceptions of royal couples' fertility. The narrative significance of reproduction in chronicles—whether used to illustrate Edward II's failings or to highlight Isabella of France's success after producing heirs—demonstrates that fertility was crucial to the roles of both king and queen, even when chroniclers only explicitly discussed it in relation to queens. The evidence suggests that contemporary concerns about royal fertility were triggered by factors beyond simply the queen's age or the passage of time, pointing to the need for a more nuanced understanding of how medieval observers evaluated royal reproductive success and failure.

Chapter 3

NARRATIVES ABOUT ROYAL CHILDLESSNESS

WE HAVE SEEN how chronicles used royal fertility to highlight the success or failure of kings and queens like Edward II and Isabella of France. This chapter narrows in on how chronicles approached royal childlessness, showing how commentary on the absence of an heir conveyed assessments of the king and the condition of the realm. The first half of this chapter examines comments about the childlessness of David II and his two queens, Joan and Margaret. Narrative sources for David's reign were significantly revised in the reigns of his successors and this chapter argues that their handling of royal childlessness shows their perspectives on David's kingship. The second half of the chapter considers claims about queens faking pregnancies. These narratives shed light on the significance of fertility for a queen. Several factors, namely, their uniqueness, the lack of coverage by any other chronicles, and the fact that the accounts were written after the queens' reigns, make these stories unlikely. Nonetheless, it is the retrospective narrative use of fake pregnancy, rather than the matter of their accuracy, which is revealing of how infertility could be perceived and ultimately weaponized against a medieval queen. The fake pregnancy claims illustrate the pressure on a queen to produce an heir, perceptions about the importance of fertility for maintaining her position, and the uncertainty surrounding pregnancy and childbirth in the Middle Ages.[1] Ultimately, these chronicles wove royal childlessness into their narratives, utilizing it as a tool for political commentary and, in so doing, reflecting the perceived significance of successful fertility for medieval kings and queens.

The King Under Scrutiny

David II spent much of his adult reign, particularly after 1357 when he was released from imprisonment in England, locked in a power struggle with his adult nephew and heir presumptive, Robert the Steward. Ultimately, when David died in 1371 without having produced his own biological heir,

1 Some of the section on fake pregnancies has been previously published as Trivett, "'Because She Pretended to be Pregnant and Was Not," in *The Art of Illness: Malingering and Inventing Health Conditions*, ed. Wendy J. Turner (Routledge, 2023), 115–37. Reproduced by permission of Taylor & Francis Group.

his nephew became King Robert II. The Scottish chroniclers' perspectives on David II versus the Steward shaped their accounts about David and his queens' childlessness. The *Gesta annalia II*, completed by 1363 during David's reign, is the most pro-David and anti-Stewart of the fourteenth-century Scottish chronicles.[2] The *Gesta annalia II*'s portrayal of the events of the 1330s–1350s preserves the contemporary criticism of Robert the Steward that existed in the 1360s, fostered in David's court.[3] Later fourteenth- and fifteenth-century chronicles, Andrew of Wyntoun's *Orygynale Cronykil*, Bower's *Scotichronicon*, and the *Liber Pluscardensis* (mostly an abridgement of Bower's slightly earlier work with the addition of some "eyewitness" accounts), were written after 1371, during the reigns of Stewart kings.[4] As such, they offer a much more favourable view of Robert the Steward's actions in the 1340s–1360s than of David's.[5] These accounts give a polarized impression of the two men and their actions, depending on whether they were completed before or after 1371.[6] Ultimately, the chroniclers who were most critical of David II were also the most outspoken about his childlessness.

David returned to Scotland after eleven years of imprisonment in England but his queen, Joan of the Tower was granted safe-conduct by her brother, Edward III, to return to England indefinitely in 1358.[7] Scholars have interpreted this as a breakdown of the royal marriage—even though Joan still supported David in diplomatic talks with her brother after 1358—because she never returned to Scotland before her death in 1362.[8] As a result,

2 *Gesta annalia II* was written contemporaneously between 1285–1363 and is preserved in John of Fordun's *Chronica gentis Scotorum*. Boardman, "Chronicle Propaganda," 23. Penman, *David II*, 253 argues that the *Gesta annalia II* was written by the Bishop of St. Andrews, a supporter of David, who died in 1363.

3 Boardman, "Chronicle Propaganda," 24–25.

4 For work on the fourteenth- and fifteenth-century Scottish chronicles, see Drexler, "The Extant Abridgements of Walter Bower's 'Scotichronicon,'" 63–64. Mapstone, "Older Scots Literature and the Court," 273–85. Boardman, "A People Divided? Language, History and Anglo-Scottish Conflict in the World of Andrew of Wyntoun," 112–29.

5 Boardman, "Chronicle Propaganda," 23.

6 Boardman, "Chronicle Propaganda," 24.

7 *Rot. Scot.*, ed. Illingworth et al., 1:822 (safe conduct). Penman, *David II*, 204, suggests that this may indicate that David was planning to have his marriage to Joan annulled.

8 Penman, *David II*, 204, 218–20, says it is not clear whether this indicates a breakdown of the marriage, but he goes on to treat it as such in his analysis. Mark

between 1358–1362, David found himself in limbo, still married but without the ability to produce a legitimate heir. Around this time, David took Katherine Mortimer as a mistress. Most extant manuscripts of the *Gesta annalia II* say nothing about Joan's return to England, her death there in 1362, nor that she was childless; however, two surviving manuscripts have an additional insertion which briefly mentions the date and place of Joan's death in England, her burial there, and that she died "without children."[9] Katherine Mortimer is not mentioned, and the account ends in 1363, with a brief note that David married Margaret Logie. As the surviving chronicle compiled closest in time to the events of David's reign, the *Gesta annalia II*'s account indicates that the king's adultery and marital separation reflected so poorly on David II that they could not be mentioned.

Andrew of Wyntoun, like the *Gesta annalia II*, does not say anything about David's adultery but he does explain that Joan went to England in 1358 and stayed there after David returned home to Scotland:

> the queen, Lady Joan, was with him, to see her mother and her brother; she was happy to be there. And within a short time, she died there. She was buried with her ancestors, and her soul passed to paradise. For she was sweet and gracious, charming, kind, pleasant, and fair.[10]

Andrew of Wyntoun was more favourable to the Stewarts than the *Gesta annalia II*, but many of the individuals on both sides of the events of the 1350s and 1360 were still living when he was writing in the early fifteenth century, which seems to have tempered his account.[11] This proximity to the events and characters of David's reign adds to the significance of Wyntoun's silence about royal childlessness and the king's adultery. Wyntoun's praise for Queen Joan's character helps to emphasize David's failings, without

---

Ormrod also suggests that David might have been trying to annul the marriage, as Joan possibly entered the Franciscan order just before her death in 1362: Ormrod, "Katherine Mortimer's Death at Soutra," 115–16. Penman, *David II*, 204, says that "divorce/remarriage was certainly a tactic which David employed later in life."

9 *Chron. Fordun*, ed. Skene, 380. Skene mentions these passages in a footnote: the two manuscripts insert two extra chapters, one on the death of Queen Joan and one on the death of Pope Innocent VI. Joan is described as "sine liberis" (without children).

10 *Wyntoun*, ed. Laing, 2:502: "Dam Johne the Quen wyth hym had he,/ Hir modyr and hir brodyr to sé:/ Than wes scho blyth thiddyr to faire./ And wythin schort tym deit thare./ Wyth hir eldrys scho beryit was./ Tyl Paradis hir sawl mot pas./ For scho wes swete, and debonare,/ curtas, hamely, plesande, and faire."

11 Penman, *David II*, 253.

needing to explicitly record his adultery, while the silence about childlessness prevents any blackening of Joan's image. Similar to the *Gesta annalia II*, but in light of his own more anti-David perspective, the way that Wyntoun handled Joan's return to England and remained quiet about David's adultery and the couple's childlessness indicates that such behaviour and circumstances were damaging to perceptions of both the king and queen.

Walter Bower's *Scotichronicon* is much more critical of David II than the *Gesta annalia II* and even Wyntoun, and his staunchly pro-Stewart perspective is reflected in his comments on David's adultery.[12] Bower mentions Katherine Mortimer and describes her murder in 1360, saying that she was "wickedly killed when she was in the king's company as he was coming from England. The king loved her more than all other women, and on her account the queen was entirely neglected while he embraced his mistress."[13] In a following line, Bower states that "[t]he gravity and danger of adultery is clear for three reasons, namely: the heavy punishment laid down in ancient law; the procreation of illegitimate offspring; the breaking of pledges of faithfulness."[14] After explaining each reason in lengthy detail, Bower finishes by stating that if adultery discredits "any simple man because he is notorious, how much do you think it is disgraceful in a king!"[15] Notably, Bower says only that Joan was in England "after seeking permission from King David her husband; and after spending a little time there as a pilgrim she died."[16] Like the earlier chroniclers, Bower makes no explicit remark about the couple's

12 Walter Bower's chronicle was composed in the 1440s. Bower used Fordun's compilation as his main source for the *Scotichronicon*, and so his mid-fifteenth-century work also preserves the much older sources *Gesta annalia I*, and *Gesta annalia II*. Bower also had access to more material than just the *Gesta annalia I* and *Gesta annalia II*, including a lost source probably written in St. Andrews in the thirteenth century which seems to have been unknown to the author of the thirteenth-century *Gesta annalia I*. Broun, "A New Look at *Gesta annalia*," 14–15; Boardman, "Chronicle Propaganda," 25–26. *Chron. Bower*, ed. Watt, 9:234–51, esp. 244–45.

13 *Chron. Bower*, ed. Watt, 7:320–21: "quam in comitiva regis venientis de Anglia… nequiter occiderunt. Quam pre ceteris mulieribus rex pretulit in amore; propter quam nimium regina fuit neclecta et complexa concubine." English translations are by Watt.

14 *Chron. Bower*, ed. Watt, 7:320–21: "Adulterii igitur magnitude et periculum patet ex tribus, vielicet: ex legis antique gravi punicione; prolis perverse procreacione; date fidei violacione."

15 *Chron. Bower*, ed. Watt, 7:322: "Et si istud vicium quemcumque simplicem dedecoret, quia infamis est, quantum putas dedeceat regem!"

16 *Chron. Bower*, ed. Watt, 7:304–5: "petitia licencia a David rege sponso suo, Angliam peciit, et ibidem aliquanto tempore commorata obit peregrina."

childlessness.[17] The resulting picture is of a good and blameless queen (she even sought David's permission before going on pilgrimage) and a dishonourable king who abandoned his wife for his mistress.

The implication from Bower is that David and Joan's childlessness was because David abandoned his queen and duty. By mentioning that Joan was entirely neglected by David, Bower absolves Joan of any blame for her return to England, while simultaneously criticizing and highlighting the consequences of David's behaviour on the fertility of the marriage. The passages about David's adultery are followed by an explanation of the king's proposal of the succession-peace deal in 1364, when he pushed the Scottish magnates to accept a son of the English king as his heir.[18] For Bower, who particularly admired individuals who "led or sustained the 'patriotic' cause" in Scotland, David's willingness to hand over his kingdom to an English prince completes the tripart condemnation of the Bruce king, who was adulterous, Anglophilic, and neglectful of his wife and reproductive duty.[19]

The late fifteenth-century *Liber Pluscardensis* author goes even further than Bower and *explicitly* attributes infertility to David's adulterous behaviour. The *Liber* states that Joan "asked permission from David to go on a pilgrimage to St. Thomas of Canterbury and to visit her brother Edward king of England...So she went away to England, and remained there some time, and died."[20] The chronicle then explains Katherine Mortimer's murder and comments on the king's adultery:

> through the keeping of that mistress [Katherine] the queen was neglected and many other evils ensued...By this may be seen what evils are brought on by that sin of adultery, as saith the Lord by the prophet, "the sword shall not depart from thy house for ever, seeing thou hast despised me in violating thy neighbour's bed."...See then how adultery displeases the Divine Majesty.

---

17 Wyntoun and Bower had access to the same source for their histories. Known as the *Anonymous Chronicle*, covering 1324–1390 and finished during the reign of Robert III, it gives a favourable portrayal of the Stewart family in the 1350s and 1360s. Bower used it to add to the *Gesta annalia II* in Fordun's *Chronica*, his main source for the *Scotichronicon*. The *Anonymous Chronicle* seems not to have been known or used by Fordun. Boardman, "Chronicle Propaganda," 25–26, 29.

18 *Chron. Bower*, ed. Watt, 7:323.

19 Boardman, "Chronicle Propaganda," 23 describes Bower's sympathy for the "patriotic cause."

20 *Liber Pluscardensis*, ed. Skene, 1:302: "Regina vero Scociae, petita licencia a rege David, marito suo, ut peregre apud Sanctum Thomam' de Canterbury proficisceretur, et ut fratrem suum Edwardum regem Angliae...ubi remanendo pro aliquo tempore, mortua est."

> King David, who was an open fornicator, never could have peace or happiness or prosperity or favour during his life, or secure the throne in the lineal succession of his body, or have fruitfulness or plenty in his time.[21]

In case there was any doubt about why David had failed to produce a child after reading Bower's account, the *Liber* chronicle makes it clear that the king did not produce a legitimate heir because he was an adulterer. The explanation that Joan was only in England for a pilgrimage removes any sense that she had abandoned her duty as wife and queen by returning to England. The silence about childlessness in relation to Joan, as in Bower's account, helps to portray the queen as blameless while bolstering the impression that David was an immoral king who was responsible for his own childless fate. At the same time, the Scottish chronicles' silence about Joan's childlessness may also reflect heightened sensitivity to the Scottish succession crisis of 1290 and the Anglo-Scottish warfare that followed in the fourteenth century. Laura Barefield has argued that women's roles were submerged in narratives in order to demonstrate the "smooth passing of generations, the accomplishment of narrative itself and the creation of patriarchy." [22] Glossing over Joan's childlessness creates a narrative about the passage of time and smooth transfer of power down to the Stewart kings in the fifteenth century.

The sources closest to David's reign are vague about the king's second marriage to Margaret Logie. The *Gesta annalia II* ended in 1363, with a short passage about David's marriage to Margaret, and it therefore contains nothing about the breakdown of the marriage five years later.[23] Andrew of Wyntoun wrote that "King David married Margaret Logie in the month of April.

---

21 *Liber Pluscardensis*, ed. Skene, 1:305: "quia, licet in retencione illius concubinae regina neclecta fuit, et multa alia mala consecuta sunt...Per hoc poterit apparere quanta mala in illo peccato adulterii perveniunt, dicente Domino per prophetam: Non recedet de domo tua gladius in aeternum, eo quod despexisti [me] violando thorum Christi tui. ...Videte inquantum adulterium ergo displicet Divinae majestati; quod rex David, qui fornicator publicus erat, nuncquam in vita sua pacem vel felicitatem, prosperitatem aut graciam, vel regnum successione liniali sui corporis potuit praemunire, sive fertilitatem aut habundanciam in tempore suo." English translation by Skene, *Liber Pluscardensis*, ed. Skene, 2:232. In this same passage, the chronicler notes that David's nephew, John of Sutherland, was killed by the plague. Penman, *David II*, 115, suggests that David was likely hoping to make John his heir instead of Robert the Steward.

22 Barefield, *Gender History in Medieval Chronicle and Romance*, 8. On the narrative function of women in the Scottish chronicles, see Royan "Some Conspicuous Women," 131–44.

23 *Chron. Fordun*, ed. Skene, 382. Although Fordun's *Chronica* was continued until 1385 in several manuscripts, the *Gesta annalia II* ended in 1363, discernible because

But they were together only a short while."[24] He says nothing else about Margaret, perhaps because many who knew and were related to her were still alive when he was writing.

However, as the chroniclers gained more distance from the fourteenth-century events that they described, the depictions of David and Margaret's marriage worsen. Walter Bower claims that

> with the aim therefore of providing for the succession to the kingdom from the fruit of her womb (if God granted it), King David chose a most beautiful lady, Margaret Logie, the widow of John Logie, perhaps not so much for the excellence of her character as a woman as for the pleasure he took in her desirable appearance.[25]

This is followed by six and a half chapters about the traits of a good wife and how to choose and manage her, implicitly illustrating all the ways that David went wrong.[26] Bower wraps up the lesson with a note about the end of David and Margaret's marriage, stating that "[David] lived with her for a short time, [but following animosity that arose between them] he divorced her about the beginning of Lent 1369."[27] Distinctly, Margaret and David's childlessness is at the centre of Bower's assessment of their marriage: he bookends his account of their marriage with the introductory statement that its purpose was to provide for the succession and concludes by stating that it ended in failure, which implies that the marriage was valued by fertility and subsequently ended by their infertility.[28]

---

there is a gap in the narrative from that year until the report of David's death in 1371, and then it continues until 1385; See Boardman, "Chronicle Propaganda," 24–25.

24 *Wyntoun*, ed. Laing, 2:506: "King Davy/ weddit Dame Mergret off Logy/ In the moneth off Aprile./ Thai ware togiddyr bot schort quhile."

25 *Chron. Bower*, ed. Watt, 7:332: "Volens igitur rex David previdere pro successione regni de fructu ventris sui, si Deus dederit, elegit unam speciossimam dominam, Margaritam Logy relictam [Johannis Logy], forte non tam bonitate virtutis feminee quam voluptate forme appertitive."

26 *Chron. Bower*, ed. Watt, 7:332–59.

27 *Chron. Bower*, ed. Watt, 7:358: "cum qua parvo tempore habitavit, et sed propter quasdam simultates inter eos conceptas] divorcium celebravit. The inserted section is only included in one extant manuscript."

28 Bower seems particularly anti-Margaret, because these passages about the end of Margaret and David's marriage are followed by the claim that David had previously arrested three of Robert the Steward's sons, at Margaret's instigation, but after the "divorce," the king "restored them to favour as before." *Chron. Bower*, ed. Watt, 7:358: ad pristinam graciam recepit.

The late fifteenth-century *Liber Pluscardensis* unsurprisingly repeats most of Bower's description about David and Margaret's marriage and "divorce" but with a crucial additional detail. The *Liber* states that David "did not, however, stay very long with [Margaret] before again getting a divorce, because she pretended to be pregnant and was not."[29] There is no evidence that David tried to formally divorce Joan, except perhaps their possible separation after 1358, so the *Liber*'s claim that the king was "again getting a divorce" is the author's (mis)understanding.[30] The accusation that Margaret faked a pregnancy takes Bower's veiled comments about the marriage's failure one step further and attributes the breakdown specifically to the absence of a biological heir (and Margaret's desperate attempt to supply one). Infertility was not grounds for divorce, but the fact that the *Liber* depicts it as such shows the perceived effect that childlessness had on the royal marriage, David's actions in the late 1360s and the immense pressure for fertility experienced by his second queen.

A substantial narrative source for David II's reign, Sir Thomas Gray's *Scalacronica* offers an entirely different perspective from the other chronicles and serves as an illustrative point of comparison for the Scottish (monastic) chronicle accounts of David and his queens' childlessness. Gray was an English knight who was captured by the Scots in 1355 and imprisoned in Edinburgh Castle for two years, during which time he started his Anglo-Norman chronicle, completed around 1363.[31] Given this context, Gray's account of David II is hardly filled with flattery, but it does show how a different purpose and perspective from the pro-Bruce or pro-Stewart Scottish chroniclers alters the narrative on royal fertility and David's marital fidelity. Gray's account of Joan's return to England and David's adultery is arranged more chronologically than in the Scottish chronicles. He first mentions Katherine, David's mistress, under the year 1358, which is probably when their relationship began; Gray states that David "loved passionately" the wife of

---

29 *Liber Pluscardensis*, ed. Skene, 1:307: "Sed cum ea non tempore multo perduravit quin iterum divorcium celebravit, eo quod ipsa impregnatam finxit et non fuit."

30 Penman, *David II*, 219 suggests that David had been "putting out feelers" to Pope Clement VI about annulling his marriage to Joan, but there does not seem to be any documentary evidence of this, except that Joan joined the Franciscans shortly before her death.

31 Thomas Gray, *Scalacronica*, ed. and trans. King, xvii–xxxiii. For more on Gray, see King, "A Helm with a Crest of Gold," 21–36; King, "Englishmen, Scots and Marchers," 217–31; King, "Scaling the Ladder: The Rise and Rise of the Grays of Heaton, *c*. 1296–*c*. 1415," 57–73.

William de Ramsay, Earl of Fife.[32] A few passages later, still under 1358, Gray writes that Joan,

> the Queen of Scotland...came to Windsor in the same season, to speak with her brother the king, and to put forward a longer treaty for discussion; and she was with her mother, Queen Isabella, who died at Hertford in the same season [Aug 1358], who she had not seen for thirty years.[33]

Two years later in his account, Gray describes how

> Katherine de Mortimer, a young lady of London, became so intimate with Monsieur David de Bruce (who was called King by the Scots), through the acquaintance he had with her while he was a prisoner, that he could not do without her presence. In the absence of his wife, the King of England's sister, who was staying with her brother at the time, he always rode everywhere with her; and this special treatment was displeasing to some Scottish lords.[34]

The lords' displeasure was so great, according to Gray, that they had Katherine killed.[35] Gray's description of Joan's death in 1362 is brief; he states just that she died and was buried next to her mother in the Minorites of London.[36] He notes that Joan was living in England before her death, and his description that David loved Katherine Mortimer "passionately" just a few passages later might be an implied explanation for why Joan never returned to Scotland. However, Gray presents the initial reason for Joan's visit to England as a diplomatic mission and so that she might spend time with her mother.

David does not come across well in Gray's account; it was the king's insistence on keeping his mistress with him at all times, in the absence of his wife, that so provoked (according to Gray) some Scottish magnates to have Katherine murdered. Gray makes no mention of Joan and David's childlessness, perhaps to save Joan from blame but more likely because he was not particularly interested in the Scottish succession. He does not condemn

---

32 Thomas Gray, *Scalacronica*, ed. and trans. King, 147.

33 Thomas Gray, *Scalacronica*, ed. and trans. King, 151.

34 Thomas Gray, *Scalacronica*, ed. and trans. King, 189–91. Gray's remark about Katherine being from London is a strange confusion, given his initial description that she was the wife of William, the Earl of Fife in 1358.

35 Thomas Gray, *Scalacronica*, ed. and trans. King, 189–91.

36 Thomas Gray, *Scalacronica*, ed. and trans. King, 201. Herbert Maxwell, the nineteenth-century editor of Gray's *Scalacronica*, adds a layer of his own assumption here, stating in a footnote that "[Joan] had left King David because of his infidelity, receiving Hertford Castle from King Edward as a residence." See *Sir Thomas Gray's Scalacronica*, ed. Maxwell, 171.

David for adultery, nor relate it to childlessness and Gray's *Scalacronica*, unlike Bower's account, lacks any long moralistic discussion of adultery. Gray is also matter-of-fact about David's second marriage: he reports only that "David took to wife Margaret de Logie, a lady who had been married already, and who had lived with him for some time. This marriage was made solely on account of love, which conquers all things."[37] He does not mention the breakdown of the marriage in 1369. Gray died in 1369, though, the same year that David and Margaret's marriage seems to have broken down, so perhaps he did not know about it.

Ultimately, how the chronicles explained royal childlessness was shaped by their perspectives on David II. The *Gesta annalia II*, closest in time and most favourable to David, says nothing about Joan's return to and death in England or the king's mistress and avoids assigning blame for the marriage's infertility. On the other hand, the Stewart-era chroniclers, Bower and the *Liber Pluscardensis*, openly blame infertility on David's behaviour, as an adulterous and neglectful husband to Joan. Joan's reproductive record is barely mentioned by any of the chroniclers, with only two manuscripts containing the *Gesta annalia II* even noting that she died childless.[38] Generally, the chroniclers seem quite sympathetic towards her. In contrast, the pro-Stewart chronicles do not depict Margaret Logie favourably. Bower illustrates her failing as a wife based on the criteria he included for judging good wives (his claim that David married Margaret for her beauty after six-and-a-half chapters about the folly of choosing a wife based on lust). His ultimate blow to Margaret and final demonstration of David's regrettable decision to marry her was noting the infertility of their marriage. The *Liber Pluscardensis* makes this cause and effect even more explicit, with the accusation that David ended the marriage because Margaret pretended to be pregnant, blaming the marriage's failure on the failure and reproductive deception of the queen. The contextual factors of David's reign and the nature of the surviving sources are important for understanding chronicle comments relating to royal fertility; the fifteenth-century chronicles compiled furthest from David's reign held particularly harsh and retrospective views of his kingship which influenced how they depicted his accomplishments and judged his failures as king, including infertility.

---

37 *Sir Thomas Gray's Scalacronica*, ed. Maxwell, 174.

38 *Chron. Fordun*, ed. Skene, 382, does also mention the king's childlessness in the notice of David's death in 1371: "Regnavit XLVIII annis, sine liberis" (He ruled for 48 years, [and died] without children). The notice of David's death in 1371 was not part of the original *Gesta annalia II* source (completed in 1363), however.

Fake Pregnancy Narratives

Accusations that Yolande de Dreux and Margaret Logie faked pregnancies are only made in two chronicles, but these narratives require some consideration and are rich for understanding the significance of fertility and childlessness for medieval queens. According to the *Chronicle of Lanercost* and the *Liber Pluscardensis*, respectively, Queens Yolande de Dreux and Margaret Logie pretended to be pregnant at pivotal moments of uncertainty around the Scottish succession—in 1286, after the unexpected death of Alexander III without a clear, adult heir, and during the reign of David II, whose first marriage of several decades had also remained childless. These claims about faked pregnancy offer insight into medieval knowledge and perceptions of royal fertility and how that was written in narrative sources, rather than serving as accurate records of events. While the fake pregnancies illustrate the pressure experienced by queens to produce an heir, they also reveal the ambiguity surrounding pregnancy in the Middle Ages and demonstrate how queens negotiated and were affected by this.

Yolande de Dreux and Alexander III's short marriage is mainly a footnote at the end of Alexander's reign, a brief episode preceding the succession crisis of the 1290s.[39] As such, it is not unexpected that Yolande features so little in the contemporary sources. The *Chronicle of Lanercost*, however, mentions Yolande de Dreux far more than other contemporary accounts. The chronicler describes how Alexander III ignored repeated advice to wait out a storm late one night in 1286 because he was determined to travel across the Forth to be reunited with his new wife, Yolande, who was staying in Kinghorn (Fife).[40] Alexander made it to Inverkeithing (Fife) and was once again advised to delay his late-night journey to Kinghorn, due to bad weather, but he refused and, during the ride along the shore, he fell from his horse

39 Queen Margaret died in 1275 and by 1284, all three of Alexander III's adult children had died in short succession and he was left without an heir. In order to produce a legitimate heir, Alexander married Yolande de Dreux in November 1285, but he died unexpectedly in the spring of 1286, before they produced a child. There *is* some possibility and contemporary suggestion that Yolande might actually have been pregnant in 1286. The *Chronicle of Osney*, a contemporary chronicle produced at Osney Abbey records that Yolande "seemed to be pregnant" after Alexander's death, "Annales Monasterii de Osenia," in *Annales monastici*, ed. Luard, 4:306. *Chron. Bower*, ed. Watt, 6:10–11 also mentions that "it was said that [Yolande] was pregnant… [but] it ended in failure or a miscarriage" (*dicebatur reginam Joletam sive Jolandam impregnasse…Quo casu deficient sive aborsum edente*).

40 *Chronicon de Lanercost*, ed. Stevenson, 116–17.

and died.[41] Before describing the events that led to Alexander's death, the *Lanercost* chronicler noted that Alexander's marriage to Yolande was "to his own sadness, and to the everlasting damage of the whole kingdom."[42] This is followed by a description of the changeable, ambitious nature of Yolande: allegedly many people declared that before her marriage, she was pledged to become a nun but then changed her mind, "with the readiness of a woman's heart and with ambition for a kingdom."[43] These comments precede the description of Alexander's death, and so the reader is primed to see Yolande as an unpredictable and ambitious woman, even before learning that Alexander III would surely have still lived if he had not been so determined to reach his wife. The chronicler implicitly blames Yolande and her womanly wiles for Alexander's untimely death, for she was the reason he was so set on making the dangerous late-night journey in the storm.

The *Lanercost* chronicler then describes that after Alexander's death, in the absence of an obvious and mature heir, his kingdom was ruled by a group of guardians. These magnates administered the kingdom and granted Yolande her rightful dower lands as Alexander's widow.[44] Yet despite this just treatment, the widowed queen,

> resorting to feminine cunning, was pretending to be pregnant, so that the guardians would postpone their decision [about who was to be Alexander's heir] and she might more easily acquire favourable public opinion for herself. But, in the way that women's craft always turns out terribly in the end, with her deceit she disturbed the land from the day of the king's death until the Feast of the Purification [March 19, 1286 until February 2, 1287], not permitting honest women to examine her condition. And so that she could discredit those from whom she had received reverence and honour, she decided to delude the nation forever by substituting the child of another.[45]

---

41 *Chronicon de Lanercost*, ed. Stevenson, 116.

42 *Chronicon de Lanercost*, ed. Stevenson, 116: "sibi in dolerem et toti provinciae in damnum perpetuum."

43 *Chronicon de Lanercost*, ed. Stevenson, 116: "sed facilitate cordis feminei et ambitu regni retro respexisse."

44 *Chronicon de Lanercost*, ed. Stevenson, 117: "dominae reginae, relictae Alexandri, pro sua tertia protionem assignantes."

45 *Chronicon de Lanercost*, ed. Stevenson, 117–18: "At illa, astu femineo usa, impregnatam esse mentiebatur, ut suspensos animo redderet patriotas, et sibi favorem populi procliviorem faceret. Sed, quoniam semper mulieris versutia miserum vertit in exitum, cum solitasset terram suis simulationibus a die mortis regis usque ad festum Purificationis [Fe. 2, 1287], nec matronas admitteret honestas ad discernendum suum statum, ut ignominiam retribueret his a quibus receperat

As part of her elaborate plan, Yolande arranged for a baby boy to be brought to her so she could pass him off as her own; a white marble font was made for the infant's baptism and nobles and dignitaries gathered at Stirling where Yolande was confined before the birth in a lying-in of her own arranging.[46] Thankfully (indicated by the tone of the chronicler), Yolande's trickery was uncovered by William of Buchan, who revealed her scheme to all those assembled and awaiting the birth. And so "she departed from the land with shame, first attracted by the promise of wealth from across the sea and united in marriage with a king. This is what I have to say on the fidelity of a woman."[47] The implication from the *Lanercost* account is that producing an heir was critical for the queen to maintain influence and position in the wake of Alexander's unexpected death.

The *Chronicle of Lanercost* presents Yolande's calculated attempt to secure her fate after Alexander's death as a startling and unnatural response to the situation. In the narrative, not only does Yolande disrupt the reproductive process by failing to have a child and trying to substitute another baby as Alexander's, but she also disturbs the legal process for determining whether a woman was pregnant. *Bracton*'s protocol for establishing if a woman was faking pregnancy involves an examination by lawful, or wise and loyal women.[48] The *Lanercost* author explicitly notes that Yolande would

reverentiam et honorem, statuit perpetuo deludere populum supponendo sibi partum alienum." The detail about Yolande's deception lasting until the Feast of the Purification is notable. It is perhaps a further comment by the *Lanercost* chronicler on Yolande's intentions and status as an outsider, as a dowager queen without a child, given the associations of the feast of Purification with medieval women's reintegration into the community following childbirth. On the significance of the feast day and the ritual of purification after childbirth, see McMurray Gibson, "Blessings from Sun and Moon," 139–54.

46 *Chronicon de Lanercost*, ed. Stevenson, 118: "Fontem novum extrui fecit de marmore candido" (a new font was made of white marble).

47 *Chronicon de Lanercost*, ed. Stevenson, 118: "Sic recessit a terra cum verecundia, qui prius intuitu tantum eleemosinae de transmarinis adducta et associata est regi copulae. Hoc dixerim pro fide feminarum."

48 Although Yolande was queen of Scotland, the *Lanercost* was a northern English chronicle, hence the use of *Bracton* for this analysis. The practices involving examination by honest women outlined in *Bracton* were also used in other countries in the Middle Ages. See Butler, "More than Mothers: Juries of Matrons and Pleas of the Belly in Medieval England," 356–61. Similar language also appears in a miracle of St. Margaret of Scotland: A women's long-dead fetus was delivered with the help of the saint and "devout and respectable women." See *Miracles of Saint Æbbe of Coldingham and Saint Margaret of Scotland*, ed. and trans. Bartlett, 80–83; Harris-Stoerz, "Pregnancy and Childbirth in Twelfth and Thirteenth-Century French and

"not allow honest women to examine her condition."[49] Yolande is not only condemned for her reproductive failure and plotting, but also by her refusal to follow the correct legal recourse (which would have exposed her "pregnancy" as a lie). The chronicle's depiction of Yolande's transgressive actions as woman and queen seem to parallel the disrupted, unnatural fate of Scotland more generally in 1286, when the expected course of events was disrupted by the king's premature death which left Scotland without a clear or able heir.

There is also a medieval understanding about the cause of infertility wrapped up in the *Lanercost*'s account, in the emphasis on Yolande's character. The chronicler portrays Yolande's moral failing by mentioning that she had abandoned her commitment to become a nun because of her ambition for a kingdom. He also implies that it was her sexual allure that drove Alexander to risk and lose his life by travelling late at night through a storm to reach her. These depictions of her character ultimately explain why Yolande and Alexander did not produce an heir (while incidentally absolving Alexander III of any responsibility for leaving Scotland in such a situation), and thus the narrative of faked pregnancy and queenly treachery is not only a way to illustrate the unhappy state of Scotland in 1286, but on account of her sinful character, the chronicler blames Yolande personally for the lack of heir. In comparison, the late fifteenth-century *Liber Pluscardensis* has much less to say about Margaret Logie's fake pregnancy:

> King David set about espousing Margaret Logie, daughter of Sir Malcolm Drummond, a noble and most beautiful lady, at Inchmurthow; and he raised her to the throne with great magnificence as queen. He did not stay very long with her before again getting a divorce, because she pretended to be pregnant and was not. This was about the Feast of Fasten-Even in the year 1369.[50]

English Law," 277. This practice is also mentioned in Britton and the *Fleta* law books and was standard protocol for establishing things like whether a woman had had sexual intercourse, or whether a man was impotent.

49 *Chronicon de Lanercost*, ed. Stevenson, 118: "nec matronas admitteret honestas ad discernendum suum statum."

50 *Liber Pluscardensis*, ed. Skene, 1:307: "Hiis itaque stabilitis, disposuit se rex David ad disponsandum Margaretam de Logi, filiam domini Malcolmi de Drummond, nobilem [et] pulcerrimam dominam, apud Enchemarthow; et in reginam magnifice exaltavit. Sed cum ea non tempore multo perduravit quin iterum divorcium celebravit, eo quod ipsa impregnatam finxit et non fuit; et hoc circa festum Carnis Brevii, anno Domini m.cc.LXIX." English translation by Skene, *Liber Pluscardensis*, ed. Skene, 2:233. "Fasten-Even" is a Scottish festival, also called "Beef-Brose [broth] Day," on Shrove Tuesday.

The passage follows an explanation of David II's proposed plan for an English heir and his secret relief when the three estates of the Scottish political community refused (allegedly, he had only agreed to the plan originally because he was Edward III's prisoner). The *Liber* also praises David's kingly mercy in his treatment of the nobles who rebelled against him in 1364 because of the succession proposal.[51] This is immediately followed by the comment about David and Margaret's marriage, the faked pregnancy and their "divorce." The chronicler then claims that Margaret went to Rome to contest the divorce and had plans to marry the king of England (further evidence of her treachery to David and Scotland) before she died in 1369. Repeating Bower's account, the *Liber* concludes the whole discussion by claiming that David had imprisoned Robert the Steward's sons because Margaret wished it, but that he quickly righted this wrong once he was free from her influence. The *Liber* declares that "after this king David ruled his kingdom admirably" until his death in 1371.[52]

In contrast to the length and detail of the *Lanercost* comments about Yolande, the *Liber*'s passage about Margaret's fake pregnancy and the end of the marriage is short and blunt but, situated in the narrative as it is, it is part of the juxtaposition of the characters, actions and roles of Margaret and David. The *Liber*'s author reinforces Margaret's unsuitability as both wife and queen and makes the same point as Bower's wordy condemnation of marriages based on lust. The *Liber* lumps the blame for political decisions in the mid to late 1360s *and* the royal marriage's failure on Margaret while simultaneously exonerating David. The end of the royal marriage is explicitly attributed to Margaret pretending to be pregnant, which shows that the author at least *thought* a faked pregnancy was a serious enough thing to justify the end of the marriage.[53] Pretending to be pregnant indicates the

51 *Liber Pluscardensis*, ed. Skene, 1:306: "Sed tamen, considerate causa, propter distruccionem patriae et alias multas inconveniencias et dampna sequenda, rex, qui clemens et misericors erat, micius cum eis agendo, eidem hac vice misericorditer remisit, attendens quod magnae nobilitatis est regi miserere cum ulcisci poterit" (But, thinking over the matter, and because of the destruction of the country and many other troubles and losses that would follow, the king, who was kind and merciful, dealt with them mildly, mercifully giving them this time, thinking that it is more noble for a king to have mercy when he could have revenge).

52 *Liber Pluscardensis*, ed. Skene, 1:307: "Post hoc autem rex David regnum suum optime rexit."

53 Infertility was not legal grounds for divorce in the fourteenth century. *Bracton* has five chapters on substituting a false heir and the legal protocol for when a woman was suspected of faking pregnancy, but divorce is not cited as a consequence and the queen's desperation at a pivotal moment when the royal marriage seems to have been crumbling, and the startling way that she tried to fix the situation. Margaret's supposed actions indicate the *Liber* author's perception of the significance of fertility for a queen's position, the pressure for fertility that she experienced and the lengths she might go to try to supply an heir.

It is worth noting the singularity of both the chronicle comments. Yolande's fake pregnancy is only mentioned by the *Lanercost* chronicle, and the *Liber Pluscardensis* alone declares that Margaret and David II's marriage ended because Margaret pretended to be pregnant. The *Lanercost* chronicle was written in the late thirteenth or early fourteenth century, and the *Liber* was composed at the end of the fifteenth century, and so it could be that the later *Liber Pluscardensis* chronicler confused and misattributed an earlier rumour about a queen's fake pregnancy.[54] However, the significant difference in the texture of the accounts suggests otherwise. The *Lanercost* chronicler describes Yolande's deception in lengthy detail. He carefully works to establish her ambitious and changeable nature and her pivotal role in causing Alexander's premature death, before describing her attempt to manipulate the legitimate succession. In contrast, the *Liber Pluscardensis* passage is short, just one line, and we are given no details beyond the fact that Margaret pretended to be pregnant and her marriage to David ended as a result. Furthermore, the differences between how the fake pregnancies are worked into the chronicle narratives indicate that the two accounts are distinct and deliberate rather than some confusion of queens by the later *Liber Pluscardensis* chronicler.

Considering the specific implications of a faked pregnancy is important for analyzing the claims about the queens and what they tell us about perceptions of royal fertility. The attention to fake pregnancy in medieval legal sources was a response to fears about inheritance.[55] Fiona Harris-Stoertz argues that in medieval England and France, there was societal concern

laws are concerned with inheritance rather than marriage: *Bracton: On the Laws and Customs of England*, ed. Woodbine, trans. Thorne, 2:201–4.

54 On the composition of the chronicles, see: McGladdery, "Liber Pluscardensis," *Encyclopedia of the Medieval Chronicle Online*, eds., Dunphy and Bratu; Gransden, *Historical Writing in England*, 2:494–501.

55 Harris-Stoertz, "Pregnancy and Childbirth," 263–65. However, there is no mention of fake pregnancy in the *Regiam majestatem*, the medieval compendium of Scots law: *Regiam majestatem*, ed. Cooper (1947). On Scots law and the *Regiam majestatem* see Taylor, *Shape of the State*; Simpson, "The Scottish Common Law: Origins and Development, c. 1124–c. 1500"; McQueen, "'Regiam majestatem,' Scots Law, and National Identity," 1–25.

about what women might do to manipulate the reproductive process, whether mothers themselves or the midwives and women who attended births, and this is reflected in the emergence of laws relating to pregnant women and childbirth from the twelfth and thirteenth centuries.[56] The legal requirement of hearing the infant cry from the birthing chamber was established in England in Edward I's reign to combat fear that a false heir might be smuggled in when the men were not looking.[57] There is also a protocol in *Bracton* for determining whether a woman was faking pregnancy.[58] Such procedures indicate the contemporary fear about women substituting heirs, but also the risk associated with faking a pregnancy. The emergence of legislation to protect against women substituting heirs, even though men might have been just as motivated to present a false or illegitimate heir, is particularly striking because it makes supplying a fake heir a uniquely gendered crime.[59]

While fake pregnancies appear in legal sources, adultery was a more common accusation against medieval queens.[60] For instance, the eleventh-century *Encomium Emmae Reginae* commissioned by Emma of Normandy, claims that Harold, son of her husband Cnut and his first wife, Ælfgifu of Northampton, was fathered by a priest.[61] In a later medieval example, it was rumoured that Margaret of Anjou's son was not fathered by

56 Harris-Stoertz, "Pregnancy and Childbirth," 266. This distrust of mothers appears in laws concerning abortions and infanticide, and in the emergence of legislation that addressed substituted children and faked pregnancies.

57 Hearing the heir cry is also cited in the *Regiam majestatem*, bk. II, cap. 58, no. 1, p. 168: "si ex eadem haeredem habuerit auditum, vel brayantem inter quatuor parietes" (if by her he has an heir who lives long enough to be heard crying within four walls). On hearing the infant cry: Seabourne, "'It Is Necessary That the Issue Be Heard to Cry or Squall Within the Four [Walls],'" 44–68.

58 *Bracton: On the Laws and Customs of England*, ed. Woodbine, trans. Thorne, 2:201–4: the woman was to "be examined by responsible matrons, by feeling her breasts and abdomen, in order to discover the truth." If the woman was thought to be pregnant after this humiliating and invasive examination, or even if there was some uncertainty about her condition, she was to be confined in the king's castle until she gave birth, or until she could be shown to have been faking pregnancy. While confined, she was to be kept away from any pregnant maids and potential collaborators. Harris-Stoertz adds that if it was found that the woman was not pregnant, she would be imprisoned or fined, Harris-Stoertz, "Pregnancy and Childbirth," 277.

59 Harris-Stoertz, "Pregnancy and Childbirth," 277, notes that men had equal reason to wish to substitute fake heirs.

60 Harris-Stoertz, "Pregnancy and Childbirth," 277.

61 Stafford, "Ælfgifu of Northampton," *ODNB* [online], published September 23,

Henry VI.[62] These claims, made by rival claimants to the throne, use adultery to discredit a royal heir and open up the succession for another—in Queen Emma's case, her own son, and in Margaret's, the Yorkist faction in the fifteenth century. The adulterous queen character is also a recognisable trope in medieval French romance literature. Peggy McCracken argues that the adulterous queen's body was split between two men (the king and the lover), which challenged contemporary ideas about property and proper succession in medieval France. Notably, the adulterous queen character is always remarkably childless, and therefore is a careful disassociation of reproduction from sexual (mis)conduct. This conflicts with the reality of a queen's body, in which her female sexuality and the political future of the realm were intertwined.[63] McCracken argues that the character of the adulterous queen existed in the context of courtly love literature but that it developed from deeper societal worry about dynastic reproduction, inheritance, and succession, which were threatened by a sexually transgressive female body.[64] There is a core similarity between adultery and faking pregnancy because the queen also manipulated her reproductive role and jeopardized the legitimate succession when she pretended to be pregnant.

There are significant differences between adultery and pretending to be pregnant though. First, there is no sexual transgression involved in a fake pregnancy. In the models of romantic and historic queens accused of adultery, the legitimate inheritance was threatened by the woman's sexual exploits and her attempt to cover it up. In the examples of Ælfgifu of Northampton and Margaret of Anjou, adultery is implied by suggesting that their sons were fathered by someone other than the king. In contrast, the claims that Yolande de Dreux and Margaret Logie pretended to be pregnant highlight that neither queen actually had a child; there is no insinuation that they were really pregnant, with someone else's child, and so they are not accused by the chroniclers of a sexual transgression. The alleged faked pregnancies specifically hinge on the *absence* of children, rather than accusing the queens of trying to pass off a lover's child as the king's heir.

2004. Harris-Stoertz, "Pregnancy and Childbirth," 278. There is a visual reference to this in the Bayeux Tapestry. See Stephenson, "Where a Cleric and Ælfgyva," 71–74.

62 Dunn, "Margaret of Anjou," *ODNB* [online], published September 23, 2004; Geaman, "A Bastard and a Changeling?," 15–17.

63 McCracken, "The Body Politic," 44.

64 McCracken, "The Body Politic," 46–47.

The chronicle charges against the two Scottish queens are based precisely on their childlessness, *not* sexual misconduct.

Fake pregnancy was also a particularly gendered condemnation of the queen and her fertility which left the king's masculinity completely untarnished. Accusing a queen of adultery implicated the king's masculinity because it implies that he was bested by another man and unable to maintain control of his wife. However, a king's manhood was not at stake if a queen pretended to be pregnant and he is left blameless by her manipulation of her reproductive role and dynastic duty to provide a legitimate heir. Preserving the king from blame is a significant part of the chronicles' comments about Yolande and Margaret's fake pregnancies. The *Lanercost* chronicler attributes the turmoil in Scotland in 1286 specifically to Yolande but is careful not to blacken Alexander III's image. In the *Liber Pluscardensis* too, the chronicler blames Margaret for David's lapse in judgement when he imprisoned the Steward's sons, and the assertion that she pretended to be pregnant places the blame for the "divorce" solely on the queen. Simultaneously, David's character is redeemed, and he is absolved of any responsibility for bad judgement *or* the marriage's end because of reproductive failure.

The claims about fake pregnancies also show the realities of knowing and writing about royal pregnancy and fertility in the Middle Ages. Whether or not Yolande or Margaret actually pretended to be pregnant in order to provide an heir, the chroniclers thought it was reasonable to make these claims about the queens as explanation for the events that followed. As part of the didactic purpose of historical writing, chronicles needed to be trusted by medieval audiences.[65] As such, chroniclers took care to assure their audience of their reliability and the sources of their information.[66] Accounts like the *Lanercost* and *Liber* were only useful if they were close enough to the "facts." They could only describe what might *reasonably* have happened, as far as it fell within what could be accepted as the truth by their audiences. In this respect, chronicles are particularly valuable as sources, not for their "facts" but for their preservation and testimony of contemporary perceptions and understanding.[67]

65 Given-Wilson, *Chronicles*, 65–78.

66 Van Houts, *Memory and Gender in Medieval Europe*, 21. Given-Wilson, *Chronicles*, 1–20.

67 Strohm, *Hochon's Arrow*, 4.

In this light, the confusion and uncertainty about whether Yolande was pregnant in the *Chronicle of Lanercost* shows us some contemporary understanding about pregnancy. Harris-Stoertz investigated the "somewhat shaky notions" about the length of the gestational period in the twelfth- and thirteenth-century legal sources.[68] *Bracton* concluded that an infant should be deemed illegitimate if the husband was dead, away, or somehow incapacitated as much as a year before the child's birth, thus making the gestational period fifty-two weeks.[69] Another legal text advises a more realistic forty-week wait for a birth after a husband's death before declaring the child to be illegitimate.[70] According to the *Lanercost* chronicler, Yolande pretended to be pregnant from before March 19, 1286, until the Feast of Purification (February 2, 1287), when her deception was uncovered before all the court assembled at Stirling.[71] Remarkably, after about fifty weeks of "pregnancy," it was only the discerning William of Buchan, rather than the length of her pregnancy, which alerted the gathered nobles to Yolande's plot in the *Lanercost*'s account. This seems not only to reflect the chronicler's difficulty knowing the details about a royal pregnancy, but the actual ambiguity and uncertainty about pregnancy in the medieval world.

Furthermore, this difficulty in determining pregnancy in the early stages and the different understandings of the reproductive process could give a queen some influence in the time of "unpregnancy"; the phase of uncertainty before a pregnancy was, or could be, known.[72] Just Yolande's claim that she was pregnant after Alexander III died was enough to buy her a year of influence and support from the Scottish magnates. The desire for a Bruce heir also seems to have allowed Margaret Logie political influence throughout the 1360s. In 1368, she confronted the earl of Ross in Inverness over a dispute about a land grant and arranged for his arrest and the seizure of his lands.[73]

---

68 Harris-Stoertz, "Pregnancy and Childbirth," 270, the thirteenth-century *Britton* was based on *Bracton*, as was the *Fleta*, which was also a thirteenth-century text, but less popular than *Britton*.

69 Harris-Stoertz, "Pregnancy and Childbirth," 280.

70 *Britton*, see Harris-Stoertz, "Pregnancy and Childbirth," 280.

71 Alexander III died on March 19, 1286, so he and Yolande could have not been together for at least a day or two before that, as the king was in Edinburgh just before his death, while Yolande was in Fife.

72 See the research project by Isabel Davis and Anna Burel, *Conceiving Histories*, which uses the term "un-pregnancy" and explores the time of waiting, without knowing, for pregnancy or infertility: www7.bbk.ac.uk/conceivinghistories/.

73 Penman, *David II*, 364.

Michael Penman noted that such political actions were not unusual for Margaret during her tenure as queen, and he argues that her power derived from her ability to exert pressure as "the woman who might give [David] a child," which also seems to have protected her from the repercussions of her actions, at least for a while.[74]

Whether Margaret had actually pretended to be pregnant like the *Liber* asserts, or because David II had decided that the marriage would never produce a child and was already planning to marry Scottish noblewoman, Agnes Dunbar, Margaret's time of "unpregnancy" ended in 1369.[75] Given what was at stake if she was found out, pretending to be pregnant seems like something only a queen who felt particularly immense pressure for fertility might attempt. In reality, David's efforts to put Margaret aside in favour of a new, younger, queen indicates that he had lost hope in the fertility of the marriage by 1369.[76] What changed, from the time of hope and potential earlier in the 1360s? It might have just been time; perhaps after five years of marriage, it seemed like David and Margaret would never have a child. It might also have been Margaret's age (rather than a fake pregnancy), which signaled that the marriage was infertile. By 1369 she was between about forty and forty-five, perhaps perimenopausal or already experiencing menopause.[77] Similar to the *Liber*'s claim that Margaret was to blame for the end of the marriage, David's apparent faith in his own ability to produce an heir with a new queen implies a perception that it was not him, but Margaret who was infertile by 1369.[78] The allegation that Margaret pretended to be pregnant preserves the reality that there was a point of change in the royal marriage, from "unpregnancy," when there was hope for an heir and Margaret was able

74 Penman, *David II*, 364.

75 For David hoping to marry Agnes Dunbar in 1369: Penman, *David II*, 271.

76 A queen under enormous pressure to produce a child might also have pretended to be pregnant until it actually happened. Conversely, faking a pregnancy could also be an indication that she believed for some reason that she would never conceive a child.

77 Beattie, "The Life Cycle: The Ages of Medieval Women," 21; Gilchrist, *Medieval Life*, 46, 59–63; Shahar, *Growing Old in the Middle Ages*,18–19; Cooke, "Nice Young Girls and Wicked Old Witches," 219–28; Grauer, "Life Patterns of Women from Medieval York," 407–13; Post, "Ages at Menarche and Menopause," 83–87; Amundsen and Diers, "The Age of Menopause in Medieval Europe," 605–12.

78 Due to the fact that Margaret had a son from her first marriage, it is difficult to suggest that she would have been understood as infertile or considered *solely* responsible for the childlessness of her marriage with David.

to exercise significant political influence as David's consort, to when David sought to end the marriage because of continued childlessness.

Ultimately, the fake pregnancy narratives in the chronicles demonstrate the consequences that failing to produce an heir had for a kingdom and a queen. These stories emphasize and critique the women's failure to execute their reproductive role and, crucially, both depictions of fake pregnancies lay the blame for the events that followed, whether the succession crisis of the 1290s or the end of the royal marriage, on the queens by accusing them of the gendered crime of trying to substitute an heir. The circumstances and consequences of both fake pregnancies demonstrate how the queens' positions hung in the balance of their fertility when they faced uncertain, precarious futures and how the blame for infertility was disproportionately placed on the queen. The chroniclers frame the queens' deception as the reason for their downfalls and, in so doing, they reflect the exceptional pressure on both queens to produce heirs.

* * *

The chronicle narratives about royal childlessness shed light on medieval perceptions of the importance of fertility for kings and queens. The perspectives of the Scottish chroniclers on David II are present in what they wrote about the childlessness of David and his two queens. Chroniclers' critiques of David—for taking a mistress while neglecting his reproductive duties and pointed explanations about his controversial marriage and possible divorce from Margaret Logie—demonstrate that producing legitimate children was central to perceptions of good kingship. Ultimately, the sources most critical of the king were most outspoken about royal childlessness.

The chronicle accusations that two queens faked pregnancies to secure their futures also indicate the significance of fertility for medieval queenship. The *Chronicle of Lanercost*'s description of Yolande de Dreux's fake pregnancy plot reflects the gravity of Alexander's unexpected death without an heir. That Yolande supposedly took the extreme risk of pretending to be pregnant and plotted to pass off someone else's baby as her own in order to secure her uncertain future shows the danger of being a childless queen, and therefore the significance of fertility for a queen. Fertility was equally essential for Margaret Logie's position, according to the *Liber Pluscardensis*, which attributes the breakdown of the royal marriage to Margaret's attempt to fake pregnancy. The claim that she took the risk of pretending to be pregnant in order to provide an heir preserves a sense of the immense pressure that Margaret experienced to produce a child and implies that *not* being pregnant was enough to cost her position as David's wife and queen.

Additionally, the fact that chroniclers reasonably claimed that two queens faked pregnancies illustrates the reality of knowing about royal fertility in the Middle Ages. That faking pregnancy was even a possible recourse by a queen shows how difficult actually determining pregnancy was in the thirteenth and fourteenth centuries. We can also see understandings of reproduction in the claims of fake pregnancies, particularly in the fact that the impossibly long gestation period of Yolande's "pregnancy" did not (allegedly) raise any alarm bells for the Scottish magnates. Remarkably, for both Yolande and Margaret, the uncertainties that existed around pregnancy and reproduction created a time of "unpregnancy," before it was possible to know whether the queen was pregnant or not and which gave them both unique influence for a limited time.

Chapter 4

CAUSE FOR CONCERN

THE KING'S AGE, GENDER, AND CHILDLESSNESS

THIS CHAPTER RETURNS to a fundamental question: when and why did couples and their contemporaries begin to worry about delayed conception? Matthew Paris's claim that there were fears about Eleanor of Provence's fertility in 1236–1238 is an oddly timed concern; she was barely in her teens and married for just two years. Compared to the examples of other medieval queens like Isabella of France or Eleanor of Castile, there was nothing exceptional about Eleanor's age or the delay before the birth of her first child. Indeed, a survey of Plantagenet marriages has shown that the women of the English royal family did not usually give birth at such a young age and generally were not expected to have their first child until their late teens or early twenties.[1] While Paris's comments ostensibly concern Eleanor's fertility, the following analysis reveals that the underlying anxiety was driven more by Henry III's age and masculine status.

There is a discernible pattern in the pious behaviours of Henry III, Alexander II, and David II when each king reached an age associated with masculine perfection. Between 1236 and 1238, at the age of twenty-nine to thirty-one, Henry III first cultivated a new spiritual intercessor—St. Edward the Confessor—whose cult became central to his piety for the rest of his life. Comparable, marked shifts in devotional practice can be identified for Alexander II and David II: in each case, the king turned to new saints and orders, suggesting a perception that their earlier religious strategies had failed to deliver. Strikingly, all three kings were still childless when these changes occurred, and each was about thirty years old. This chapter argues that these broader shifts were not incidental but related to pressures surrounding the production of an heir.

First, this chapter argues that the early thirties for kings marked a point at which concerns about royal childlessness were activated. The second section of this chapter examines how pressure for fertility was rooted in the association of chronological age with social maturity and the anticipation of masculine behaviour when a king reached the age of perfection in the male life course. Ultimately, the behaviours of all three kings contextualize Paris's

1 Parsons, "Mothers, Daughters," 68.

focus on Eleanor of Provence's fertility and illuminate how ideas about age and masculinity influenced both contemporary perceptions of a royal couple's childlessness and the responses it elicited from the rulers themselves. The final part of this chapter considers the queen in light of the significance of the king's age, because Matthew Paris's comments about fertility were still centred on the queen. This investigation shows that there was no comparably significant age or stage in the female life course when the achievement of motherhood was as critical for queens as fatherhood was for adult kings.

A Common Pattern: Three Kings in Their Thirties

Something crucially changed in the period between Matthew Paris's first comment about the queen's fertility in 1236, when it was uncertain whether Eleanor of Provence would be fertile or barren, and his second comment in 1238, when "it was greatly feared" that she was barren. Paris's initial contemplation about the new queen's *future* reproductive ability in 1236 had transformed into worry that she was infertile by 1238. Such an outright expression of concern about a queen's fertility in a chronicle is unique, yet in 1238, Eleanor of Provence was a fairly typical young queen. Earlier discussion showed that, although probably barely pubescent, she was not unusually young for a royal bride, and some delay before having a child was not unusual, perhaps it was even expected.[2] We need to look at the king to help understand what changed between 1236 and 1238. At precisely this time, a decade into his majority rule, there is a noticeable shift in Henry III's devotional activities. He began seeking new and more effective spiritual support in the mid-1230s, when he first cultivated his devotion to St. Edward the Confessor. The timing of this shift in devotional practice coincides with Paris's concerns about Eleanor's fertility and suggests a link between the king's pious behaviours and anxieties about the couple's childlessness.

The significance of Henry's devotion to Edward the Confessor, in this instance, lies not in the meaning of St. Edward's cult but in the *timing* of the king's early and sustained devotion to the saint, which began in the years that Matthew Paris recorded the scrutiny of Eleanor's fertility. Indeed, St. Edward the Confessor's *vita* emphasizes the royal saint's vow of chastity in marriage, and he and his queen, Edith, were childless.[3] However, the

2 Parsons, "Mothers, Daughters, Marriage," 67–68. Phillips, *Medieval Maidens*, 26. For comparison, Eleanor of Castile was thirteen and Isabella of France was twelve when they were married to Edward I and Edward II, respectively.

3 Binski, *Westminster Abbey and the Plantagenets*, 52–89.

Confessor did hold significance for Henry's reproductive hopes: Edward represented the ancient Anglo-Saxon royal bloodline that had been severed by the Norman Conquest. Henry's devotion to the saint symbolically reconnected his dynasty to the older, pre-Norman English kingship, emphasizing his future children's claim to a unified English crown. The purpose of this chapter is *not* to argue that Henry turned to the Confessor as a model for childless marriage or because the saint was specifically known to remedy infertility.[4] Rather, I argue that Henry sought Edward's intercession for divine help with reproduction because of the saint's royal status and spiritual authority. Additionally, I do not suggest that fertility concerns were Henry's sole motivation for this devotion, but rather one significant factor among multiple reasons for his intensified veneration of the saint in the 1230s. Medieval devotion to saints was shaped by a complex interplay of factors and was not determined solely by the narrative content of a saint's *vita*; local customs, political contexts, personal needs, and the obligations of royal patronage played equally significant roles in directing rulers' focus and intensity of veneration.[5] Henry's attention to the cult of the Confessor and the institution of Westminster was multifaceted and prolific; his efforts installed the saint as an important royal spiritual ally for subsequent generations of his successors.[6] It is the timing of Henry's interest in St. Edward that is significant because it shows him cultivating a new spiritual intercessor at a point in his reign when he faced considerable pressures as king, including Paris's explicit scrutiny of his new queen's fertility.

It was Henry's focused attention, not a commitment inherited from his royal predecessors, which promoted St. Edward's cult and established Westminster Abbey as a lasting recipient of royal patronage.[7] David Carpenter has shown that Henry's interest in St. Edward took hold between 1233 and 1238.[8] In the early 1230s Henry made no special attempt to travel to Westminster to celebrate St. Edward's important feast days; in 1231, he called for the feast of St. Edmund, not St. Edward, to be celebrated throughout English Cistercian abbeys.[9] It was not until 1235 that he called for the celebration

---

4 See Chapter 6 for consideration of this argument.

5 Webb, *Pilgrimage in Medieval England.*

6 Carpenter, *Henry III*, 167.

7 David Carpenter, "King Henry III," 866. Binski, *Westminster Abbey and the Plantagenets.*

8 Carpenter, "King Henry III," 866.

9 *Statuta capitulorum generalium ordinis Cisterciensis Tomus II*, ed. Canivez, 101 (no. 51), 141 (no. 15). The name of the saint was left blank in the 1231 entry (no. 51),

of St. Edward's Translation.[10] From 1235 onwards, Henry consistently travelled to Westminster every year to celebrate Edward's Translation feast on October 13. The king first marked St. Edward's death, January 5, at Westminster in 1238, and from that year, he almost never missed celebrating both St. Edward's translation and death days at Westminster.[11] This shift in devotional practice closely aligns with the period of rising anxiety over the royal couple's childlessness.

Significantly, Henry's observance of the Confessor's Translation-day feast at Westminster was established in 1235, coinciding precisely with the final negotiations for his marriage to Eleanor of Provence. Henry's first effort to attend St. Edward's Translation at Westminster happened after he received the news in early October 1235 that the marriage to Eleanor was to go ahead; presumably to give thanks, Henry rushed to Westminster to mark the Confessor's feast on October 13, 1235.[12] Once married, Henry wasted no time introducing his queen to his much-loved saint: at Eleanor's coronation in January 1236, Henry gave her "a great cope" to place at the Confessor's shrine.[13] In September 1236, the king had already made arrangements for joint offerings to be made by himself and his queen at Westminster on St. Edward's Translation.[14] Henry appears to have been praying to the Confessor for help with the marriage negotiations and felt his faith had been rewarded.[15]

While Henry showed devotion to the Confessor from 1235, his observance of *both* the Translation and death feasts—displaying his intensified attention to the saint—did not happen until 1238.[16] In the first years of their marriage, Henry may also have commissioned a text about the Confessor for Eleanor.[17] The surviving Anglo-Norman manuscript, dated ca. 1250–1260 and

---

but Carpenter, "King Henry," 868, argues that it refers to St. Edmund because it mentions a martyr king, which could not have been St. Edward, as Canivez inserted.

10 Carpenter, "King Henry," 868.

11 Carpenter, "King Henry," 868–69. In January 1252 for instance, he missed the feast because he was in York for his daughter's marriage to Alexander III of Scotland.

12 Carpenter, "King Henry," 876.

13 *CCR* (1234–1237), 278, 309. Howell, *Eleanor of Provence*, 24.

14 Carpenter, "King Henry," 885.

15 Carpenter, "King Henry," 885.

16 Carpenter, "King Henry," 868. Carpenter notes that in the ten years since Henry had assumed power in maturity (1227–1237), he had not once been at Westminster for January 5.

17 Binski, "Reflections on *La estoire de Seint Aedwardi le rei*," 333.

known as *La estoire de Seint Aedward le rei* is a copy of a now lost original text which was possibly written and illustrated by Matthew Paris.[18] Paris's original was probably produced prior to 1239, as the preface in the surviving copy declares that Henry and Eleanor were St. Edward's *only* special devotees, which would not make sense once their son, Edward, named for the saint, was born in 1239.[19] Indeed, as Carpenter asserts, "Eleanor surely no longer needed to be told to love her husband's saint" after the first few years of marriage.[20] If Henry felt that the Confessor had helped bring about his marriage to Eleanor in 1236, he was perhaps now looking for saintly support for the continuation of his dynasty by the end of the decade.[21]

The timing of Henry's devotion to St. Edward is significant when compared to Matthew Paris's comments about Eleanor's fertility: the suggestion and then fear about Eleanor being barren coincided with the full development of Henry's devotion to St. Edward, between 1236 and 1238. While Carpenter suggests that Henry's interest in St. Edward in the mid-1230s was the result of pressures facing his reign (including the threat of excommunication, civil war, marriage negotiations, and the betrayal of a chief mentor from his minority reign), which left him feeling socially and politically isolated by 1233–1234—-the timing suggests other motivations. Significantly, the king's observance of both feast days began *after* his marriage had taken place and the turmoil of the early 1230s had somewhat subsided, suggesting that Henry's new devotional practices were related to events later in the 1230s.

The potential connection becomes clearer when considering that Matthew Paris may have authored the *La estoire de Seint Aedward le rei* text that Henry commissioned. If Paris was indeed closely connected to the royal court, he may have been reflecting the king's own anxieties when he reported the concern that the queen was barren. The coincidence of Paris's comment on the queen's fertility with Henry's intensified devotion to

18 Cambridge, University Library, MS Ee. 3.59. The text is thirty-seven folios. Binski, "Reflections on *La estoirede Seint Aedwardi le rei*," 333–38: Binski speculates that Matthew Paris was the author of the original manuscript of *La estoire* based on the style of the illustrations in the surviving copy and a line in the text which says the poet also did the drawings (which was not a common practice, and we know that Paris illustrated his chronicles). Additionally, a note in a flyleaf of another manuscript mentions that Paris wrote and illustrated a life of St. Thomas and a life of St. Edward for ladies of the royal court.

19 Binski, *Becket's Crown*, 139; Carpenter, "King Henry," 886.

20 Carpenter, "King Henry," 886. *Lives of Edward the Confessor*, ed. Luard, lines 84–86, p. 27: St. Edward "has none but you two, the king and you who are his wife."

21 Carpenter, "King Henry," 890.

Edward the Confessor suggests a possible link between the king's search for spiritual intercession and contemporary worries about royal reproduction.

Henry's personal circumstances made childlessness particularly concerning. Having turned thirty in 1237 with a decade of majority rule behind him, he was still struggling to differentiate his reign as an adult king from his minority. The absence of an heir only emphasized his continued political vulnerability and failure to achieve the dynastic security expected of a mature monarch.

Changes in the piety of two other childless kings around the age of thirty suggest that the connection between Henry III's actions, age and concerns about fertility was not unique. When both Alexander II and David II reached their early thirties without yet having produced heirs, they also looked in new directions for spiritual support and directed their patronage towards different saints and institutions than those they had called upon earlier in their reigns, as will be demonstrated below. The contention is that their behaviours were, as with Henry III, related to their age and worry about childlessness.

David II began to seek spiritual support in a markedly new way from 1357, when he was thirty-three. David and Joan of the Tower spent their childhood exiled in France and, when they returned to Scotland in 1341, David's piety was typical of a young Scottish king; he issued grants and confirmations to the Dominican and Cistercian houses across Scotland and the Augustinian abbey of Holyrood.[22] While imprisoned in England between 1346–1357, there was no indication that David was any more pious than he had been previously, nor that he was especially devoted to particular saints.[23] However, towards the end of his imprisonment, in late 1357, David made his first pilgrimage to Canterbury to visit St. Thomas Becket's tomb.[24] This was the beginning of a lasting habit.

David made at least five requests of Edward III to visit Becket's tomb in the 1360s: Edward granted the Scottish king safe-conduct in 1364, twice in 1365, in 1366, and in 1368.[25] Of the five grants to visit Canterbury, two were for David and his attendants, and the other three were for both David and

22 Penman, "Christian Days and Knights," 253–54.

23 Penman, "Christian Days and Knights," 253.

24 *CDS*, ed. Bain, 3:no. 1672. Balfour-Melville, "Papers Relating to the Captivity and Release of David II," 29; Penman, "The Bruce Dynasty," 361–62.

25 *Rot. Scot.*, ed. Illingworth et al., 1:884b, 887b, 892a, 899a, 900b, 917a. Queen Margaret was also granted safe-conduct to Canterbury with her own retinue in 1364: *Rot. Scot.*, ed. Illingworth et al, 1:881.

his second queen, Margaret Logie. David's devotion also extended beyond Becket, and there were additional requests, beginning in 1358, for safe-conduct to England, including at least one visit to the shrine of Our Lady of Walsingham in Norfolk.[26] Jean Froissart, a fourteenth-century Flemish chronicler (who lived with David's court in 1365) also mentions that, in 1363, David visited the shrine in Walsingham.[27]

It was specifically from 1357 that David II began making new religious dedications and pilgrimages. Penman suggests that the shift in David's behaviour at this point might have been due to several reasons: "[the result of] a far more religiously pious and contemplative lifestyle" which he adopted while captive in England with so much time on his hands, or an attempt to win Edward III's approval and "sweeten the deal" for his release, which was being negotiated in 1357.[28] Furthermore, David may also have been inspired to visit Becket's shrine by his English queen, Joan, or to ease the pain from an arrow wound that he received at the Battle of Neville's Cross in 1346.[29] Penman concludes that David's attention to Becket's shrine shows:

> that he was acting, at this juncture [in 1357], out of sincere piety, not merely convention or political expediency: numerous factors including his captivity, his domestic political predicament, his apparent infertility, recurrent illness and the backdrop of plague epidemics after 1348–9, may have precipitated such a spiritual shift.[30]

However, Penman did not use gender as a category of historical analysis and David's behaviour beginning in 1357 needs more careful consideration. The *timing* of the shift in David's piety is the crucial detail in this present analysis. When David first visited Becket in 1357, talks were already underway for his release; he had also endured any residual pain from his arrow wound for over a decade by 1357, and plague epidemics had devasted Britain for nearly as long. If these factors caused David to seek spiritual support, why did he wait until 1357?

26 *Rot. Scot.*, ed. Illingworth et al., 1:828b, 872a, 881a, 928a, 937a. Penman, *David II*, 303, notes that the other safe-conducts in 1364 (*Rot. Scot.*, ed. Illingworth et al., 1:877, 881), for Canterbury and Walsingham went unused.

27 *Chronicles of England, France, Spain and the Adjoining Countries by Sir John Froissart*, ed. Johnes, 1:306.

28 Penman, *David II*, 189; Penman, "Christian Days and Knights," 256.

29 Penman, "Bruce Dynasty," 361.

30 Penman, "Bruce Dynasty," 361.

David expanded his devotional interests in Scotland after 1357, too. In 1361, he asked the pope for approval to appoint a confessor to accompany him for his personal use.[31] Beginning in 1362, he pledged his support for St. Monan, an obscure (perhaps sixth-century Irish) saint about whom little is known.[32] A shrine to the saint had already existed in the East Neuk of Fife, and David planned a new chapel there in 1362.[33] There was some near-contemporary confusion over David's interest in St. Monan. Walter Bower, writing in the fifteenth century, declared that St. Monan responded to the king's prayers to remove the arrow barb that supposedly remained in his head after battle in 1346.[34] There is also a legend from an unknown source which says that St. Monan saved David from shipwreck while crossing the Forth, and so the king founded a church on the shores where he found safety.[35] In contrast, Jean Froissart claimed that David suffered from headaches at full moon because of arrow barbs that remained in his skull from 1346. After praying to St. Monan, the king was relieved of his headaches when the barbs dropped out of his nose.[36] Froissart had spent time with David's court, which perhaps lends some credibility to his account about the healing miracles of St. Monan.[37] David remained devoted to St. Monan throughout the 1360s.[38] In 1363, he made a pilgrimage to the chapel in Fife and it seems that throughout the 1360s he observed the saint's feast day there.[39] Additionally, by 1365, a street which ran to the south of St. Giles Cathedral in Edinburgh was named "St. Monan's Wynd," perhaps because of David's influence.[40]

---

31 *Calendar of Entries in the Papal Registers*, ed. Bliss, 1:365. Penman, *David II*, 407.

32 Lamb, "David II's Chapel Royal at St. Monans," 118: Lamb reasonably suggests that David II likely knew St. Monan as a ninth-century companion of St. Adrian, from the Isle of May, who survived a Danish raid by going to mainland Fife as a missionary. This narrative is the one recorded by Bower and Wyntoun.

33 *ER*, eds. Stuart and Burnett, 2:114; Lamb, "David II's Chapel at St. Monans," 119.

34 *Chron. Bower*, ed. Watt, 7:261.

35 Watt mentions this in a footnote, *Chron. Bower*, ed. Watt, 7:261n464.

36 *Chroniques de Jean Froissart*, ed. Luce, 1346–1356, 4:xi.

37 Penman, *David II*, 340–43. But Penman also states at another point that Bower's account is more reliable than Froissart's: Penman, *David II*, 261.

38 He made regular payments for chaplains at St. Monans in 1364, 1365, and 1367: *ER*, eds. Stuart and Burnett, 2:121, 133, 190, 141, 265.

39 Penman, *David II*, 264, 283.

40 Miller, "The Mercat Cross of Edinburgh," 379; Penman, "Christian Days and Knights," 260–61.

Beginning in the late 1350s, David also developed a newfound interest in St. Katherine of Alexandria. The cult of St. Katherine had widespread popularity in the later Middle Ages and had associations with multiple groups and roles in medieval society.[41] In 1358, David II and an Edinburgh burgess named Roger Hogg dedicated an altar to St. Katherine in St. Giles Cathedral, Edinburgh.[42] In addition to the altar in St. Giles, David may also have supported several other sites that were dedicated to St. Katherine in this period: a Dominican friary in Ayr, an altar in Holyrood, a chapel, hospital and altar in Dunfermline, an altar in Cambuskenneth, a house of the Blackfriars in Edinburgh, and the Priory of Beauly.[43] There is no explicit evidence which connects David to these dedications other than timing, although his illegitimate nephew was prior of Beauly, and Dunfermline and Holyrood had longstanding royal significance and favour.[44]

The timing of David's devotional shift becomes significant when considered alongside his complex political circumstances in the same period. David faced considerable issues as king by the late 1350s. Crucially, despite brushing it aside as "apparent infertility," childlessness was a significant underlying factor which directly impacted several of the concerns highlighted by Penman, namely, the king's captivity and domestic political predicament. From 1352, David had pushed the Scottish council to accept a succession-peace deal for his release.[45] When he failed again to have the plan accepted in 1357, he continued promoting versions of the succession proposal in the 1360s.[46] David's failure to have a child also contributed to the ongoing political power struggle in Scotland between the king and his nephew in the late

---

41 Penman, "Christian Days and Knights," 260–61, describes her as a "crusader saint." However, Lewis, *The Cult of St. Katherine of Alexandria in Late Medieval England*, 13, 80–84, 88, argues that by the late Middle Ages, St. Katherine was the most popular of the Virgin martyr saints and her popularity derived from her multifaceted appeal. See also: Lewis, "A King, Not a Servant," 397–416; Walsh, *The Cult of St. Katherine of Alexandria in Early Medieval Europe*; Lewis and Jenkins, eds., *St. Katherine of Alexandria: Texts and Contexts in Western Medieval Europe*; Jotischky, "Saints' Cults and Devotions on the Norman Edge,"191–218; Sands, *The Company She Keeps*; Simon, *The Cult of Saint Katherine of Alexandria in Late-Medieval Nuremberg*.

42 *RRS*, ed. Webster, 6:no. 204; *CPL*, ed. McGurk, 300.

43 MacKinlay, *Ancient Church Dedications in Scotland*, 2:418 (Cambuskenneth and Dunfermline), 420 (Beauly), 424 (Holyrood and Blackfriars); Penman, "Christian Days and Knights," 261n34.

44 Penman, "Christian Days and Knights," 261.

45 Penman, *David II*, 170–74.

46 Penman, *David II*, 308–25.

1350s and 1360s; producing his own heir would have substantially diminished the Stewart family's claim to authority in Scotland. David's childlessness created a strategic paradox: it enabled him to propose the unique solution to his crippling ransom, while simultaneously forcing him to contend with his adult nephew, Robert the Steward, as heir presumptive.

Uniquely, childlessness offered David a creative diplomatic tool: if the Scots accepted his succession plan, he could resolve England's massive reparation demands while still preserving Scottish autonomy under John of Gaunt's future rule. From 1357, David was unmistakably using his childlessness to negotiate a particularly creative, if politically unpopular, solution to his domestic and foreign diplomatic predicament. Ultimately, the comparative evidence of his political agenda in 1357 shows that childlessness was certainly on David's mind at the same point that he started looking for new forms of spiritual support in his early thirties.

Henry III and David II were not the only ones who sought new spiritual intercessors when they reached their early thirties without producing heirs. In the thirteenth century, Alexander II's piety underwent a similar shift just as he reached his early thirties. Alexander became king of Scots in 1215 when he was seventeen, and at first his devotional habits reflected the interests of his family before him; his father, William the Lion, dedicated Arbroath Abbey to Thomas Becket, and Alexander made a pilgrimage to Becket's tomb in Canterbury in the early 1220s.[47] The Cistercian abbey of Melrose also received regular support from Scottish kings and queens and Alexander II was no exception.[48] However, at the end of the 1220s (he was 30 in 1228), Alexander's pious practices distinctly changed.

The two biggest religious foundations of Alexander's thirty-five-year reign date from this period: the Cistercian abbey of Balmerino (Fife) was founded and dedicated to St. Edward the Confessor by Alexander and his mother in the late 1220s.[49] Then in 1230, he founded the abbey of Pluscarden, near his lands in Elgin, populated by the newly founded Valliscaulian Order.[50] Alexander continued his support for the Cistercians during the 1230s and

47 *Foedera*, ed. Rymer, 1.1:167.

48 Hammond, "Queen Ermengarde and the Abbey of St. Edward, Balmerino," 2–3.

49 *Statuta Capitulorum*, 63 (Item 39); *The Chartularies of Balmerino and Lindores*, ed. Turnbull, 8 (no. 1); *Chronica de Mailros*, ed. Stevenson, 140. This Scottish interest in St. Edward predates Henry III's attention to the saint by almost a decade so it cannot be easily attributed to Henry III's influence on his brother-in-law, Alexander II. See Hammond, "Queen Ermengarde," 4.

50 *Chron. Bower*, ed. Watt, 5:145 (Pluscarden). *Charters of Priory of Beauly*, ed.

it was in 1235–1236 that he made the most substantial royal endowment to Melrose Abbey since David I's reign in the twelfth century.[51] In addition to his two foundations, Alexander seems to have supported the new Dominican order in Scotland during the 1230s. Richard Oram suggests that it may have been Alexander who brought the order to Scotland and he possibly set up and supported the new Dominican convents in Aberdeen, Ayr, Perth, Stirling, Berwick, Edinburgh, Elgin, and Inverness, which date from this period.[52]

Remarkably, Alexander's interest in the new monastic orders only lasted for the 1230s. Oram argues that the king felt increased need for an heir during this period, and his patronage of new orders was a quest for more effective spiritual intercession because of his and Queen Joan's continued childlessness.[53] Significantly, Joan's death in 1238 and Alexander's marriage to Marie de Coucy in 1239 coincided with his return to more traditional forms of royal patronage for the remainder of his reign. Oram's argument is compelling, and it strengthens the present identification of a similar pattern of new devotional habits by Henry III and David II and the link between all three kings' behaviours and concerns about their childlessness.

The connection between a king's age, pious practices, and childlessness is clearer when compared to Alexander III's behaviour. Although Alexander and Margaret waited about six years from consummation until their first child's birth in 1261, Alexander was only twenty in 1261 and showed no markedly new or unusual piety during this period of childless marriage.[54] Significantly, Alexander never demonstrated comparable shifts in devotional practice at any point in his reign. This suggests, crucially, that it was a king's age, specifically reaching the age of thirty, which sparked a shift in devotional practice because the wait for an heir became concerning.

Henry III, David II, and Alexander II were each in their early thirties when their pious practices shifted, all facing conditions that called into question

---

Chisholm Batten, 16–17; Cowan and Easson, *Medieval Religious Houses in Scotland*, 84; Oram, *Alexander II*, 158–60.

51 *Liber Sancte Marie de Melros*, ed. Innes, 234–36 (nos. 264, 265); *Chronica de Mailros*, ed. Stevenson, 147; Oram, *Alexander II*, 161. Alexander granted the forest of Ettrick to Melrose Abbey.

52 Oram, *Alexander II*, 161. Cowan and Easson, *Medieval Religious Houses in Scotland*, 116–21.

53 Oram, *Alexander II*, 216–23.

54 Penman describes Alexander III's piety in this decade as the result of Henry III's influence in Scotland during Alexander's minority: Penman, "Royal Piety in Thirteenth-century Scotland," 23–24.

their maturity, masculinity, and effectiveness as rulers. Ongoing childlessness formed part of a broader challenge to their masculine identities as kings. With a decade of majority rule behind him by 1238, Henry III was still struggling to differentiate his reign as an adult king from his minority. Similar to Henry, in the late 1350s David II had yet to demonstrate his masculine maturity as an adult king; he had been defeated in battle, held prisoner by Edward III, and when he was finally able to return to Scotland, his authority was challenged by his adult heir who already had several grown sons of his own. At thirty, Alexander II looked like a more successful adult king than Henry or David, but his achievements were threatened by his failure to secure the succession and produce an heir. It is also worth noting that other thirteenth- and fourteenth-century kings, such as Alexander III and Edward I, had no such comparable shifts in their devotional practices, but they had also produced children before reaching their thirties. It was the king's age, specifically reaching the age of thirty, which activated concerns over childlessness.

Royal Masculinity, Maturity, and Fertility

To understand why the king's age might have sparked concern about childlessness, it is relevant to consider the significance of thirty in the male life course as well as the broader contexts of the three individual kings at the moments when their devotional practices changed. This section considers political maturity, marriage, and producing illegitimate children for the formation of a king's masculine identity and argues that the concerns about a couple's fertility were related to the king's demonstration of social maturity. The circumstances of Henry III, Alexander II, and David II differed when they reached their thirties and the effect of childlessness was not the same for all three, but their failure to produce an heir at the age associated with perfection and the pinnacle of male adulthood caused concern because it affected perceptions of their masculine maturity.

The age of thirty was significant in medieval conceptualizations of the male life course and achievement of mature masculinity. Medieval "Ages of Man" schemes divided life into stages and attributed particular functions and characteristics to childhood, adolescence, adulthood, and old age.[55]

55 The number of stages in these schemes varied. Many were based on three, four, or seven life stages; sometimes derived from humoral medical theory, while some seven-stage schemes were based on the seven cardinal virtues. Isidore of Seville's influential scheme (discussed below) has six stages. Aristotle describes only three

Generally, these schemes define the period between the mid-twenties to about fifty as male adulthood.[56] After youth and before decline into old age, adulthood was the peak of a man's developmental life when he had all of the physical ability of youth and the rationality of old age but without the weaknesses of either—the excessive and hot-headed qualities of youth or the deterioration of old age.[57] Isidore of Seville, in his *Etymologies*, imagined man's life in six distinct stages spanning from infancy to death.[58] He marked "adolescence" by the ability to reproduce, with the first emission of semen at about fourteen.[59] For Isidore and the generations of medieval scholars who followed, there was no such obvious physical sign that distinguished the passage from adolescence to adulthood. The only physical indication that a man had reached adulthood was his age: Isidore described the stage of *iuventus* ("youth," but not to be confused with adolescence) as mature adulthood, beginning at twenty-eight.[60] Isidore's scheme of man's development was widely known in the Middle Ages, but there were many variations of these schemes that described man's life. Some place the threshold of maturity at slightly earlier than twenty-eight, while others did not anticipate it until the mid-thirties.[61]

In these schemes, adulthood was generally the peak of man's life, but within this phase there was an even more specific high point. Man's physical perfection in his thirties was described by Aristotle, who considered the

stages—youth, maturity, and old age—and so does the thirteenth-century physician, Bernard of Gordon. Other authors, for instance, Dante, added a fourth stage: youth, maturity, old age, and extreme old age ending with death. See Shahar, *Growing Old*, 15–17. Beattie, "The Life Cycle: The Ages of Medieval Women," 16.

56 Dove, *The Perfect Age of Man's Life*, 28–29; Burrow, *The Ages of Man*, 5–54; Shahar, *Growing Old*, 15–17; Sears, *The Ages of Man*, 9–37.

57 Youngs, *The Life Cycle in Western Europe*, 129.

58 Isidore of Seville, *Etymologies*, ed. Barney et al., bk. 11, section 2, pp. 241–43.

59 Isidore of Seville, *Etymologies*, ed. Barney et al., bk. 11, section 2, p. 241 (nos. 1–8). Peter of Auvergne, a medieval commentator on Aristotle, places marriageable age for boys at fourteen because generation was (theoretically) possible from that age. See Biller, *The Measure of Multitude*, 337.

60 Isidore of Seville, *Etymologies*, ed., Barney et al., bk. 11, section 2, p. 241 (nos. 1–8).

61 Dove, *The Perfect Age*, 26–37; Shahar, *Growing Old*, 15–17; Moss, *Fatherhood and Its Representations*, 43. Avicenna believed adolescence lasted until thirty, for Isidore of Seville it was until twenty-eight, but twenty-five according to Dante. A distinction was clearly being made based on age, roughly the late twenties to thirties, but it was not an age that was based on the timing of physical adolescence.

body to be "most fully developed from thirty to thirty-five years of age."[62] This zenith of a male's life also had a parallel in Christ's life. Jesus was thought to have been baptized at thirty and crucified at thirty-three, and Christian eschatology speculated that at the end of the world, souls would be resurrected at the perfect age of thirty-three.[63] Balanced between the development of youth and the decrepitude of old age, and comparable to the perfection of Christ's body, in theory, thirty or thirty-three was the peak of a man's adult life, his most perfect age in body and soul.

However, male adulthood was not marked by age alone, but ultimately achieved by socially demonstrating maturity. Adulthood was the time of balance, and this characterized the behaviours associated with maturity. Rachel Moss argues that fathering a legitimate heir was a key function for signalling male maturity, while "infertility [was] an inhibitor to social maturation."[64] Fatherhood demonstrated a man's readiness and ability to take on the responsibilities of leading a family and providing for the future, a distinct maturation of the physical ability to reproduce that characterized the stage of adolescence. Henry III, Alexander II, and David II had not fathered legitimate children by the time that they reached the peak age of adulthood in the male life course and, while producing an heir was not a panacea for a problematic reign, it was an important function that could help to establish a king's masculine identity and maturity.

In the patriarchal structure of medieval society, demonstrating the qualities of adult, hegemonic masculinity was particularly integral for medieval kingship. In fact, the English coronation ceremony explicitly includes functions of masculine maturity by emphasizing the king's obligation to rule with restraint and balanced judgement, and prayers for him to produce children for the future of the kingdom.[65] The appropriate behaviours of masculine adulthood were essential to the role of medieval king, on a larger scale than for other medieval men. The ability to lead a family, in particular, was a role

62 Aristotle, *Rhetoric,* ed. Freese, bk. 2.14, section 14.

63 Youngs, *The Life Cycle*, 129; Dove, *The Perfect Age*, 56–57.

64 Moss, *Fatherhood and Its Representations*, 41, 44, 48.

65 A prayer in the English coronation rite probably first used for Edward II (it had many continuities with the earlier recension, used in the thirteenth century) mentions kingly fertility: "Reges quoque de lumbis eius per successions temporum futurorum egrediantur" (May there also come kings from his loins for the succession in future times; to rule the whole of this kingdom). *English Coronation Records*, ed. Legg, 92. A prayer after the king was bestowed with the rod and sceptre also asks God to "visit him with the increase of children," *English Coronation Records*, ed. Legg, 263.

writ-large in kingship, as the mature king headed not just a family but also a kingdom. Since childlessness thwarted demonstration of the responsibilities of fatherhood and leading a family, it could have significant implications for perceptions of a king's rulership.

Henry III's early adult reign illustrates how a king's struggle to demonstrate mature masculine authority could heighten concerns about his childlessness. Henry III assumed his role as adult king in 1227, but by the early 1230s he still had not decisively demonstrated the key behaviours of a socially adult man, despite his age and political maturity. In light of theories about age, and the need to demonstrate masculine maturity, Henry's childlessness looks significant when he reached the peak age of adulthood at thirty.[66] In his majority, he continued to rely heavily on the guidance of the men who had steered him through his minority, notably Hubert de Burgh.[67] In 1230, Henry was persuaded to reclaim lands in France and challenge Louis IX, but he returned to England having avoided a battle and accomplished very little.[68] In 1232, Henry's mentor, Hubert de Burgh, was ousted from power by his long-standing rival, Peter des Roches. Installed at the head of Henry's government, des Roches set out to strip his foes (de Burgh's followers) of the lands that they had accumulated over the previous decades. Nobles baulked at this and accused Henry of failing to protect their rights which had been established in the charters from 1225. Ultimately, in 1234, the archbishop of Canterbury advised Henry to dismiss des Roches. Carpenter argues that de Roches's behaviour must have left the king "feeling alone, betrayed by ministers of his youth and minority."[69] In the first years of his adult reign, then, Henry had failed in battle (by avoiding confrontation), relied too heavily on others to make the decisions for his government, and faced the threat of serious revolt from his nobles because he had followed poor advice. Ultimately, Henry had yet to distinguish his mature kingship from his adolescence and minority reign.

While holding a political position and responsibility was associated with masculinity, kingship itself could not demonstrate Henry III's maturity because he had assumed the role as a child. He struggled to shake off the

---

66 Carpenter argues that Henry's minority seems to have ended in 1227–1228, when he was twenty. Carpenter, "King Henry," 867.

67 Ridgeway, "Henry III (1207–1272)," *ODNB* [online].

68 He arrived in Brittany in 1230 but avoided engaging in battle with the French and when he made it to Gascony, he and Louis IX agreed on a truce until 1234 without fighting.

69 Carpenter, "King Henry," 878.

influence of mentors from his minority and failed to prove himself as a great warrior-king in the early 1230s. He had therefore not assumed a position of responsibility or achieved anything that signalled his adulthood when he approached the critical peak age in the male life course. As such, the roles of husband and father became crucial for differentiating Henry's adulthood and mature kingship from his minority and childhood.

The path to marriage was also not smooth for Henry. Alexander II's sister, Margaret of Scotland was suggested as a possible bride in the early 1230s but she was ultimately decided to be unsuitable.[70] In 1234–1235, negotiations with Jeanne de Ponthieu were abandoned too and, despite its invalidity because the couple were too closely related, every care was taken to carry out a formal annulment of the marriage even though it had only been celebrated by proxy.[71] This suggests that Henry and his advisors were concerned about ensuring that when Henry *did* marry, the match would be protected against accusations that his proxy marriage to Jeanne de Ponthieu was valid, which might jeopardize the legitimacy of his future heirs.

The delays securing a royal marriage likely contributed to impressions of Henry's immaturity. The king's earlier unsuccessful marriage plans and attention to securing a formal annulment help to explain the heightened pressure on Queen Eleanor to produce an heir. The delay in marrying ultimately delayed Henry's production of an heir—contributing to the concern about the still unsecured succession in the 1230s—and perhaps prolonged impressions of Henry's immaturity too. In the context of Henry's masculinity, marriage on its own would not have signalled the king's social maturity but it was one of the roles expected in adulthood and fundamental for producing an heir.

David II also struggled to establish his social maturity as king; marriage and the assumption of a leading political position did not demonstrate David's masculinity and maturity because they were associated with his childhood. When David returned from exile in France at the age of seventeen, he began cultivating a powerbase in Scotland.[72] Despite a strong start, he was unable to develop his kingship and exercise his authority as a mature king because he was captured in battle in 1346 and imprisoned in England for eleven years. When he finally returned to Scotland in 1357 at the age of thirty-three, he lacked clear signs of maturity. He was unsuccessful in battle against the English, his autonomy as king was curbed by the massive ransom

---

70 Oram, *Alexander II*, 116.

71 D'Avray, *Papacy, Monarchy and Marriage*, 92–93.

72 Penman, *David II*, 81–115.

that Scotland owed England for his release, and he had still not proven his virility by producing an heir. The personal contrast between David and his adult nephew and heir, Robert the Steward, could not have helped impressions of the king's maturity, as the Steward was nine years older than David, battle-hardened, and supported by his four adult sons.

Furthermore, the Scottish chroniclers describe David's youthfulness, suggesting that the perception of his maturity was an issue throughout his reign. David was seventeen when he returned from France in 1341, and the *Liber Pluscardensis* claims that in the 1340s, the king was only interested in celebrating with his friends, and "carried out little mature deliberation with wise counsel," a distinctly immature behaviour that a medieval audience associated with bad kingship.[73] Andrew of Wyntoun similarly emphasized David's youthful nature when he returned to Scotland in 1341, remarking that the king spent his time "jousting, dancing, and playing. He loved well, for he was young."[74] Under 1346, Wyntoun describes David as "young, courageous, and right jolly," with a yearning for fighting that suggested youthful rashness rather than mature judgment.[75] The *Chronicle of Lanercost* also emphasized David's youth, describing his fight at the Battle of Neville's Cross in 1346 as a dance, contrasted with a description of Sir Henry Percy as "a fine fighter," a juxtaposition that highlighted David's frivolous, immature approach.[76]

Despite having reached physical maturity, David was characterized as "youthful" long after the 1340s.[77] Bower commented that David was "a king who was scarcely approaching mature manhood" when he died in 1371 at the age of forty-seven.[78] His condemnation of David's decision to marry Margaret Logie, by claiming that they married for lust in 1363 also perpetuates an image of David as a reckless, passionate adolescent, not a king in his mid-thirties.[79]

---

73 *Liber Pluscardensis*, ed. Skene, 1:291: "pauca matura deliberacione cum consilio sapientum peregit."

74 *Wyntoun*, ed. Laing, 2:466: "justyng, dawnsyng, and playnge/ He luwyd welle, for he wes yhyng."

75 *Wyntoun*, ed. Laing, 2:470: "yhowng, stowt and rycht joly."

76 *Chronicon de Lanercost*, ed. Stevenson, 350: "et sic ad tripudium (tripudiet si voluerit David) eduxerunt" (and so they led off from the dance, leaving David to dance as he wished). "Dominus Henricus de Percy...bonus proeliator."

77 A similar observation is made by Smith, "Assessing Gender in the Construction of Scottish Identity," 144–52.

78 *Chron. Bower*, ed. Watt, 7:361.

79 *Chron. Bower*, ed. Watt, 7:333. This evidence and David's decision to marry Margaret are discussed above in Chapter 3.

The conditions of David's reign were stacked against him. When he was five, he inherited a kingdom which really needed a decisive adult and capable warrior king. He then grew up in France, distanced from his kingdom and the men who would have demonstrated the qualities necessary for a Scottish medieval king (like his nephew, Robert the Steward). Moreover, David's father, Robert I, had a legacy that was formidable and likely an impossible act to follow.[80] David's difficulty establishing his maturity as king, and the chroniclers' emphasis on his youthfulness, were not the direct result of his childlessness, but fathering an heir would have been an unmistakable way for David to demonstrate his masculine maturity when he returned to Scotland, in 1357, as a man in his early thirties.

Alexander II also perceptibly changed his devotional practice when he reached his thirties without producing an heir but, unlike Henry III and David II, he *had* demonstrated his maturity with other key behaviours of masculine adulthood. Indeed, by the early 1230s when Alexander was in his early thirties, he was quite a successful adult king. He had focused on asserting royal authority throughout mainland Scotland in the 1220s, specifically in the areas which were ruled more autonomously and farthest from the traditional reach of royal power in the lowlands.[81] Between 1228 and 1230, Alexander crushed the final uprising by the MacWilliams, a family based in the north of Scotland who had challenged the authority of the kings of Scots for several generations.[82] A powerful display of Alexander's ruthless determination to consolidate his power across the kingdom and eradicate any challengers to his throne came in 1230 when the last MacWilliams heir—a baby girl—was killed at the market cross in Forfar.[83] Richard Oram writes that Alexander established overlordship across more of mainland Scotland than any previous king. He had also challenged the Norwegian interest in the west coast, regained possession of the Western Isles and reformed succession and inheritance laws in Scotland.[84] Alexander successfully eliminated the most substantial threats to his power and established his kingship throughout much of Scotland by the 1230s.[85] A strong and decisive military

80 Lewis, *Kingship and Masculinity*, 257, suggests that Henry VI's masculinity was doomed to a similar impossible comparison with his father's, Henry V.

81 Oram, *Alexander II*, 72.

82 Oram, *Alexander II*, 72–73.

83 Oram, *Alexander II*, 75.

84 Oram, *Alexander II*, 118.

85 Oram, *Alexander II*, 257.

leader, strategist and legislator, Alexander displayed all the signs of mature masculine kingship *except* securing the succession.

Alexander II and Joan's childlessness was the most pressing threat to his reign by ca. 1230. In 1233, Alexander demonstrated his desire to secure his newly centralized Scottish kingship by trying to earn papal dispensation for a Scottish coronation ceremony that equalled the rite received by English and French kings.[86] His efforts were unsuccessful, but the attempt shows his resolve to cultivate and safeguard the kingship which he had developed. He also promoted linear succession in inheritance disputes, supporting the claims of children and grandchildren over siblings.[87] Producing an heir to leave the "enhanced royal inheritance" was the ultimate step for preserving the political stability that he had established in Scotland.[88] As such, Oram proposed that after Alexander's military and political success and efforts to secure his kingdom for his heir, the king turned to saintly intercessors and new monastic orders who claimed a more direct line to God because his childlessness was a sign of divine displeasure.[89]

Building on Oram's interpretation, the correlation between the behavioural shifts of Alexander, Henry III, and David II suggests that it was reaching the perfect age which activated Alexander's fear that his childlessness was a sign of divine punishment. Additionally, failing to have a child by the time of his physical peak might have implied that he suffered from some bodily imperfection or illness. Both divine displeasure and physical failing significantly threatened perceptions of Alexander's kingship *and* masculinity at a high point in his life and reign.

For comparison, Prince Edward, before he acceded as Edward I, highlights the connection between age, political maturity, and the pressure upon fertility. For the first decade of Edward and Eleanor of Castile's marriage, when he was about fifteen to twenty-five, Edward was still officially a political minor in his father's government. He also demonstrated the behavioural traits that were characteristic of adolescence, such as arrogance and changing allegiances, and he was seemingly "incapable of self-discipline."[90] After Edward and Eleanor

86 Oram, *Alexander II*, 102–4. He had tried already in 1221 but attempted again in 1233.

87 Oram, *Alexander II*, 118.

88 Oram, *Alexander II*, 116, notes Alexander's desire for an heir in the 1230s: "almost every one of his key acts as king to that point [1233] had been designed to enhance the royal inheritance which would be passed to his heir."

89 Oram, *Alexander II*, 223.

90 Prestwich, *Edward I*, 63, quoting historian Treharne, *Baronial Plan of Reform*, 164.

were married in 1254, he became involved in a factional dispute between two local families in Gascony and he acted directly against his father's policy of mediation in the region.[91] In the late 1250s, he sided with the barons, led by Simon de Montfort, in their opposition to Henry III and attempt to reform his government. Edward and his followers also brutally attacked a man in 1259, which caused Matthew Paris to ask, "if he does these things when the wood is green, what can be hoped for when it is seasoned?," showing a contemporary recognition of Edward's immaturity in the late 1250s.[92]

Edward continued to behave as an adolescent and show his social immaturity through his political inconsistency and disobedience in the first half of the 1260s. In 1260, Edward's insubordination to the royal cause had developed to the point that Henry III feared a coup d'état. Henry therefore sent Edward abroad for a couple of years and then on a campaign to Wales in 1263. Around this time, Edward had a change of heart when Simon de Montfort reignited baronial opposition to Henry III. When the king seemed about to capitulate to the barons' demands, Edward joined with some of his supporters and took Windsor Castle from the rebel barons.[93] From this point, Edward remained dedicated to defending his father's position and rights. His support culminated in the Battle of Evesham in 1265, when royal forces fought against Simon de Montfort. Before the battle began, Michael Prestwich argues that Edward showed leadership and strategic ability, and during the battle he displayed his courage against the formidable de Montfort.[94]

Edward's involvement in the Battle of Evesham in 1265 marked his transition into adulthood by demonstrating his skilled reasoning and capable leadership in battle. In the years after Evesham, Edward was made steward of England and, in 1269, Henry gave him lands and new castles around England.[95] Prestwich concludes that in the late 1260s, Edward took a leading role in the royal council, although he was still subject to some of the controls that had been placed on him by his father in the late 1250s at the peak of his rebelliousness.[96] Edward's political decisions and actions in the mid-1250s to 1260s displayed his immaturity and were the deeds of an adolescent

91 Prestwich, *Edward I*, 15–16.

92 *Chronica majora*, ed. Luard, 5:598: "Et haec facit in viridi, in arido quid sperandum?" Discussed by Prestwich, *Edward I*, 3.

93 Prestwich, *Edward I*, 41.

94 Prestwich, *Edward I*, 64.

95 Prestwich, *Edward I*, 61–62.

96 Prestwich, *Edward I*, 62.

prince, acknowledged as such by contemporaries like Paris. His shifting allegiances and hot-headedness contrasted with how he later handled the barons' rebellion and Simon de Montfort in the battle of Evesham in 1265 and this maturation is reflected in his reward of authority and political office by Henry III at the end of the 1260s.

Edward's socio-political adolescence helps to explain the lack of interest in his and Eleanor of Castile's fertility in the years when his position and behaviours were characterized by youthfulness. Recognized as "green wood" by Matthew Paris, a king-in-waiting, fatherhood and producing a legitimate heir would not have been necessary or critical functions expected of him in those years. In 1261, Eleanor of Castile gave birth to Katherine, and then Joan, in 1264.[97] However, neither daughter was shown any attention by contemporary chroniclers, suggesting that fatherhood was not a crucial part of Edward's role at that point. Coinciding with his demonstration of maturity in battle in 1265, Edward and Eleanor's first son, John, was born in 1266. In contrast to the silence about his sisters, John's birth was recorded by the Bury St. Edmunds chronicler. It is plausible that the birth of a son helped to establish Edward's social maturity and led to his assumption of a more adult role and set of responsibilities in his father's government in the late 1260s. Furthermore, Edward had turned thirty in 1269, which coincided with the grant of his new role as steward of England. At the peak age of the male life course, Edward demonstrated his social adulthood through his leadership, fatherhood and approach to justice, just as his behaviour in the previous decade had demonstrated his youth. Edward's age *and* socio-political adolescence helps to explain why there was no contemporary interest in his and Eleanor's fertility in the 1250s and 1260s.

By the time that they reached their thirties, and the age of physical perfection, Henry III and David II had difficulty demonstrating their maturity as kings in multiple ways, not just because of, but including childlessness. On the other hand, Alexander II had successfully established himself as a highly capable warrior king, a contemporary ideal, and brought stability to Scotland by the time that he reached his thirties. Having demonstrated other key behaviours of manhood, childlessness on its own was not a barrier to his social maturity in the 1230s, but it jeopardized his hard-won accomplishments as king. For all three kings, remaining childless when the male body was at its most perfect sent a worrying message about their social and reproductive abilities; if they had not produced a legitimate heir by now, then when?

---

97 Parsons, *Eleanor of Castile*, 24.

Illegitimate Children

It is worth considering whether producing an illegitimate child had a similar effect as legitimate fatherhood for the establishment of a king's social maturity. Indeed, Edward I, Edward II, and Alexander II each had, or were rumoured to have had, an illegitimate child. In the "age of man" schemes, adolescence was distinguished from childhood by the capacity for generation, a transition marked by puberty.[98] Adolescence was characterized as a period of excess, both socially and sexually. Rachel Moss notes that the production of illegitimate children was for a man perhaps "an expected part of the young male life cycle, [and] an aspect of his growing up, not of his having grown up."[99] In adolescence, a male might show he was *able* to sire a child, but maturity was ultimately demonstrated by founding a family and ensuring the future security of his lineage by producing and raising an *heir*. Simply producing a child did not signal maturity because it did not carry the same responsibilities as fatherhood.[100]

Edward II had an illegitimate son sometime before or shortly after he married Isabella of France in 1308.[101] Knowledge that Edward had produced an illegitimate son does not seem to have mitigated the concern about his and Isabella's initial childlessness, as the chroniclers still expressed their relief when Isabella gave birth to a son in 1312. Indeed, the contemporary concern about royal childlessness perhaps partly derived from the fact that Edward *had* already proven his fertility but continued to neglect his duty to produce a legitimate heir with Isabella. Edward's illegitimate son actually accentuated the childlessness in the first four years of his and Isabella's marriage. Also, Edward's extra-marital fertility was distinctly linked to his youth, as Adam was probably born around the time that Edward became king and married Isabella. As Edward transitioned into social adulthood, marked by his accession as king and marriage in his twenties, his illegitimate son belonged to the previous stage of his life.

It was rumoured that Edward I had illegitimate children before he was king, but he never acknowledged any and the sources are vague.[102] Despite

---

98 Sears, *Ages of Man*, 66; Youngs, *The Life Cycle*, 97–98; Moss, *Fatherhood and Its Representation*, 42.

99 Moss, *Fatherhood and Its Representations*, 49, quote from 71.

100 Moss, *Fatherhood and Its Representations*, 71.

101 Phillips, *Edward II*, 102n144.

102 The *Chronicle of Bury St. Edmunds* reports the *rumour* of Edward's indiscretions. Given-Wilson and Curteis, *The Royal Bastards of Medieval England*, 136.

the lack of evidence, just the rumour that he had an illegitimate child in the decades before he became king shows that reproduction alone was not associated with maturity. There were accusations that he had an affair with the countess of Gloucester in the late 1260s, but these rumours were likely unfounded.[103] A John Botetourt is listed as an illegitimate son of Edward in a genealogical table of Edward I's family in a manuscript of the Hailes Abbey chronicle, although his name is added over an erasure and Prestwich suggests that the scribe perhaps meant to put the name of the husband of Edward's daughter Elizabeth.[104] The very plausibility of such rumours implies that siring illegitimate children was understood as characteristic youthful behaviour rather than evidence of adult masculine responsibility. Significantly, the emergence of rumours that Edward produced an illegitimate child or pursued someone else's wife in the 1260s demonstrates that medieval contemporaries specifically associated such sexual behaviours with adolescent lack of restraint, not maturity.

Alexander II had an illegitimate daughter, probably born before 1221. Oram states that this daughter, Marjory, was proof of Alexander's fertility before he married Joan Plantagenet in 1221, which contributed to a gulf between the royal couple in the 1230s.[105] However, the shift in Alexander's piety in the 1230s suggests that he, at least, was not convinced that his illegitimate daughter was proof that he would sire a legitimate heir. Alexander's extra-marital fertility might actually have accentuated the lack of legitimate fertility. His illegitimate daughter was born before his marriage, perhaps before he became king too, so his show of fertility belonged to his youth. Ultimately, knowing that he was *able* to reproduce but yet still had no legitimate biological heir as an adult king might have contributed to the sense that something was wrong by the late 1220s.

---

103 *Chronicle of Bury St. Edmunds*, ed. Gransden, 45: "Orta est discordia inter Eadwardum filium regis et G[ilbertum] comitem Glouernie ob nimiam [amoris] familiaritatem quam idem Eadwardus erga uxorem dicti comitis dicebatur havere" (A quarrel broke out between Edward, the king's son and Gilbert, earl of Gloucester, because of excessive intimacy which Edward was said to have with the earl's wife). English translation by Gransden. For argument that the rumours were unfounded, see Given-Wilson and Curteis, *Royal Bastards*, 136; Prestwich, *Edward I*, 60–61, 131.

104 Prestwich, *Edward I*, 132, 136: John Botetourt was born sometime in the 1260s and was a knight in Edward's household, a member of the royal council and favoured by the king for his military service but Given-Wilson argues that while he was of uncertain parentage, Botetourt's coat of arms shows "no hint of royal blood."

105 Oram, *Alexander II*, 117.

In contrast, there is no evidence that Henry III or David II had illegitimate children. Although adolescence was distinguished by the ability to reproduce, actually siring a child was not necessary for marking the transition from childhood to adolescence. While Alexander II's fertility outside of marriage does not seem to have mitigated his concern about childlessness in the 1230s, Henry and David's failure to demonstrate their reproductive ability in youth perhaps contributed to the pressure for fertility when both kings reached the peak age of adulthood. Ultimately, though, reproduction alone without the commitment of raising an heir does not seem to have been a behaviour that marked a king's maturity. In fact, it seems to have been distinctly associated with their adolescence.

In sum, the shift in the three kings' devotional behaviours around thirty seems significant in light of contemporary thought about maturity and masculinity. As they reached the theoretical perfect age of manhood, Henry III and David II had not clearly distinguished themselves as adult men nor differentiated themselves from their minorities. Short on other markers of adulthood, producing a legitimate heir would have been particularly meaningful indications of Henry and David's masculine maturity when they reached the perfect age. Alexander II's success as king in the late 1220s and 1230s coincided with reaching his thirties. At a physical and political high point in his reign, he demonstrated his maturity through his effective kingship, but he still had no clear heir to leave his hard-won legacy to. Although failing to produce an heir was not a barrier to social maturity for Alexander, as it was for Henry and David, remaining childless at the age of perfection likely reflected uncomfortably on his masculinity and suggested a worrisome divine assessment of his achievements as king.

Fertility and the Queen's Age

This chapter has highlighted a connection between the king's age, pious behaviours, and responses to royal childlessness, but Matthew Paris only mentioned the queen's fertility. How does the queen factor into the argument that the king's age was central to the pressure for fertility? If reaching the anticipated age of fatherhood prompted fertility concerns among childless kings, was there a comparable point or circumstance in queens' lives which contributed to the concerns about a couple's fertility? The following discussion of medieval practice and theory about the female life course indicates that motherhood was not anticipated in the perfect age of woman, as it was for men. Furthermore, consideration of medieval thought about the compatibility of partners in marriage suggests that contemporary understanding of marital ages and fertility meant that royal fertility was perceived in relation to the royal couple, not the king or queen in isolation.

Female Perfect Age

Balmerino Abbey, near the banks of the River Tay (Fife), was founded in the late 1220s by Alexander II and his mother, the dowager Queen Ermengarde.[106] This foundation has interested scholars because it was dedicated by the Scottish king and his mother to St. Edward the Confessor, a particularly English saint.[107] Matthew Hammond argued that, in Scotland, St. Edward served as a reminder of the lineage and dynastic significance of Alexander II and Joan's future children: Aelred of Rievaulx's *Vita* of St. Edward, which led to the saint's canonization in the twelfth century, contains a prophecy about a tree branch being reunited with the main trunk, symbolizing the return to the English throne of Edward's royal bloodline. The bloodline had been severed by the Norman Conquest but preserved in the Scottish royal family through the sainted queen Margaret (Edward the Confessor's grand-niece) in the twelfth century.[108] Hammond asserts that the foundation of Balmerino "coincided with the coming of age of Joan" at sixteen, and that St. Edward was Queen Ermengarde's "wisely chosen intercessor to help the young English wife of the Scottish king to conceive an heir to the kingdom."[109] Does this explanation hold up in light of medieval ideas about the female life course? Was sixteen a significant age for a childless queen, comparable to the early thirties for kings? If Balmerino was intended to encourage royal fertility, was it in response to concern about the couple's childlessness activated by Joan's age?

In contemporary theory, twelve was a more significant "coming of age" point for girls than sixteen. The onset of menstruation was generally expected around this age, though medical writers acknowledged variation between individuals, with menarche usually occurring between twelve and

106 *Statuta Capitulorum*, 63 (Item 39); *The Chartularies of Balmerino and Lindores*, ed. Turnbull, 8 (no. 1). Alexander II confirmed the foundation in 1231: *Handlist of the Acts of Alexander II, 1214–1249*, ed. Scoular, no. 145.

107 Hammond, "Queen Ermengarde," 4–6; Carpenter, "King Henry," 867–68; Nelson, "Queens and Queenship," 155–56. The dedication is even more unusual because it predates Henry III's interest in and promotion of the Confessor.

108 Hammond, "Queen Ermengarde," 5; Oram, *Alexander II*, 113, accepts Hammond's interpretation.

109 Hammond, "Queen Ermengarde," 3, 5.

fifteen.[110] Canon lawyers, drawing on the timing of puberty, set the legal age of consent for marriage and consummation at twelve for girls. In medieval "ages of man" schemes adapted for women, the transition from childhood to youth, signalled by the beginning of reproductive capacity, was placed at twelve. As with men, both medical and legal authors recognized that these ages were theoretical markers; physical capacity and function were considered just as important as chronological age in determining maturity or life stage. Compared to the schemes for men, female age divisions tended to be fewer, usually only four, with emphasis placed on physical development, marital status, and reproductive ability rather than specific chronological age.[111] Based on the evidence of medieval practice and theory, there is no reason to believe that reaching sixteen was particularly meaningful for expectations of Joan Plantagenet's fertility or maturation. Sixteen might have been significant for Joan personally, if she began menstruating then, but no evidence on this survives. Sixteen, specifically, was not an important milestone in medieval understandings of female life stages, reproduction, ageing or maturity.

The explanation for the foundation of Balmerino Abbey not only assumes that sixteen was a meaningful age for medieval women, but that there was enough real concern about Joan's fertility by that point to prompt the expensive and labour-intensive process of building, populating and supporting a new abbey to invite royal fertility. Alexander II's mother, Ermengarde, had married William the Lion in 1186 and they did not have a child until 1193. Based on her own example, sixteen-year-old Joan's fertility would not necessarily have concerned Ermengarde when she founded Balmerino in the late 1220s.[112] Admittedly, it is not decisive evidence, but there are no signs in the chronicles that contemporaries were particularly anxious about Joan's fertility by the late 1220s either. The timing of the Balmerino foundation and dedication to St. Edward the Confessor *does*, however, align with the shift in Alexander II's devotional practices around age thirty, when he was increasingly focused on securing the royal inheritance.

The foundation and dedication of Balmerino Abbey to St. Edward the Confessor can still be interpreted as an effort to boost royal fertility, but it seems prompted by Alexander's age rather than Joan's, as Hammond's analysis presumed. Alexander confirmed the foundation in 1231 but, after

110 See Chapter 2.

111 Beattie, "The Life Cycle."

112 Nelson, "Queens and Queenship," 145.

Ermengarde died in 1233 (and was buried at Balmerino), the king's interest dwindled and the association with St. Edward faded from the abbey by the late 1230s; the saint had completely disappeared from the abbey's dedication by 1238–1241.[113] This change caused Hammond to argue that the foundation and attention to the Confessor was really Ermengarde's endeavour and Alexander was merely giving formal approval for his mother's wishes.[114] Oram suggested that Alexander lost interest in Balmerino because of his mother's death and Joan's continued failure to produce a child.[115] However, the Balmerino association with St. Edward ended not in 1233–1234 when Ermengarde died, but around 1238–1241. This timing aligns with the pattern of Alexander's devotional practices, which only lasted for the 1230s when *his* age, rather than Joan's, made their childlessness particularly concerning. The abandonment of St. Edward around 1238 coincides with Joan's death, Alexander's second marriage and his return to earlier forms of royal devotion.

There was a "perfect age" in the female life course, but it was not sixteen and motherhood was not its defining function. Women's perfect age was not the "middle age," as it was in the schemes for men, but maidenhood.[116] Maidens, virginal but sexually developed young women, were far younger than thirty and representations of perfect women are depicted in medieval art with the characteristics of maidenhood. Virginal saints—for instance, Margaret, Lucy, and Agnes—were all between the ages of twelve and eighteen but characterized by their sexual maturity because each virgin's martyrdom and sanctity resulted from her sexual attractiveness and refusal to marry her suitor-turned-tormentor.[117] Medieval writers believed that Christ had died at thirty-three because he would have experienced physical decline after that point, so Phillips proposed that "the virgin martyrs died in their teens because that was the peak of the lives of their feminine bodies."[118] This suggests that the perfect age for women spanned from puberty, around twelve, to around eighteen, based on the ages of the virgin martyr saints. According to Giles of Rome, these years coincided with the end of growing (reminiscent

113 Hammond, "Queen Ermengarde," 14–21.

114 Hammond, "Queen Ermengarde," 2–7.

115 Oram, *Alexander II*, 158.

116 Phillips, *Medieval Maidens*, 43–47; Phillips, "Maidenhood as the Perfect Age of Woman's Life."

117 Phillips, *Medieval Maidens*, 47.

118 Phillips, *Medieval Maidens*, 47.

of the descriptions of thirty for men), and the perfect time for intercourse and producing children.[119] Sixteen falls in the middle of this span, but it was not significant in its own right, as Hammond presumed. Distinctly, the defining quality of maidenhood was *not* motherhood, but sexual maturity coupled with virginity. While legitimate fatherhood was an important function of man's perfect age, motherhood was not especially associated with woman's age of perfection.

Thinking more broadly than just about Joan and Balmerino, the queens of Henry III, Alexander II, and David II were not the same age when the kings' devotional habits shifted. Joan Plantagenet, Eleanor of Provence, and Joan of the Tower had few discernible similarities except for their status as queens when their husbands' devotional practices changed. Eleanor of Provence was in her early teens, while Joan Plantagenet was twenty in 1230 when Alexander II pursued new kinds of religious support. In 1357, when David's piety changed, Joan of the Tower was thirty-six and well beyond the ideal few-year-delay advised between menarche and childbearing. She and David had lived apart for over a decade, when he was imprisoned, and they continued to live separately when he returned to Scotland and Joan stayed in England. These dissimilarities suggest that the kings' devotional shifts were not triggered by their queens reaching a particular age or stage in life, but by other concerns surrounding the absence of heirs.

Compatibility of Ages and Fertility

While there is no sign that it was a specific age for the queen that activated concerns about childlessness and caused the kings to change their pious practices, the queen's age was still relevant to perceptions of royal fertility. Medical texts and works on canon law also consider the reproductive compatibility of the couple. At the end of the thirteenth century, Pope Boniface VIII issued his ruling on underage marriages, declaring that, among many other impediments, a marriage was not valid if only one of the partners had reached puberty.[120] This makes sense: in the absence of puberty, one partner was still a child and therefore lacked the physical ability to reproduce and intellectual capacity that was essential for marriage. It also highlights how both partners (in theory) were considered equally integral in marriage. Both Giles of Rome and Peter of Auvergne, in discussions about the age of marriage, advised against intercourse and reproduction by very young

119 See discussion in Chapter 2.

120 D'Avray, *Papacy, Monarchy and Marriage*, 132.

couples, despite ability, because it was harmful for *both* sexes and the health of their future children.[121] In addition to demonstrating that sex and child-bearing were believed to affect negatively men *and* women's growth if experienced too young, it also implies that intercourse and procreation should be postponed until both partners were sufficiently old; *both* partners needed to reach a suitable phase of maturity.[122]

The importance of mutual maturity of partners is implied in Matthew Paris's anecdote about the delayed consummation of Alexander III and Margaret of England's marriage in 1255. Paris explains that the property of Robert de Ros, one of the original protectors of Alexander III and Margaret, who had been appointed by Henry III in 1251, was seized in 1255 because of his treatment of the royal couple. De Ros allegedly defended his actions by declaring that he "did not permit the king and queen to sleep together because of *their* youth, until a certain time should come which had not yet proved to have arrived."[123] This "certain time" presumably referred to the onset of puberty. Paris's account underscores the contemporary belief that consummation, and therefore, potential for fertility, should wait until both partners were mature.

Based on more than mutually achieving maturity, medical writers considered the incompatibility of partners to be a cause of infertility. Fourteenth-century medical texts attribute sterility to multiple causes in men and women, including anatomical and physiological problems and behavioural and lifestyle "bad habits" in both sexes, but they also advised that "sterility may reside in the couple" because of some physical or complexional incompatibility or lack of mutual attraction.[124] Therefore, both partners were equally integral for fertility and fertility resided in the couple. When a childless king reached the perfect age of male adulthood, he faced a heightened need to produce an heir because of the implications for his masculinity and, with the ensuing attention on the *couple's* fertility, this implicated the queen too. The queen's age mattered in the respect that she needed to have reached a point of maturity when sex and reproduction were possible and not harmful to herself or her future children, but, at least for the royal

121 Biller, *Measure of Multitude*, 334.

122 *Chronica majora*, ed. Luard, 5:569.

123 *Chronica majora*, ed. Luard, 5:569.

124 Cadden, *Meaning of Sex Difference*, 240. See the anonymous fourteenth-century treatise on sterility from Montpellier: Pagel, "Raymundus de Moleriis und seine Schrift de impedimentis conceptionis," 530–37.

couples discussed in this book, it was not specifically her age that initiated concerns about fertility or problematized royal childlessness.[125]

Henry III's devotional behaviour in the 1230s also suggests that fertility was associated with the couple not the individual. When he cultivated his faith in St. Edward the Confessor and support for the monks of Westminster, Henry included Queen Eleanor. We saw this with *La estoire de Seint Aedward le rei*, which he commissioned for Eleanor in the first few years of their marriage. Henry also founded several new chapels for the queen before and during Eleanor's years of childbearing which were dedicated to St. Katherine of Alexandria.[126] Lewis suggests that St. Katherine may have been cultivated as Queen Eleanor's patron saint from the beginning of the couple's marriage, and so Henry developed not only his own new personal saintly intercessor in the mid-1230s but also one for his young queen.[127] Both chosen saints have associations that were significant for the couple's fertility too: St. Edward was an important dynastic saint for the English monarchy, tying Henry's post-conquest family to the ancient Alfredic kings, while one textual version of St. Katherine's miracles feature cures for sterility, and, as will be discussed later, her circulating image also had associations with milk, a substance which had spiritual associations with fertility.[128] It was Henry's age that made the couple's childlessness concerning, but royal fertility was inseparable from himself *and* Eleanor.

* * *

We can now understand why, according to Matthew Paris, there was concern about Eleanor's fertility in 1238. As Paris mentioned fears that the queen was barren, Henry III developed his devotion to St. Edward the Confessor in

125 The assertion that Margaret and Alexander III were *unjustly* kept from consummating their marriage in 1255 might reflect the English attention to ensuring that the marriage was fully legalized once Alexander III turned 14 in 1255. Boniface VIII's ruling on underage marriage from 1298 specifies that "a marriage which was invalid because of an impediment of age" was only validated by reaching the age of consent (14 for Alexander, but 12 for Margaret) and having intercourse to show that they had "reached the ages of puberty without any change of mind." Quoted from D'Avray, *Papacy, Monarchy and Marriage*, 132.

126 Between 1227–1247, Henry founded about twenty new chapels, and at least ten were perhaps intended for Eleanor: Brown, Colville and Taylor, *The History of the King's Works I*, 124n.

127 Lewis, *The Cult of St. Katherine of Alexandria in Late Medieval England*, 64.

128 Morrison, *Women Pilgrims in Late Medieval England*, 10, 16. This is discussed in Chapter 6 below.

1235–1238. Something had prompted the king to seek a new spiritual intercessor at this time. In those years, Henry III reached what was considered to be the prime age in the male life course, his late twenties to early thirties. This detail became more conspicuous when we observed similar shifts in the reigns of two other kings. Alexander II and David II also altered their pious practices when they reached their thirties, seeking new and different forms of spiritual intercession. Despite few similarities beyond childlessness, all three kings adopted markedly new spiritual strategies at the same age. The common thread is that the king's age sparked these spiritual behavioural shifts and triggered concerns over childlessness.

The king's age was significant because it carried expectations of behaviour. The peak age for men was associated with the end of growing in the male life course and the achievement of maturity, which was demonstrated by social functions such as legitimate fatherhood. Producing a child was *possible* in adolescence, but fathering an heir was dependent on marital status and position as head of the family, both functions that distinguished an adult man from an adolescent boy. Distinctly, it was not reproduction alone, as consideration of kings' illegitimate children showed, which contributed to perceptions of a king's maturity. Rather, a king had "an obligation to the country he inherited [to] provide future rulers for it, [which was] a necessary part of demonstrating...that he [was] a real man."[129]

This chapter explored the three kings' contexts and achievements when they reached their thirties and argued that childlessness was concerning for the kings in light of their social maturity at the perfect age of adulthood. Henry III and David II, when they reached the age associated with the peak of masculinity, struggled to differentiate their rule as mature kings from their earlier minority reigns. Short on other markers of adulthood, continued childlessness also impeded Henry III's and David II's demonstration of social maturity at the peak of the male life course. In contrast, Alexander II had demonstrated his capability as a king and displayed his maturity in his success as a leader in the late 1220s. However, at his physical peak, his successes highlighted his continued failure to produce a legitimate heir. Childlessness was not a barrier to social maturity for Alexander as it was for Henry and David, but not producing an heir at the age of physical perfection threatened existing perceptions of his manhood by suggesting divine punishment for his actions as king. Ultimately, the kings' age seems to have activated concerns about childlessness because of the significance of

129 Moss, *Fatherhood and its representations*, 60.

reproduction and fatherhood for perceptions of masculine maturity at the zenith of the male life course.

The initial lack of concern about adolescent royal couples' fertility helps to illustrate the fundamental role of the king's age in shaping perceptions of royal fertility. Both Eleanor of Castile and Margaret of England were married as very young teenagers and, like Eleanor of Provence, these queens did not have (surviving) children until their mid-teens, or later. Unlike Henry III in his thirties, Margaret's husband, Alexander III (aged ten to twenty), and Eleanor's husband, Prince Edward (aged fifteen to twenty-two), were both still in their teens during their respective waits for an heir. The silences surrounding Eleanor of Castile and Margaret's respective fertility contrasts sharply with the anxiety expressed about Eleanor of Provence's fertility at the same age. This suggests that worries about a couple's fertility did not stem from a specific number of childless years—both adolescent couples were childless for longer periods than Henry III and Eleanor—but rather from the king reaching the chronological age of masculine perfection without producing a legitimate heir.[130] It is important to note that by their early thirties, Alexander III and Edward had already assumed several mature, masculine roles, including producing heirs, and neither significantly altered their pious practices when they reached thirty.[131]

While the king's age seems to be the crucial element in determining when royal childlessness prompted concern, Paris's comment about Eleanor of Provence, not Henry III, ties the concerns to the queen too. There was no specific age for the queens which seems to have activated concern about childlessness, nor was the age of female perfection defined by motherhood in contemporary theory about the female life course. Instead, when their husbands tried to support fertility with new spiritual intercessors, the differences between the queens highlight how perceptions of her fertility were not separable from that of the king's. The point at which the queen was expected to reproduce was relational to the king; in the instances discussed

130 It must be noted that Eleanor of Castile and Edward had already proven their ability to conceive, with the early pregnancy and stillbirth in 1255, so presumably no contemporary would have questioned if Eleanor was infertile, as Paris did for Eleanor of Provence.

131 Edward I became king in 1272, when he was thirty-three so he assumed a significant role of social maturity as king when he reached the perfect age of manhood. His accession at this age disqualifies him as a comparative case study here because his new royal status required such significant changes in religious patronage that it becomes impossible to identify comparable patterns in his devotional behaviour that might relate to fertility anxieties.

above, that point looks determined by *his* age. Significantly, the spiritual practices employed by Alexander II and Henry III also involved their queens, like the foundation and dedication of Balmerino Abbey to St. Edward, and Henry's efforts to cultivate a saintly intercessor for Eleanor of Provence in St. Katherine, as well as his inclusion of the queen in the veneration of St. Edward. Ultimately, the king's age might have determined whether royal childlessness became a concern, but royal fertility was nothing without both partners.

Chapter 5

ROYAL HEALTHCARE AND REPRODUCTIVE MEDICINE

CONCERNS ABOUT FERTILITY were activated because of the king's age, but what did royal couples actually do to encourage fertility? Looking at evidence of royal healthcare, this chapter focuses on how kings and queens managed their health, and reveals factors that shaped the medical care, and therefore fertility medicine, practised in royal households.

This chapter addresses two key questions, building on the previous chapter's insight that kings were central to both activating concerns about royal fertility and shaping contemporary perceptions of it. To what extent were royal health-seeking efforts gendered, in terms of who initiated and received treatment? And does the timing of couples' traceable health-seeking efforts align with the concerns about childlessness that emerged due to the king's age?

The first question considers to what extent queens bore the brunt of responsibility for remedying infertility. To answer it, this chapter examines surviving evidence for royal couples' general healthcare. It is possible to identify several of the physicians and apothecaries who served in the English and Scottish royal households. There are also fragments of herbal medicines preserved in an apothecary list of ingredients purchased for Isabella of France in 1313, and both she and Eleanor of Provence had connections to *regimen sanitatis* texts, a genre of medical texts intended for personal and practical use. These documentary breadcrumbs show connections to practitioners and texts which illustrate the different roles of king and queen in the management of health and receipt of treatments. Even though the king's behaviour was important for determining perceptions of royal fertility, medical aids for reproduction and fertility were focused on treating the queen's body. However, queens also ultimately influenced the healthcare and medical knowledge that circulated in royal households. This chapter then turns to the second question and considers whether the evidence for medical treatment aligns with the concerns about childlessness that emerged when kings reached their thirties.

In the absence of more explicit documentary evidence for royal reproductive medicine, this chapter traces evidence of royal medical care, and questions how we might infer promotion of fertility from the sources that we *do* have. Applying a novel approach which has not been used in scholarship on medieval medicine or royalty, the key, as the chapter illustrates, is to understand the broader patterns of healthcare for kings and queens.

The Queen's Medical Network: Practitioners, Texts, and Roles in Royal Healthcare

Scholars have argued that, despite theoretical discussion about sterility in medieval men, it was usually the woman who was blamed and treated for fertility problems in practice.[1] This section examines the medical care dynamics between kings and queens, revealing a more complex picture. While kings initiated medical care for their wives in some instances, and the treatments for miscarriages, stillbirths, and complications of childbirth focused squarely on the queen's body, the dynamic was not entirely one-directional. Queens also played active roles in shaping royal medical care through their personal preferences and connections. By analyzing the networks of medical practitioners in royal households and the couples' connections to medical texts, this section argues that the queen influenced the medical care available to the royal couple, and so ultimately, how they accessed reproductive medicine.

Initiating and Receiving Medical Care

Three separate cases demonstrate how medical care for queens was initiated and directed either by the king or the queen's natal family. Both kings and queens had their own personal practitioners and dedicated medical staff, but the request for care and decision-making power was not necessarily held exclusively by the patient. First, evidence for Margaret of France, Edward I's second wife, sheds light on this dynamic, when the king made the ultimate decisions about the queen's treatment. Margaret arrived from France in 1299, probably with her own physician, John of Fountains.[2] In May 1305, John wrote to Edward I twice about the queen's ill health.[3] Margaret's physician advised the king that the queen's worsening condition indicated that she needed to be bled, but seemingly, neither he nor the queen wanted the responsibility for making such a decision.[4] Edward replied in support of the procedure, and encouraged the physician to bleed Margaret "as soon as

1 Cadden, *The Meanings of Sex Difference*, 228–58; Rider, "Men and Infertility in Late Medieval English Medicine"; Toulalan, "'Elderly Years Cause a Total Dispaire of Conception'"; Oren-Magidor, *Infertility in Early Modern England*, 49–84.

2 Talbot and Hammond, *The Medical Practitioners in Medieval England*, 145.

3 Chaplais, "Some Private Letters of Edward I," 83, 85.

4 TNA, SC 1/12/203. The letter is dated May 1, 1305, at St. Albans. It is printed in Chaplais, "Some Private Letters of Edward I," 83.

the queen had a great deal of bad blood."[5] John subsequently made a diagnosis of measles and wrote to tell Edward, who instructed that the queen should not travel until she had recovered.[6] Margaret was not being treated for a fertility-related condition in this instance, but the letters from John to Edward and the fact that Margaret was unwilling to make the decision about, and accept responsibility for, her own health suggests an important dynamic in royal medical treatment. The decisive power about Margaret's care was held by the king. Or, conversely, responsibility for her health and medical care was considered by her physician to be Edward I's business.

Edward's decision-making power over the queen's health was likely shaped by the dynamic between the royal couple. At the time he was directing her care, Edward I was in his mid-sixties and had reigned successfully as king of England for more than three decades. By contrast, Margaret, his second queen, had only recently arrived in England and was still in her mid-twenties. The balance of power between them was thus heavily weighted in Edward's favour. A similar dynamic is visible in another case: when Eleanor of Provence first came to England in 1236 at the age of twelve, Henry III appointed the physician Nicholas of Farnham to oversee the health and wellbeing of his young queen. These examples highlight how differences in age, experience, and standing shaped the respective roles of kings and queens in matters of healthcare, particularly influencing who determined medical decisions.[7]

Another example illustrates how a queen's mother could exercise decisive influence over her daughter's medical care and reproductive life. In 1255, Eleanor of Provence sent her personal physician, Reginald of Bath, to Scotland to assess Margaret's wellbeing. He reported that the fifteen-year-old queen was unhappy and frustrated because her marriage to Alexander III had not yet been consummated.[8] Acting on Reginald's report, Henry III travelled to Scotland, removed Robert de Ros and John Balliol from their positions, and reversed the policy keeping the young couple apart.[9] Henry III's concern was not merely fatherly: consummation confirmed the marriage

5 Chaplais, "Some Private Letters of Edward I," 83. English translation quoted from Talbot and Hammond, *Medical Practitioners*, 145.

6 TNA SC 1/12/204.

7 *Chronica majora*, ed. Luard, 4:158. Howell, *Eleanor of Provence*, 23; Talbot and Hammond, *Medical Practitioners*, 223–25.

8 *Chronica majora*, ed. Luard, 5:501–6.

9 *Chronica majora*, ed. Luard, 5:501–6.

and ensured Margaret's entitlement to her dower should Alexander die prematurely. By sending her physician, Eleanor intervened directly in decisions that linked healthcare, reproductive management and political diplomacy. This case demonstrates how medical oversight could function as a means for a queen's family to exercise authority while also advancing political and dynastic objectives.

This episode also preserves the extent of parental authority over a royal daughter's health and reproductive life. Rather than the Scottish minority council, the fourteen-year-old King Alexander III, or Margaret herself making decisions about her medical care and marital consummation, it was Margaret's English parents who controlled these intimate aspects of her life. Eleanor of Provence's appointment of a physician with such considerable investigative power, and the swift political action that followed his report, demonstrate that the decisive authority over not only healthcare but also when Margaret and Alexander might consummate their marriage—and potentially conceive an heir—remained firmly in the hands of the queen's birth family during the early years of the Scottish royal marriage.

In a final example, Eleanor of Provence and Eleanor of Castile were influential in deciding when their granddaughter and daughter (respectively) were married. In early 1282, Edward I and Eleanor of Castile's daughter, Eleanor, was betrothed to Alfonso of Aragon.[10] Young Eleanor was about twelve or thirteen at the time of the betrothal and, a few months later, her mother and grandmother together urged Edward I to delay the marriage until she was older.[11] Edward wrote to request the delay of Eleanor and Alfonso's marriage for a couple of years, citing that it was at the insistence of his wife and mother.[12] As a result, the marriage did not take place until Eleanor was seventeen.[13] This seems like a joint effort by mother and grandmother to protect young Eleanor from the reproductive demands of marriage in her early teens. This presumably stemmed from the queens' personal experiences: Eleanor of Provence and Eleanor of Castile were both married at twelve or thirteen, and both faced the pressure and consequences of marital and reproductive roles from this young age. Eleanor of Provence had faced concerns about sterility soon after her wedding, while Eleanor of Castile had

---

10 Howell, *Eleanor of Provence*, 289.

11 Howell, *Eleanor of Provence*, 290. The letter is printed in Chaplais, *English Medieval Diplomatic Practice*, pt. 1, ii, no. 248.

12 Parsons, "Mothers, Daughters," 68–69; Phillips, *Medieval Maidens*, 40.

13 Phillips, *Medieval Maidens*, 40.

fallen pregnant immediately and braved the premature birth of a stillborn or short-lived daughter when she was fourteen. Remarkably, none of Eleanor of Castile's daughters who survived infancy left for their marital homes before the age of fourteen, perhaps a reflection of the impact that Eleanor's early and unsuccessful pregnancy had on both her and Edward I. The desire of the two queens to protect the health of young Eleanor shows the influence and involvement of royal families—particularly queens as mothers—in medically based decisions about royal health and reproduction.

The Queen's Body and Reproductive Medicine

A second dynamic at play in medieval royal medicine is the centrality of the queen's body in treatments for fertility. A list of herbs from Isabella of France's apothecary, Odinet, survives from November 1313 and offers a rare insight into medicines administered to a queen.[14] Scholars have previously argued that the herbal substances were prescribed to treat bad burns on Isabella's arm after a fire.[15] However, the following reinterpretation of this list (Table 2) suggests that she had a miscarriage or stillbirth and highlights how the fertility problems and concerns of couples who had children have been overlooked by historians. The list also shows how the medical treatment for reproductive issues was disproportionately experienced by the queen.

Edward II and Isabella's first child, Edward, was born in 1312, followed by John, in 1316, so Odinet's list dates from the four-year gap between the births of the royal couple's first two (documented) children. While this list of medicines for the queen has been studied before, it has not been seriously considered in the context of royal fertility medicine. The first transcriber of the list, G. E. Trease, suggests off-handedly that Isabella had a miscarriage in November 1313 but does not explain the reason for this observation.[16] Jeffrey Hamilton published the list in his chapter on royal medicine but admits to using it mostly for comparison with the ingredients contained in another, unrelated apothecary list.[17] Hamilton remarks that Trease was mistaken about a miscarriage in 1313 and reads the ingredients on the list as remedies for sleep and treatment for burns that Isabella received from a fire in the spring of

14 Printed in Trease, "Spicers and Apothecaries of the Royal Household," 46 (Document J); also printed in Hamilton, "Some Notes on Royal Medicine," Appendix I.

15 Hamilton, "Some Notes on Royal Medicine," 36–37; Woolgar, *The Senses*, 243. Weir, *Isabella, She-Wolf of France, Queen of England*, 112–13.

16 Trease, "Spicers and Apothecaries of the Royal Household," 46n184.

17 Hamilton, "Some Notes on Royal Medicine," 37n34.

1313.[18] However, the following analysis contends that the queen suffered a miscarriage or stillbirth at the end of 1313 because the ingredients supplied by her apothecary were common substances in reproductive medicine.

Isabella does seem to have suffered burns in early 1313, but the timing does not match up with Odinet's supply of medicinal ingredients for the queen in November of that year. A French chronicle, *Chronique de St. John Victor*, reports that one night, while Isabella and Edward II were in Paris in the spring of 1313, "the wardrobe of the king of England caught fire, much of the furniture was ruined, and the king and queen fled in nothing but their undershirts."[19] The event is not mentioned by English chroniclers and the *Chronique de St. John Victor* says no more about it.[20] Apparently though, Edward rescued Isabella from the fire and her arm was burned when she was trying to save some of her belongings.[21] Hamilton claims that she was still suffering from this injury in November 1313 when she was prescribed treatment by her apothecary, Odinet.[22] He also claims that "her condition rendered her unable to attend the Paris *parlement* and it is likely that she continued to have skin problems related to these burns for the rest of her life."[23] This interpretation needs reconsideration; the time between Isabella's injury and Odinet's provision of medicines was about five months.[24] Second-degree burns generally heal in weeks, and third-degree burns would at least have significantly improved by the autumn of 1313.[25] It also seems

18 Hamilton, "Some Notes on Royal Medicine," 36–37.

19 "Chronique John St. Victor," ed. Bourquet, 21:657: "Sed quadam nocte, ignis in gardaroba regis Angliae est accensus, et multam supellectilem perdiderunt rex et regina, nudique in camisiis de incendio aufugerunt."

20 I have found no mention in any English chronicles, and Hamilton does not cite any other sources.

21 *Chronique métrique de Godefroy de Paris*, ed. Buchon, 196–97.

22 Hamilton, "Some Notes on Royal Medicine," 36. Initial treatment for the burns: TNA E101/375/9, fols. 22r–v, 24r–v.

23 Hamilton, "Some Notes on Royal Medicine," 36, cites *Foedera*, ed. Rymer, 2.1:238. Hamilton also cites London, BL, Cotton MS Galba E XIV, fol. 42, which contains a payment to apothecary Nicholas Thomasyn in 1358 for "various spices and unguents and diverse medicaments for the dowager queen's body." He interprets this as evidence that Isabella received care for her burns for the rest of her life. Perhaps she did, but this order from Thomasyn seems much more likely to be related to the preparations of Isabella's body for burial when she died in 1358. The list itself specifies "for the dowager queen's body," which is strange phrasing if she was living.

24 June to November 1313.

25 Classified medically as "partial-thickness burns," second-degree burns typically

strange that even a partially healed arm injury would have prevented the queen from sitting in on the November *parlement*, particularly given that she and Edward II were in Paris for diplomatic reasons. Plasters and ointments would have been supplied initially to help with the healing, but there is no specific evidence to connect the burn injuries from early 1313 with the November apothecary list.

To properly interpret the herbal substances that Odinet supplied for Isabella, we must understand the humoral framework that guided medieval medical practice. Medieval physicians, following Hippocratic tradition, believed that health depended on balancing four vital fluids or "humours"—blood, phlegm, black bile, and yellow bile—each associated with specific qualities of heat, cold, wetness, and dryness.[26] Additionally, individuals had a unique complexional makeup determined by their particular humoral proportions: sanguine (hot and moist), phlegmatic (cold and moist), choleric (hot and dry), or melancholic (cold and dry). Illness arose when these humours fell out of balance or one became excessive, disrupting the body's natural equilibrium. Generally, physicians preserved health and treated illness by regulating the six non-naturals—external and behavioural factors including air, food and drink, exercise and rest, sleep and wakefulness, secretion and excretion, and emotions—to maintain or restore complexional balance. Physicians diagnosed patients by examining symptoms, urine, pulse, and physical characteristics, and treatments for illness included methods like bloodletting, purging, dietary changes, and herbal remedies to restore balance.[27]

---

heal in two-three weeks, with minimal scarring and a full return of function. Healing time of "deep-layer," or third-degree burns depends on how far it extends into the muscles, perhaps even down to the bone. Generally, healing takes three weeks up to two months, usually leaving scars. Fourth-degree burns, burns that extend to the bone (when all skin, subcutaneous fat and muscle layers are burned), will not heal on their own and require skin grafts. It seems unlikely that the tent fire would have caused such significant burns to Isabella's arm; if it had, it is strange that such life-changing injury was not mentioned by any English chroniclers and only received passing comment from a French chronicler. Problems with infection could have occurred while any thickness burn healed, but if Isabella's arm was still infected five months after she received the injury, it seems unlikely that she would have survived without antibiotics. For a medical overview of burns, see Tintinalli et al., *Tintinalli's Emergency Medicine*, 1400.

26 Nutton, "Medicine in the Greek World," 23–30; Nutton, "Medieval Western Europe," 141; O'Boyle, *Art of Medicine*, 85.

27 Getz, *Medicine in the English Middle Ages*, 85; Rawcliffe, *Medicine and Society in Later Medieval England*, 32–36.

Table 2. Medicines for Queen Isabella, November 1313.
Source: TNA E101/375/11, printed in Hamilton, "Royal Medicine," 39–40.

Odinet's List	English Translation
demi lb de pewle	½ lb pennyroyal
i li de mastiz	1 lb mastic
ii li de diquilon	2 lb lead plaster
demi li de diaute	½ lb *dialthea*[28]
ii li de eurose	2 lb rose water
demi li de populion	½ lb poplar bud ointment
camamille	chamomile
Milelott	melilots
Sauge	sage
Mauves	wild mallow
guimmaubes	marshmallow
volveus	convolvulus
calamenti	calamint
Poveri miauti	Perhaps *Teucrium polium*[29]
i li de diaqulon	1 lb lead plaster
i li de diaute	1 lb *dialthea*
ii li de eurose	2 lb rose water
i li de populion	1 lb poplar bud ointment
demi li de tamarinde	½ lb tamarind
i quartier de casafiscul	¼ [lb] cassiafistula
Roses et camamille	roses and chamomile
ceue	hemlock
reysuns	raisins
i li doile rosat	1 lb rose oil
i li de ceruse	1 lb white lead
i li d'ensens	1 lb incense: frankincense or olibanum
i li de litarge	1 lb lead oxide

28 *Trotula*, 194–95: "dialthea" (also spelled "dialtea) was made from marshmallow root, linseed, fenugreek, and several binding agents, like Greek tar and resin.

29 Trease, "Spicers and Apothecaries," 46 suggests *Teucrium polium*. Perhaps "mountain germander," see *Trotula*, 287.

Odinet's List	English Translation
demi li de sire verge	½ lb virgin beeswax
v maneres de erbes	5 kinds of herbs
xii boistes de plusur de maneres	12 boxes of other kinds [of herbs]
ii unce de mastic	2 oz mastic
i unce de boile armeniche	1 oz *Armenian bole*[30]
vi maneres derbes	6 kinds of herbs
Oile roast et violet et camomille	rose, violet and camomile oils
ii li de eurose	2 lb rose water
i li de sire verge	1 lb beeswax
Let de femmes a plusour fois	breastmilk
Plusur maneres derbes	more herbs
vii maneres de erbes	7 kinds of herbs
Oile rosat	rose oil
Fleur de fewes et pour fluer de orge	bean flour and barley flour

Medieval, university-trained physicians drew upon a core set of learned medical texts that provide the crucial context for understanding Odinet's prescriptions. Medical education at medieval universities (particularly at Paris and Montpellier) was based on five or six core texts compiled in the twelfth century (the compendium was known as *Ars medicinae* or *Articella*) and augmented with several newer texts in the thirteenth century.[31] Two key additions in the thirteenth century were Platearius's *Liber simplicibus medicine* (it became known by its incipit, *Circa instans*) and the *Antidotarium Nicholai*, both practical pharmacological works compiled in twelfth-century Salerno.[32] The *Circa instans* lists herbs with descriptions of their degrees of heat/coldness and wetness/dryness, indicating their ability to treat humoral imbalances, while the *Antidotarium* served as a pharmacopoeia of common medicinal ingredients and became the most popular text of its kind from the twelfth to sixteenth centuries.[33]

Alongside these texts, the *Trotula* ensemble—comprising the *Liber de sinthomatibus mulierum*, *De curis mulierum*, and *De ornatu mulierum*—formed

30 Green describes Armenian bole as a "kind of medicinal earth," *Trotula*, 274.

31 O'Boyle, *The Art of Medicine*, 105–7.

32 O'Boyle, *The Art of Medicine*, 106, 108–11.

33 O'Boyle, *The Art of Medicine*, 106, 111.

the point of reference for women's medicine from at least the thirteenth century.[34] The three books in the *Trotula* were likely compiled in twelfth-century Salerno and, although never formally part of the medical curriculum at medieval universities, were frequently used alongside the foundational texts of medicine which were taught in the academic curriculum.[35] The *Liber de sinthomatibus mulierum* and *De curis mulierum* are the two gynaecological texts in the compendium, while the *De ornatu mulierum* is concerned with cosmetic recipes.[36] As royal physicians were almost exclusively university-trained, the *Trotula* likely defined their understanding of women's medicine.

Against this backdrop of medieval medical knowledge and foundational texts, the ingredients on Odinet's list (Table 2) suggest that Isabella had a miscarriage or stillbirth in late 1313.[37] The nature of herbal therapy in humoral medicine did mean that an herb—sage for example—could be taken for various and unrelated problems, and the inclusion of a single substance on a list of medicines does not necessarily indicate treatment for miscarriage. However, the inclusion of multiple substances which were commonly used in reproductive remedies suggests that Isabella was prescribed them following a miscarriage or stillbirth, given the similar approach and multi-faceted application of ingredients for managing these events. A pregnancy loss also fits in the timeline of the births of Isabella and Edward's children. There is a four-year gap between the birth of the couple's first child in 1312, and their second in 1316, while their third and fourth children were born in *slightly* quicker succession, in 1318 and then 1321.[38] The gaps between births might reflect a rhythm of conception and pregnancy without loss, but the four-year break between 1312–1316 at least gives space to suggest that Isabella had an unsuccessful pregnancy in late 1313. Recovery from a miscarriage or stillbirth would also explain Isabella's absence from the November *parlement*.

---

34 *The Trotula*, ed. Green, 2–3, 17–48; Green, *Making Women's Medicine Masculine*, 75.

35 Green, *Making Women's Medicine Masculine*, 75–76.

36 Green describes *De curis mulierum* as the "less bookish" of the two gynaecological works in the *Trotula,* and its primary focus seems to be promotion of fertility: *Trotula*, ed. Green, 39–41.

37 Geaman, "Anne of Bohemia and Her Struggle to Conceive," 232–33: Geaman applies a similar approach in her analysis of an apothecary list for Anne of Bohemia who was struggling to conceive. She argues that these herbs are an indication that Anne was actively employing medical therapies to aid conception because several of the herbs on the list were commonly used to promote fertility and aid conception.

38 Isabella and Edward had also spent most of the spring and summer of 1313 together, so the possibility that Isabella was pregnant by late 1313 is reasonable. For Isabella's itinerary in 1313, see Warner, *Isabella of France*, 77–81.

There are two items on Odinet's list which were specialized ingredients in fertility medicine. The first is pennyroyal; from the mint family, pennyroyal was a potent emmenagogue and common element in multiple remedies for fertility problems.[39] According to the *Circa instans*, pennyroyal's natural quality was warmth in the third degree and so it could be used to combat excessive complexional coldness and dryness (enough moisture and heat were considered the necessary complexional characteristics for fertility).[40] The *Antidotarium Nicholai* specifies that pennyroyal could be used for expelling dead fetuses and retained placentas.[41] Pennyroyal also features extensively in treatments for fertility-related issues in two of the *Trotula* texts: in the *Liber de sinthomatibus mulierum* it is prescribed for retention of the menses, and menstruation was understood to be fundamental to fertility.[42] It is mentioned three more times in the *Liber de sinthomatibus mulierum*, all for conditions related to fertility: twice for treating "paucity of the menses" and also in a remedy for "sterility on the part of the man."[43] In *De curis mulierum*, the text in the Trotula which is predominantly focused on encouraging fertility, pennyroyal is mentioned twenty-one times, all in remedies related to fertility, pregnancy and childbirth, with the exception of a treatment for strangury (retained urine).[44] *De curis mulierum* prescribes pennyroyal for menstruation problems, vaginal lesions, constriction, and swelling, as well as for pain in the womb, "exit of the womb after birth" and for pain after birth.[45] Pennyroyal is also listed as an ingredient for aiding conception in the text: it could be added to a bath with several other herbs to help a woman conceive, particularly if she was

---

39 It is a known emmenagogue, or a substance which stimulates menstrual flow and can cause an abortion if consumed during pregnancy. See Romm, "Pregnancy and Botanical Medicine: Use and Safety," 323–24.

40 Matthaeus Platearius, *Liber de simplici medicina* (1512), 23, under "Caput XVI: 'Pulelgium'"; Bernard of Gordon, *Practica seu Lilium medicinae* (image 362).

41 *Incipit antidotarium Nicholai* (1471), fol. 12v.

42 *Liber de Sinthomatibus mulierum*, section 14 (*Trotula*, 76–77). For medieval thought about the necessity of menstruation for fertility: Cadden, *The Meanings of Sex Difference*, 173; *Trotula*, 40.

43 *De curis mulierum*, sections 14, 19, 21, 131 (*Trotula*, 77–79; 114–15).

44 *De curis mulierum*, section 157 (*Trotula*, 131): "Strangury." See n29 above: Green discusses how the conditions and remedies in *De curis mulierum* are primarily concerned with promoting fertility.

45 *De curis mulierum*, sections 136, 161, 190, 196, 206, 209, 214, 227, 229 (*Trotula*, 118–19, 132–33, 144–45, 146–47, 150–51, 152–53, 156–57, 158–59, 160–61).

"phlegmatic and fat."[46] The inclusion (and primary position) of pennyroyal on Odinet's list is significant because of its centrality in fertility medicine in *Liber de sinthomatibus mulierum* and *De curis mulierum,* the first two texts of the *Trotula*—the foremost medieval compendium for women's reproductive medicine.[47] Although impossible to know for certain, Isabella might even have been prescribed the herb to help her conceive again, after a miscarriage.

Isabella was also supplied with "let de femmes a plusour fois," or breastmilk, by Odinet. Hamilton supposed that it was the breastmilk on the list which led to Trease's conclusion that Isabella had a miscarriage in late 1313. He disagrees with Trease and links the "let de femmes" to a remedy for sleep called "God's Grace," a mixture of breastmilk and poppies advertised as "good for the arms."[48] However, Hamilton's source is a fifteenth-century recipe that has no particular connection to Isabella or her medical practitioners. Even with the versatility of ingredients in medieval medicine, Hamilton's explanation is unconvincing, particularly as there is no reference to poppies on Odinet's list.[49] Instead, breastmilk had several medicinal uses in remedies for fertility problems: it is mentioned in the *Liber de sinthomatibus mulierum* for treating excessive heat of the womb (too much heat caused sterility), lesions of the womb, and for healing an "ulcerated womb" after miscarriage.[50] It could also be used as a remedy for difficult birth, especially for delivering a dead fetus.[51] The inclusion of pennyroyal, a powerful emmenagogue, and breastmilk, both common ingredients recommended in medieval medical remedies for reproductive problems, strengthens the hypothesis that Isabella had a miscarriage or stillbirth in late 1313.

---

46 *De curis mulierum*, section 142 (*Trotula*, 121).

47 Pennyroyal is not mentioned in *De ornatu mulierum* which contains cosmetic recipes for women and was usually the third text bound in the *Trotula*.

48 Hamilton, "Some Notes on Royal Medicine," 37. Hamilton's dismissal of the miscarriage seems to come from a misinterpretation of the medicinal uses for the ingredients on the list. He thinks that Trease's suggestion of miscarriage was because of the inclusion of breastmilk, but it makes more sense that Trease was at least referring to the pennyroyal too. On the medicinal use of breastmilk, see Buck, "Woman's Milk," 467–85, esp. 478.

49 Warner, *Isabella of France*, 79, also suggests that Isabella perhaps had a miscarriage in November 1313 because of the inclusion of pennyroyal on the list.

50 *Liber de sinthomatibus mulierum*, sections 64, 65,70 (*Trotula*, 88–89, 90–91, 92–93).

51 *Liber de sinthomatibus mulierum*, sections 64, 68, 70, 91, 100 (*Trotula*, 88–93, 100–103).

There are several other herbs on Odinet's list which were used in remedies for fertility problems. For instance, sage is recommended in *De curis mulierum,* among other ingredients, in a remedy for staunching excessive flow of blood after giving birth;[52] or to provoke the menses.[53] Another popular thirteenth-century herbal that was also frequently bound with copies of the *Ars medicinae, De viribus herbarum* (attributed to Macer), advises that sage could be used to provoke the menses and expel a dead fetus.[54] *Cassia fistula,* also on the list, was believed to help balance menstrual flow and expel a dead fetus from the womb.[55]

Admittedly, herbal substances had diverse applications in medieval medicine—for instance, "sage" is an ingredient in a compound medicine for treating cancer in *De curis mulierum*.[56] Here, it is significant that common ingredients like sage are listed together with the more specialized substances like pennyroyal and breastmilk. Many of the more generic ingredients on the list are also found clustered together or combined with specialized ingredients in fertility remedies. For instance, an oil, powdered frankincense and mastic (all on Odinet's list) could be mixed together to help prevent a miscarriage according to *De curis mulierum*.[57] Marshmallow was a remedy for swelling of the vagina and to ease pain after a miscarriage when combined with pennyroyal, while in a concoction with barley flour, also on the list, it helped to provoke the menses.[58] Marshmallow mixed with melilots, among other ingredients, helped with "lesions of the womb," too.[59] This remedy is mentioned in the same chapter of the *Liber sinthomatibus*

52 *De curis mulierum*, secion 147 (*Trotula*, 124–25). However, sage is also prescribed in *De curis mulierum* as an ingredient for treating cancer (*Trotula*, 143) and particularly cancer of the nose (*Trotula*, 151).

53 *De curis mulierum*, section 216 (*Trotula*, 153).

54 Macer Floridus, *De viribus herbarum*, 64: "XXIV: Salvia." O'Boyle, *The Art of Medicine*, 106.

55 *Incipit antidotarium Nicholai* (1471), fol. 3r.

56 *De curis mulierum*, section 183 (*Trotula*, 143).

57 *De curis mulierum*, section 233 (*Trotula*, 161).

58 *De curis mulierum*, section 135 (provoking menses), 196 (swelling), 255 (pain of the womb), (*Trotula*, 117–19, 147, 157). Marshmallow is an ingredient in several other fertility-related remedies: *De curis mulierum*, sections 154, 214, 225 (*Trotula*, 129, 153, 157). Marshmallow is also recommended in *Liber de sinthomatibus mulierum*, section 115, for a difficult birth (*Trotula*, 105). "Wild mallow," also on Odinet's list, is an ingredient used as a remedy for impeded conception: *Liber de sinthomatibus mulierum*, section 129 (*Trotula*, 114).

59 *De curis mulierum*, section 66 (*Trotula*, 91).

mulierum which recommends breastmilk and rose oil as a remedy for treating lesions of the womb.

A contemporary practical medical text supports this interpretation of Odinet's list as fertility medicine. A mid-thirteenth century *regimen* written by Aldobrandino of Siena for Eleanor of Provence's mother, Beatrice of Savoy, recommends that to ease childbirth a woman could "bathe every day in mallows, violets, linseed, fenugreek, barley, and chamomile" and, once out of the bath, she should anoint her genitals with chicken fats, butter, chamomile oil and *dialthea*—a compound medicine made from marshmallow.[60] Chamomile oil and *dialthea* are on the list from Odinet, as well as mallow, chamomile and barley flour. The inclusion of multiple substances used in reproductive medicine, notably in remedies for expelling a dead fetus and easing pain during birth, strengthens the suggestion that Isabella was receiving medical care relating to a miscarriage or stillbirth in November 1313.[61]

Additionally, Odinet's list reflects how kings and queens experienced fertility medicine differently. The nature of male and female reproductive roles and the reality of reproductive labour is represented in the focus on the queen's body in medical treatment for fertility problems. Reproduction involved much more than successfully conceiving a child for a queen, as she might face problems during pregnancy, labour or post-partum and need medical care. In particular, a significant and gendered part of reproductive medicine is the management of miscarriages. Reproductive medicine for kings was about seeking and promoting conception, but queens might need treatment for conditions after conception happened; indeed, during labour, after giving birth or having a miscarriage or stillbirth.

---

60 Wallis, *Medieval Medicine*, 494. Green describes *dialthea* (or *dialtea*) as a compound substance that was used to produce heat: *Trotula*, 194–95.

61 Other substances on the list were also used for fertility-related remedies. *Liber de sinthomatibus mulierum,* section 33 (*Trotula*, 82) prescribes Armenian bole to help with excessive flux of the menses. Section 70 (*Trotula*, 94), for ulcers of the womb. *De Ornatu mulierum*, sections 307 and 308 (*Trotula*, 189), to cause vaginal constriction, to make it seem like a woman was still a virgin, and to staunch blood flow, either menstrual or from the nose. Hemlock is also given as a remedy for retention of the menses, *Liber de sinthomatibus mulierum*, section 16 (*Trotula*, 77). Other substances on the list, like rose water and beeswax were common substances used as fillers and binding agents in herbal remedies. The oils like rose, violet and chamomile were used in humoral medicine because of their pleasant smell. For instance, *Liber de sinthomatibus mulierum*, section 48 (*Trotula*, 85) recommends that the vagina be anointed with oils that have sweet odours, like chamomile oil, to provoke the menses.

The Queen's Influence on Royal Medicine

The queen's role in royal healthcare was not limited to that of a passive patient. Scholars have shown how queens brought architectural, intellectual, and fashion trends from their natal homelands to their marital territories.[62] However, that this exchange also extended to cultures of medicine in royal courts has so far been missed.[63] As this section will show, queens brought practitioners with them to their new homes when they married, and subsequently continued to attract individuals and disseminate medical texts through their familial networks that stretched across Europe.

At least two of Eleanor of Provence's physicians were from Provence; when she arrived in England in 1236 she was probably accompanied by Peter de Alpibus, a physician from the mountainous region of Provence, indicated by the name "de Alpibus" ("of the Alps").[64] Peter was given a prebend in the chapel of Pontefract Castle by Henry III in 1241 and remained Eleanor's physician until the 1260s.[65] Eleanor was also cared for by William le Provençal.[66] He does not appear in sources for the first half of Eleanor's tenure, nor the years when the couple's five children were born, but William may have been what Charles Talbot and Eugene Hammond described as, "one of the numerous loyal servants whom the Queen had brought into England from her native land."[67] At least one other well-known royal practitioner may also have come from France. The origins of Eleanor's physician, Raymond de Bariamondo, are unclear but his name suggests that he was not originally

62 Crossley, "The Architecture of Queenship," 263–300; Bell, "Medieval Women Book Owners," 742–68; Hamilton and Proctor-Tiffany, eds., *Moving Women Moving Objects*.

63 Jennifer Borland's chapter on the transmission of *regimen* texts by royal and noble women has made a notable start: Borland, "Female Networks," 107–36. I am also currently working on an article about the transmission of royal healthcare and fertility medicine as a form of diplomacy between royal courts.

64 Talbot and Hammond, *Medical Practitioners*, 244. He is also called "Peter Provincialis" in *CPR 1232–1247*, 255. "Pierre d'Alps" in Wickersheimer, *Dictionnaire biographique*, 2:611. Wickersheimer does not mention the connection to Eleanor, but notes that Peter witnessed a charter of Raymond Berenger, Count of Provence, who was Eleanor's father.

65 Talbot and Hammond, *Medical Practitioners*, 244.

66 *CPR 1247–1258*, 376. Talbot and Hammond, *Medical Practitioners*, 411. William also served Henry III as clerk in Gascony in the 1250s: Talbot and Hammond, *Medical Practitioners*, 411; *Rôles gascons*, ed. Michel, 1:542, 543, 548.

67 Talbot and Hammond, *Medical Practitioners*, 411.

from England.[68] Furthermore, the apothecary Robert of Montpellier was one of Henry and Eleanor's most frequently used and well-known apothecaries and Leslie Matthews suggests that Robert also came from Provence with Eleanor.[69] Matthews argues that Robert must have come highly recommended by Eleanor's father, Raymond Berenger IV, Count of Provence, as he was taken on as Henry III's "speciarius."[70] All four practitioners' names appear in the administrative rolls over extended periods of time, suggesting continued trust and closeness to the king and queen. Not all of their medical practitioners had Provençal connections certainly, and Henry III and Eleanor had several long-serving and trusted medical practitioners such as Reginald of Bath and Ralph de Neketon who were English, but the preference for Provençal physicians in Eleanor's household is significant because these were the practitioners close to the queen who would also have managed her multiple childbirths and any concerns about fertility.

Isabella of France also had medical practitioners from her homeland. The most cited and well-known of the physicians who cared for Isabella throughout her marriage was Theobald de Troyes. Also called "Thibaud Rotarii de Lanis" by Ernest Wickersheimer in a register of French medical practitioners, Theobald was a clerk in the diocese of Langres, close to Troyes, before joining Isabella's household.[71] There is no indication of where Theobald trained in medicine but, given his connection to Troyes, it may have been in nearby Paris (where he later taught).[72] Theobald was first paid for his service to Isabella in 1310 and he was with her in Paris in 1313, when the tent fire occurred.[73] He was still employed when she travelled to Paris once again

68 At the end of his royal career, Raymond was granted the same prebend of the chapel in Pontefract Castle that had previously been held by Peter de Alpibus when he retired as Eleanor's physician: Talbot and Hammond, *Medical Practitioners*, 267. He was granted rewards for his service by Henry III from the mid-1250s to mid-1260s: *CCR* (1256–1259), 72, 249; *CCR* (1259–1261), 95; *CCR* (1261–1264), 53; *CLR*, 5:19. Talbot and Hammond, *Medical Practitioners*, 267.

69 Matthews, *The Royal Apothecaries*, 7–10: Several generations of the Montpellier family seem to have served as royal apothecaries.

70 "Spicer," or apothecary. Matthews, *Royal Apothecaries*, 7–10. *Rôles gascons*, ed. Michel, 1:223, no. 1670. Henry even paid the expenses of Robert and his wife when they came to England.

71 Wickersheimer, *Dictionnaire biographique*, 2:752.

72 O'Boyle, *The Art of Medicine*, 72, makes the point that people generally attended the university closest to where they were from.

73 He was paid 15*d.* a day in 1310. Hamilton, "Some Notes on Royal Medicine," 35–36: E101/374/5, fol. 32; (E404/483/10 nos. 7, 24; E101/375/9, fols. 33, 35, 37.

in 1324.[74] Theobald remained in Isabella's household at the start of Edward III's reign but seems to have ended his career teaching medicine at the University of Paris.[75] Isabella's apothecarist, Odinet, was also French, although not much is known about him. Matthews suggests that he was appointed as the queen's apothecarist when Isabella and Edward were in Paris in 1313.[76] Theobald and Odinet were specifically described as the queen's physician and apothecary and so both men would have managed reproductive medicine for the queen, including the suggested pregnancy loss in 1313.[77]

Other queens also had physicians with connections to their natal countries. Edward I specified that Nicholas of Menona was specifically Eleanor of Castile's physician, and Talbot and Hammond suggest that he came from Spain, perhaps when Eleanor married Edward in 1254.[78] Little is known about Nicholas but his nomenclature (of Menona) suggests he was not of English origins. He is not mentioned in sources before 1283 but there is little sign of Eleanor of Castile herself in sources for the first decades that she lived in England and so it is possible that Nicholas came to England with Eleanor in the 1250s.[79] A grant by the king for Nicholas also suggests that the physician had served the queen for some time, as it resembles Henry III's reward to two of Eleanor of Provence's long-serving Provençal physicians

---

74 Hamilton, "Some Notes on Royal Medicine," 35.

75 Wickersheimer, *Dictionnaire biographique*, 2:752.

76 Matthews, *Royal Apothecaries*, 24.

77 Hamilton, "Some Notes on Royal Medicine," 35, for references to Theobald and Odinet as the queen's practitioners: E101/375/9, fol. 22. When Isabella was in Paris in 1313 with Edward II, she was treated by Theobald de Troyes after the tent fire but also by Jean Pitard and Henri de Mondeville. Pitard was a well-respected surgeon of the French king Philippe (IV) le Bel, Isabella's father, and Henri de Mondeville had cared for King Philippe's children so he would have known and treated Isabella since her childhood. For Pitard and de Mondeville, see Wickersheimer, *Dictionnaire biographique*, 2:752. At that same time, Isabella was also attended by an English royal surgeon, Philip de Beauvais, and royal apothecary Peter of Montpellier: E101/375/11, E101/375/12. The desire (or perhaps need) for care from Pitard and de Mondeville possibly reflects the personal choice of Isabella because even though the English royal couple seems to have travelled in 1313 with a full medical staff, Isabella was primarily cared for by French practitioners who had known her since birth.

78 Talbot and Hammond, *Medical Practitioners*, 228: a letter by the king from 1283 specifies that Nicholas was the queen's physician.

79 I have not found any early references to him in the chancery rolls and Talbot and Hammond and Getz do not mention any sources.

at the end of their service to the queen.[80] After Eleanor of Castile died in 1290, Edward I's second queen, Margaret of France, was cared for by John of Fountains, mentioned earlier in relation to the letter he sent Edward I about Margaret's treatment for measles in 1305.[81] In addition to that care, it was probably John who attended the birth of the queen's daughter in 1306. Given that he was seemingly already a senior physician in the queen's household by 1305, John likely came from France with Margaret in 1299.[82] Margaret was also served by the physician Luke Matheu de Perrers who probably came from France with her too, as he returned there soon after Edward I's death in 1307.[83]

One of the English princesses who married into the Scottish royal house also preferred, at least initially, the care of English physicians. Reginald of Bath, who had been sent to Scotland by Eleanor of Provence, was trusted by young Queen Margaret when she confided in him about her unhappiness in Scotland and frustration at being kept from consummating her marriage to Alexander III. Then, when Margaret was pregnant with her first child in 1260, she and Alexander went to England to visit her parents. According to the *Flores historiarum*, she deceived the Scottish magnates about how soon the baby was due so, when it was time to return to Scotland, Margaret stayed behind in England and gave birth at Windsor (where she had grown up).[84] Although unusual, Margaret's plan to give birth in her childhood home, with her parents close by and attended by the medical practitioners who had probably known her since birth, emphasizes the close personal relationship between queens and their medical entourage, and the importance of the queen's trust and familiarity in the choice of royal practitioners.

Medical practitioners, knowledge and texts also circulated on the recommendations and connections of queens. Familial networks united the ruling dynasties of medieval Europe and the creation and maintenance of these

---

80 Talbot and Hammond, *Medical Practitioners*, 228: in 1283 Edward I sought Nicholas's appointment to a vacant church near Southampton, and in his letter the king specifies that Nicholas was the queen's physician. See Raymond de Bariamondo: *CCR* (1259–1261), 95. See discussion of Peter de Alpibus above.

81 Talbot and Hammond, *Medical Practitioners*, 145.

82 Talbot and Hammond, *Medical Practitioners*, 145n4. Wickersheimer, *Dictionnaire biographique*, 1:401, refers to him as "Jean de Fonte," a physician of Queen Margaret. Wickersheimer writes that Jean was canon of Rouen and rector of a church in the diocese of York (in 1309).

83 Hamilton, "Some Notes on Royal Medicine," 34.

84 Howell, *Eleanor of Provence*, 113; *Flores historiarum*, ed. Luard, 2:459–60, 461, 463.

connections by royal and elite women has been acknowledged by scholars.[85] A royal couple's connections to medical practitioners, access to texts and, ultimately, reproductive medicine was affected by these networks. There are two examples which suggest how these kinds of connections might have brought Henry III and Eleanor of Provence into contact with certain practitioners and texts. In 1235, Henry negotiated the marriage of his sister, Isabella of England, to Frederick II, the Holy Roman Emperor. Emperor Frederick sent his personal physician, Michael Scot, to England to meet and examine Isabella.[86] Scot had earned Frederick's attention in the late 1220s; before serving at Frederick's court, he had compiled a work on gynaecological diagnoses while working in Bologna. Scot seems to have studied medicine (possibly in Paris) before moving on to work in Bologna in the early 1220s, and then translating astrological texts at Toledo at the end of the decade. At the imperial court, he composed the *Liber physionomiae* for the emperor, part of his larger *Liber introductorius*, a broad introduction to astrology and his understanding of the relationship between the macrocosm and microcosm. The first three books of the *Liber physionomiae* deal with birth and generation.[87] Scot's writing was influential to later generations of scholars, inspiring parts of Vincent de Beauvais's *Speculum doctrinale* and Bartholomeus Anglicus's *De proprietatibus rerum*.[88] It is possible that through his sister Isabella, Henry III (and his royal physicians) came into contact with Scot and his work when he took part in the negotiations for Isabella's marriage in 1235.

Scot's connections to Toledo and Bologna are significant because both were medieval centres of transmission for Graeco-Latin and Arabic medical texts. Major texts by both Galen and Arabic authorities, like Avicenna and Rhazes, were translated by scholars like Gerard of Cremona in Toledo; this work not only supplied a new vocabulary for learned medicine, but it also brought Aristotelian and Arabic texts into the existing Galenic tradition.[89] The University of Bologna was also central in the development of learned medicine in the medieval world, and scholars working there were influenced by the translations produced in Spain to produce new works on medicine.[90]

---

85 Krause, "From Mothers to Daughters"; Brown, "Family Female Networking," 209–40.

86 Morpurgo, "Scot [Scott], Michael," *ODNB* [online]. Matthew Paris mentions the examination of Isabella: *Chronica majora*, ed. Luard, 3:319.

87 See Morpurgo, "Scot [Scott], Michael," *ODNB* [online].

88 Morpurgo, "Scot [Scott], Michael," *ODNB* [online].

89 Nutton, "Medieval Western Europe," 143.

90 Nutton, "Medieval Western Europe," 144.

Connecting physicians like Scot to these centres of medical learning shows that Henry III and Eleanor of Provence were in contact with physicians who were versed in the best texts and medical knowledge of their time.[91]

Eleanor and Henry's sisters also had common ties to another physician in the mid-1230s. A physician and Dominican friar, John of St. Giles, was at Henry III's court in 1236, sent as a messenger by Henry's sister, Isabella, the Holy Roman Empress. John was probably English, or at least likely studied at Oxford, before earning his Masters of Theology in Paris in 1228.[92] He joined Isabella of England's retinue at the time of her marriage to Frederick II and Matthew Paris notes that it was John who delivered the news of Isabella's pregnancy to her brother, Henry III, in 1237.[93] From this point, John of St. Giles was also linked to Henry III's other sister, Joan, queen of Scotland and wife of Alexander II: Joan was in England from 1237 and John was described as the executor of Joan's estate when she died there in 1238.[94] Finally, a thirteenth-century manuscript contains a set of recipes attributed to Ralph de Neketon, Patrick of Carlisle and "Johannis de Sancto Egidio," or John of St. Giles, which suggests a connection between John of St. Giles and medical practitioners at the English royal court.[95] Both Ralph de Neketon and Patrick of Carlisle were well-known and long-serving physicians of Henry and Eleanor, so the inclusion of John's name in the recipe collection suggests that he was operating in the same circle as their senior royal physicians.

Furthermore, Empress Isabella and queens Joan and Eleanor can all be linked to John of St. Giles, at important moments in relation to their

91 One of Henry and Eleanor's most well-known physicians in the first decades of their marriage, Nicholas of Farnham (entrusted by Henry III to oversee Eleanor's wellbeing when she arrived in England in 1236) probably studied medicine in Paris (like Scot) and by the 1220s was also in Bologna, teaching medicine. By the end of the decade, Nicholas was referred to as Henry III's physician. It is possible that Nicholas and Scot knew each other, or at least knew *of* each other from their overlapping time in Bologna. It is also possible that Nicholas knew of Scot's text on gynaecology, as Scot produced it during his time in Bologna. See Franklin, "Farnham, Nicholas of," *ODNB* [online]; Talbot and Hammond, *Medical Practitioners*, 223.

92 Morpurgo, "Scot [Scott], Michael," *ODNB* [online].

93 Jacquart, "St. Giles, John," *ODNB* [online]. Paris describes John of St. Giles as a physician in his chronicle, but not as a royal physician. This does not indicate that John did not serve Henry, Eleanor, Isabella, or Joan in a medical capacity though (see discussion below about Hector Beaton who was described as David II's clerk in 1352).

94 *CLR*, 1:318 (1238).

95 Cambridge, Peterhouse, MS 222, fols. 10v–11v.

respective fertility. It was John of St. Giles who was trusted to deliver the news of Isabella's first pregnancy to the English court. And when he arrived in England in 1236, both Eleanor of Provence and Queen Joan were childless and about to embark on pilgrimage together to Canterbury, perhaps hoping to remedy their childlessness.[96] This timing also coincides with Matthew Paris's report of fear about Eleanor of Provence's fertility. Thus, John of St. Giles was connected to all three women at pivotal moments for each queen's management of fertility: Isabella was pregnant with her first child, and Eleanor and Joan were seeking remedies for childlessness on pilgrimage.

The queens' connections to John of St. Giles suggest that the trust that was fostered in familial networks, particularly between royal female family members, facilitated contact with, and exchange of, medical practitioners; in this case, ties to a physician, John of St. Giles, who wrote texts on female physiology, birth and reproduction. This highlights how familial connections influenced the reproductive medicine available to royal couples.

Medical texts also circulated through family networks and passed between royal women. Eleanor of Provence can be connected to a *regimen sanitatis* text written by a French physician who served her parents. Aldobrandino of Siena was a physician at the court of Raymond Berenguer IV, count of Provence and Eleanor's father.[97] Sometime before 1257, Aldobrandino composed his *Régime du corps*, a health regimen manual written in French.[98] One surviving version of the text contains a prologue which declares that Aldobrandino was asked to write the text by Beatrice of Savoy, Eleanor's mother, for her upcoming visit to see her four daughters in 1256.[99]

96 There is an order (*CLR*, 1:291) for "good horses" to be found for "Brother John de Sancto Egidio" (John of St. Giles) so that he could meet Henry III at York in 1237. This was perhaps when Henry and Eleanor visited York in 1237 to meet with Alexander II and Joan. The two queens left for pilgrimage to Canterbury after this meeting and so this order shows that not only was John of St. Giles in contact with Henry III, but he was specifically requested at a meeting where both royal couples were present and when Eleanor and Joan perhaps went to Canterbury to seek remedies for childlessness. The pilgrimage to Canterbury will be discussed in Chapter 6.

97 University of Padua department of Linguistic and Literary Studies database: https://www.rialfri.eu/rialfriWP/autori/aldobrandino-da-siena. Wickersheimer, *Dictionnaire biographique*, 1:117–18.

98 Green, "The Possibilities of Literacy and the Limits of Reading," 63.

99 Paris, Bibliothèque nationale de France, MS fr. 2021. Another manuscript attributes the original ownership to Blanche of Castile, mother of Louis IX of France. Yet another copy cites Louis IX as the original patron/owner, while two other versions in the Bodleian and Vatican libraries state that the text was translated in 1234 at the request of Frederick II, Holy Roman Emperor. Monica Green believes that

Eleanor was queen of England, her sister Marguerite was queen of France, Sanchia (married to Henry III's brother, Richard) was countess of Cornwall and then queen of Germany, and Beatrice was countess of Anjou and queen of Sicily.[100] According to the manuscript copy held in the Bibliothèque nationale de France, at this momentous meeting Beatrice presented each of her adult daughters with a copy of the *regimen* by Aldobrandino.[101] In a letter sent from the physician to Beatrice of Savoy in 1256, Aldobrandino mentions that the countess commissioned the text "because he could not go with her [to meet her daughters], because she did not want him to leave the merchants from beyond the Alps who he was taking care of, and she was more attached to him than to any other. So she had him make this book to take it with her and keep it."[102] This is another indication of the close personal relationships between royal women and their physicians, and the familial networks that facilitated the sharing of medical knowledge, in this case, dissemination of a *regimen* text to the reigning couples of England, France, Germany, and Anjou.

Eleanor of Provence's connection to Aldobrandino of Siena's *Régime du corps* also gives some insight into the nature of contemporary medical theory and practical medicine available in Henry III and Eleanor's households. The connection suggests that queens did not only have sway over the choice of practitioners, but they also played an important role in the royal couple's access to medical knowledge. *Regimina* were, by their nature, intended for practical and personal use by a patient and were often written by physicians for specific individuals, as Aldobrandino did. *Regimina* deal with preventative medicine rather than treatments for specific conditions and ailments.[103] Aldobrandino's text explains how to maintain and restore health in the body,

---

the text was composed for Beatrice of Savoy, as does Wickersheimer. Green, "The Possibilities of Literacy," 63; Wickersheimer, *Dictionnaire biographique*, 1:17–18.

100 Howell, *Eleanor of Provence*, 3–12.

101 University of Padua department of Linguistic and Literary Studies database: https://www.rialfri.eu/rialfriWP/autori/aldobrandino-da-siena. For the dissemination of this text through the female network of Beatrice's four daughters, see Borland, "Female Networks," 107–36.

102 The text and translation of Aldobrandino's letter to Beatrice are available online. "A Letter From Aldobrandino of Siena (1256)," https://epistolae.ctl.columbia.edu/letter/501.html: "li fist cest livre por che k'il ne pooit aler avoec li, car ele ne vaut mie k'il laissast les marcheans d'outre les mons k'il avoit en cure, et ele tenoit plus de lui ke d'un autre. Si li fist faire che livre por porter avoec li et por garder."

103 Braekman, *Studies on Alchemy, Diet, Medecine [sic] and Prognostication in Middle English*, 58–60.

as well as including some discussion about peak physical ages and advice for childbearing. Some of these ideas, particularly the significance of age on bodily composition and health, are visible in the evidence of Henry III's approach to health and fertility. As such, it is possible to see the origins of some of the couple's understanding of fertility and relevant medical remedies in Aldobrandino's text, and thus the active role that Queen Eleanor played in disseminating this knowledge.

There is no reason to think that Aldobrandino of Siena's *Régime du Corps* was exclusively intended for the queen and not useful for Henry III also. The contents of the text are quite typical for a *regimen*.[104] *Regimina* texts were practical manuals that applied humoral theory to everyday health management, focusing on the six non-naturals (air, food and drink, exercise and rest, sleep and wakefulness, secretion and excretion, and emotions).[105] Aldobrandino's text has two chapters in Book I that deal with pregnancy, childbirth, and caring for an infant as part of the management of the non-naturals for bodily balance. The work is not directed specifically to a female reader, though; the second book covers how to care for parts of the body, like arms, eyes, and so on. The third is a guide to the humoral composition and uses of common foods substances and their medicinal effect on the body's humoral balance.[106] The final book of Aldobrandino's *regimen* is a guide to knowing the nature and complexion of a man (homme) from his outward appearance.[107] This might have been read more abstractly as "how to know a person's complexion and nature from appearance," but there certainly is no focus on women nor on the female body.[108] This makes Aldobrandino's *regimen* seem not just a book of practical medical advice for Eleanor of Provence herself, but a text that also was applicable to Henry III. This is an important detail because it indicates that a queen like Eleanor of Provence was not only active in managing her own medical care; it was through her that

104 Sotres, "The Regimens of Health," 291–318.

105 Sotres, "The Regimens of Health"; Getz, *Medicine in the English Middle Ages*, 85; Rawcliffe, *Medicine and Society in Later Medieval England*, 32–36.

106 *Le régime du corps* , eds. Landouzy and Pépin, bk. 3, p. 110.

107 *Le régime du corps*, 193: "C'est li commencemens comment on puet connoistre le nature de cascun homme par dehors, et se complexion."

108 In his letter to Beatrice of Savoy, Aldobrandino of Siena says that the fourth book covers the nature of men and women (*l'oume et le femme*), but the printed edition of the dietary by Landouzy and Pépin does not include women in this section: "A Letter From Aldobrandino of Siena (1256)," https://epistolae.ctl.columbia.edu/letter/501.html.

the king was introduced to particular texts, medical thought and practical approaches to healthcare.[109]

It is impossible to tell how closely Eleanor and Henry might have structured their lifestyle around recommendations about diet, bathing and bloodletting from *regimina* like *Le régime du corps*, but Aldobrandino's description of the body at different stages of life does align with Henry III's change in behaviour when he reached his thirties.[110] In Book I of Aldobrandino's text, he explains how to care for the body and includes a chapter on the different life stages.[111] He describes four (male) life stages between adolescence and death: *adolescentia, juventus, senectus, senium*. In the first, *adolescentia*, the body was complexionally warm and moist, defined by growth which lasted until age twenty-five or thirty.[112] The *juventus* body was warm and dry, seemingly defined by its peak physical condition (vigorous and strong), and lasted until age forty or forty-five.[113] In the last two stages, the body descended into a cold and dry state before becoming cold and moist in *senium*, which ended with death.[114] It could not have been specifically Aldobrandino's discussion that influenced Henry in the 1230s, but it is a sample of the kind of medical thought which the royal couple engaged with.

The humoral characteristics of the life stages that Aldobrandino discussed relate to contemporary theories about infertility too. Another thirteenth-century physician and author, Bernard of Gordon, describes "fecundity" as a combination of "warmth, windiness and moisture" and "so a deficiency causes sterility."[115] According to this theory, in Aldobrandino's life stages the growing *adolescentia* body (lasting until twenty-five or thirty)

---

109 See Jennifer Borland's work on the transmission of medical texts through female networks: Borland, "Female Networks," 108–36.

110 Discussed in Chapter 4.

111 *Le régime du corps*, 79: "Comment on doit le cors garder en cascun aage."

112 *Le régime du corps*, 79: "De le premiere dient qu'ele est caude et moiste et en cest aages croist li cors, et dure jusques à xxv ans ou à xxx."

113 *Le régime du corps*, 79: "Li seconde est caude et seche, et dure li cors en se vigeur et en se force juskes à xl ans ou xlv."

114 *Le régime du corps*, 79.

115 Bernard of Gordon writes that "warmth, windiness and moisture [are necessary for intercourse]…and therefore one who has all of these is fertile" (*caliditas, ventositas et humiditas…et ideo qui habet omnia ista fecundus)*. A few lines later, Bernard explains that "as the combination of all these things causes fecundity, so a deficiency causes sterility" (*Sicut igitur ex cursu omnium istorum ca[usa]tur fecunditas ita ex defectu istorum causat sterilitas*). Bernard of Gordon, *Practica seu Lilium medicinae* (image 362). This passage is also translated in Demaitre, *Medieval Medicine*, 302.

was the most naturally fertile, if it was correctly balanced and healthy. The *juventus* body (until forty-five or fifty) was drier, now fully-grown and strong, but still warm. The humoral complexions associated with these stages and Aldobrandino's ages suggest why childlessness around thirty, the shift point from physical *adolescentia* to *juventus* was concerning for Henry III. Childlessness in *adolescentia*, the stage of complexional warmth and moisture, might have been a symptom of humoral imbalance and thus some behavioural failing (in terms of lifestyle) on Henry's part. Continued childlessness when his body reached its physical peak in *juventus*, beginning around age thirty, could have signalled weakness in Henry III's natural body and his behavioural management of health.

The lifestyle advice contained in a *regimen* text like Aldobrandino's encapsulates a royal couple's practical and even self-directed approach to managing their own humoral balance, and as part of that, their understanding of reproductive health and fertility. The first book of Aldobrandino's text covers how to support the body during pregnancy and care for an infant after birth. While Henry and Eleanor did not have this particular *regimen* during the pregnancies and births of their children, Aldobrandino's *regimen* captures the kind of medical advice that was accessible to Eleanor's natal family and transmittable through family networks. Beatrice of Savoy's commission of the text preserves what she considered valuable and worth passing on to her daughters. But it was not only relevant for her daughters, as the contents of Aldobrandino's *regimen* show how a king and queen might use the same text, if not the same parts of that text. The text gives a glimpse of the kind of medicine in a royal household and how a king and queen engaged with medical knowledge and texts; it is a practical guide which demonstrates Eleanor and Henry's interest and involvement in the management of their own health, and ultimately, fertility.[116]

Isabella of France is associated with a different health guide, a dietary text that lists the effects of food and drink on the humoral balance of different parts of the body. The text survives in different versions and many manuscript copies, both in Latin and Middle English. The Latin version, usually known as *De conferentibus et nocentibus*, is typically attributed to Arnald of Villanova, a fourteenth-century author and physician in Montpellier.[117]

---

116 The text was in French, rather than Latin adding to the sense that it was meant to be accessible and for practical use.

117 Voigts and Payne, "Medicine for a Great Household (c. 1500)," 219. eTK lists 39 Latin versions, and eVK2, 9 Middle English copies. eTK is an electronic catalogue derived from a print catalogue by Thorndike and Kibre, *A Catalogue of Incipits of*

While surviving manuscripts of the Latin text do not mention Isabella, later English derivatives do, which suggests that some dietary text in Isabella's possession may have derived from Arnald of Villanova's work or a connection between the queen and physician. Significantly, Monica Green argues that the early fourteenth-century medical faculty at Montpellier had a reputation for diagnosing and treating infertility, citing that Arnald of Villanova was known for successfully treating a childless couple who had sought his expertise.[118] Perhaps a dietary was created for Isabella by Arnald, one of the most well-known physicians of Montpellier in the fourteenth century.[119]

The earliest extant Middle English version of the text is probably from the late fourteenth century, with most surviving manuscripts dating from the fifteenth century.[120] The Middle English version is known as the *Dietary of Queen Isabella* because the author states in the preface that it was written "by the physicians of Montpellier [sometimes substituted with "Salerno"]

Mediaeval Scientific Writings in Latin (Cambridge, MA, 1963). eVK2 is an electronic catalogue created from an earlier version produced as a CD-ROM: Voigts and Deery Kurtz, *Scientific and Medical Writings in Old and Middle English: An Electronic Reference* (known as eVK). Both electronic catalogues are available online: https://www.nlm.nih.gov/hmd/indexcat/index.html.

118 Monica Green suggests that by the fourteenth century, the medical faculty at Montpellier was associated with curing infertility. She describes a story in which Arnald was called by a childless couple's family to investigate—and cure—the pair's fertility problems sometime around 1304 or 1307. The couple had been married in ca. 1300, when the groom (Elzéar) was fifteen and the bride, Delphine, eighteen. Arnald examined the couple and found that they had made a secret pledge of chastity (which ultimately led to their canonization, as the story comes from their *vitae*), but Arnald reported to his medical colleagues in nearby Marseille that Elzéar suffered from three impediments to conception and Delphine suffered from four. Green, *Making Medicine Masculine*, 86–87; Green cites the saints' lives from James Campbell, *Vies occitanes de Saint Auzias et de Sainte Dauphine*.

119 The authors of the dietary are described in the text's preface as "physicians of Montpellier" or "leeches of Montpellier." See an edition of the dietary printed in Braekman, *Studies on Alchemy*, 67–76. I previously produced a transcription of Isabella's Dietary from London, Wellcome Library, MS 5262: Trivett, "Intercessor, Patron and Medical Authority?" Wellcome MS 5262 contains a fifteenth-century Middle English version of Isabella's Dietary and has an image of a swaddled infant in a cradle on fol. 7v, the Table of Contents, which perhaps implies an association with reproductive medicine. The manuscript has been photographed and is available on the Wellcome image catalogue online, under the references L0064445 to L0064580. It is also described in Wellcome Library Catalogue: https://search.wellcomelibrary.org/iii/encore/record/C__Rb1955383__SMS.5262.__Orightresult__U__X3?lang=eng&suite=cobalt.

120 Braekman, *Studies on Alchemy*, 61–62.

and sent by the king of France to Dame Isabel, queen of England."[121] There is another text, a short collection of recipes arranged *a capite ad calces*, "from head to foot," and prefaced with the same introduction and assertion of Isabella's ownership.[122] Both the dietary and recipe collection's origins and authenticity are uncertain.

If Isabella had not exactly owned a copy of the extant Middle English dietary text, the attributions of her ownership may still have been based on an element of truth. It is possible that the fifteenth-century Middle English manuscripts of the dietary which survive were based on an earlier copy that *was* actually sent to Isabella by her father or brother, both kings of France. W. L. Braekman suggests there are indications that two of the extant Middle English manuscripts—one of which is from the fourteenth century and is the oldest known copy of the text—were based on an earlier French source, as intimated by the inclusion of French words in the English versions.[123] There are many textual variants between the extant copies, even among the six surveyed by Braekman, which indicates that the text was widely copied *and* adapted from an older source. It is also possible that Isabella was known to have had an interest in medicine and to have owned practical medical texts.[124] Braekman declares that she did, stating that "this Queen Isabel must have enjoyed the reputation of being deeply interested in medical and pseudo-medical lore...borne out by the fact that her name is also connected with the elixir of youth."[125] Braekman also specifies that Arnald's Latin *De conferentibus et nocentibus* was *a* source for the Middle English "Isabella's Dietary," but not *the* source, as there are variations between the two.[126] Therefore, it is possible that the late fourteenth/fifteenth century Middle English *Dietary of Queen Isabella* was based on Arnald's Latin *regimen* and an earlier French text really owned by the queen.

An alternative explanation for the attributions is that Isabella's name was used because she was the queen when the Middle English texts were produced. Braekman asserts that Queen Isabella would be a peculiar

121 Wellcome MS 5262, fol. 54r.

122 Green, "The Possibilities of Literacy," Table 2, 65. Braekman, *Studies on Alchemy*, 65.

123 Braekman, *Studies on Alchemy*, 63.

124 Braekman suggests this, *Studies on Alchemy*, 65. Voigts and Payne allude to it, "Medicine for a Great Household," 219.

125 Braekman, *Studies on Alchemy*, 64. He cites Talbot, "The Elexir of Youth," 33–34. Braekman remarks that Talbot did not cite his source, but Braekman located the quotation in BL, MS Sloane 964, fol. 93.

126 Braekman, *Studies on Alchemy*, 64

owner for this particular dietary (he does not explain why), but it was not unusual for the name of an English royal to be attached to a medical text.[127] Another dietary text was supposedly given by Sigismund, Holy Roman Emperor, to Henry III.[128] In some of the Latin manuscript versions of *De conferentibus et nocentibus*, the text is attributed to authors other than Arnald of Villanova.[129] In particular, in London, British Library (BL), MS Sloane 282, the text's author is cited as "W. de provincial."[130] As we saw, Eleanor of Provence had several physicians from Provence, including one called William of Provence. Given that Eleanor of Provence's mother, Beatrice, commissioned a dietary text in French from her own personal physician, Aldobrandino of Siena, it is plausible that Eleanor might have done something similar and had William of Provence compile a *regimen* text for her. The Middle English dietary's claim of Queen Isabella's ownership might be the result of some confusion by the fourteenth century about which queen of England was the original owner, so it was associated with the queen at that time, Isabella of France.

For the purpose of understanding the management of royal healthcare by kings and queens, the association of the Middle English dietaries with Queen Isabella is significant. In a basic sense, it shows that her name added credibility, value and authority to the dietary text and recipe collection, both medical texts intended for practical use. It also demonstrates contemporary awareness that queens disseminated medical knowledge and texts to their marital lands through their familial networks. Despite the uncertain authenticity of the Middle English dietary and recipe collection, the claimed connection to the queen shows that there was some wider perception that queens owned practical medical texts and actively managed their own healthcare. Attributing the texts to Isabella could have only been a worthwhile choice for the scribes if it was based on existing belief that this sort of text *could* have belonged to the queen. More broadly, it suggests that management of royal healthcare was an associated function of queenship.

---

127 Braekman, *Studies on Alchemy*, 63.

128 Braekman, *Studies on Alchemy*, 64. Braekman describes him as "Emperor of Rome," but he must be referring to the later fourteenth-century Holy Roman emperor, Sigismund (r. 1387–1437). That would make "Henry III" a confusion for Richard II, whose reign overlapped with Sigismund's.

129 Braekman, *Studies on Alchemy*, 66.

130 Braekman, *Studies on Alchemy*, 66.

Royal Reproductive Medicine Reconstructed: Finding Fertility Medicine in Fragmentary Sources

We have seen that royal childlessness earned attention because of the significance of fatherhood for the king's demonstration of mature masculinity. When three kings remained childless in their early thirties, it affected perceptions of their social maturity as adult kings. The evidence suggests that Henry III and David II also employed medical therapies at the same moments when they refocused their pious practices in their early thirties. This section argues that David II's increased employment of medical practitioners in his early thirties demonstrates his deliberate effort to promote health and fertility through regular physician oversight. The second part of this section interprets decisions about herb gardens and interior designs in Henry III and Eleanor of Provence's living spaces as part of their management of health. It is significant that the surviving evidence for both David II and Henry III's health-seeking behaviours involves behavioural adjustments and lifestyle factors rather than obvious medicinal remedies for illness. This approach allowed the kings to address fertility concerns while avoiding any suggestion of disease or bodily weakness—a crucial distinction given that illness would have further undermined their masculine authority. By focusing on moderation, self-control, and lifestyle management, these kings could pursue fertility treatments within a framework that actually reinforced rather than compromised their demonstration of mature masculine kingship. Their childlessness may have inhibited their masculine maturity at the perfect age, but their chosen health-seeking practices aligned with the very principles of restraint and self-governance that defined ideal manhood and successful kingship.

Patterns of Medical Care

When David II reached his early thirties and his devotional behaviour shifted, he also began to receive far more regular medical care than at any earlier time in his life. The Scottish exchequer accounts are complete for David's reign, unlike for earlier medieval kings and they show different concentrations of medical practitioners employed over the course of his reign. From 1328 to 1346 there are no references to any practitioners.[131] This is partly a reflection of the Scottish government at least until 1341, as the Scottish crown was briefly held in the 1330s by Edward Balliol and, even

131 *ER*, 1264–1359, eds. Stuart and Burnett, vol. 1.

when Bruce supporters regained control, David and Queen Joan remained in France until 1341.[132] Therefore, the expenditure recorded for the 1330s does not really contain many details about David and Joan's lives. However, the sense that the couple required few medical practitioners in these years need not be discounted. Generations of scholars' work has produced registers of known physicians and surgeons who came from and/or studied medicine at universities in medieval Britain and France and these sources contain no mention of any practitioners associated with David and Joan during their childhood and adolescence.[133] If the couple received medical attention during those years, it was likely infrequent, involved few practitioners or was perhaps administered by a practitioner who was not university-trained.

However, after two arrows were lodged in his face and head in the Battle of Neville's Cross in 1346, David understandably needed medical attention.[134] Initially, he was cared for by Edward III's trusted personal practitioners: one of the surgeons was William of Bolton who probably attended Queen Philippa in childbirth shortly before David was wounded.[135] This suggests that the English king had sent one of the most senior practitioners from the English royal households to save the Scottish king. After ten weeks, David was well enough to be transported from Bamburgh—where he had received the initial medical care after the battle—to the Tower of London.[136] He was treated there by another trusted English royal surgeon, Roger de Eyton.[137] There are no other mentions of additional or ongoing treatment for the wounds in the English chancery accounts (as comparison, they do contain payments for other things for David, such as new clothes), which suggests

132 Penman, *David II*, 55–76.

133 Talbot and Hammond, *Medical Practitioners*; Wickersheimer, *Dictionnaire biographique*; Getz, "Medical Practitioners in Medieval England," 245–83.

134 Penman, *David II*, 133.

135 Talbot and Hammond, *Medical Practitioners*, 386, describe William of Bolton's career and his care of David. Purey-Cust, *The Heraldry of York Minster*, 2:404: The first payment for David's treatment is to William of Bolton and Hugo de Kilvington, barber-surgeons from York, paid £6 for healing David Bruce at Bamburgh, who "lay there, having been wounded with an arrow." Purey-Cust, *Heraldry*, 2:406: Philippa was confined at York for the birth of Princess Margaret who was born July 30, 1346, and David was wounded in October 1346.

136 Balfour-Melville, "Papers Relating to the Captivity," 3.

137 TNA E101/25/26; Balfour-Melville, "Papers Relating to the Captivity," 3. The payment for David's transfer to London is also recorded in *CCR* (1346–1349), 186.

that David's wounds had been successfully or at least sufficiently treated by early 1347.[138]

After the treatment for the arrow wound in 1346, David received minimal medical care during his imprisonment. In 1352 his Scottish physician, Hector Beaton, was granted safe-conduct by Edward III for travel back to Scotland, indicating that he had probably been with David in England since 1346.[139] Hector is styled as "le leche"—"leech" or "doctor"—in both the Scottish exchequer rolls and the accounts from the last year of David's captivity.[140] Beaton is never described as *magister*, and John Bannerman argues that he was not a university-trained physician but a member of the Beaton family (Clan MacBeth), known in Scotland since at least the fourteenth-century for their medical expertise.[141] Hector is mentioned three times in the accounts during David's captivity in England and, after the king was released, the Scottish exchequer accounts record payments to Hector in 1358–1359.[142] In the eleven-year period of David's imprisonment, he seems to have needed only minimal medical attention managed by just his personal physician.

This changed in 1357, though, and beginning in that year David received considerably more medical care than at any previous point in his life, apart from the arrow wound in 1346. Just before he returned to Scotland in

---

138 The absence of any further medical treatment for David in the sources likely reflects reality because there are still orders for provisions for the Scottish king during his imprisonment, like new clothes in July 1356: *CDS*, ed. Bain, 3:294 (the order is for a new tunic, jerkin, hose, a lined robe, three pairs of boots and more). There is evidence that David was visited by his own Scottish physician, Hector Beaton (discussed below), but there are no other indications that English royal practitioners attended the Scottish king, and no explicit reference to the arrow wound after 1347.

139 Talbot and Hammond, *Medical Practitioners*, 70, mention the safe conduct. *Foedera*, ed. Rymer, 3.1:250; *Rot. Scot.*, ed. Illingworth et al., 1:751, 755: Hector is described as David's "vallettus" (valet?) in the body of the text, but *medico* in the entry's heading. For Beaton's stay in England from 1346, see Bannerman, *The Beatons*, 61.

140 *ER*, eds. Stuart and Burnett, 2:562; Balfour-Melville, "Papers Relating to the Captivity," 13. The other references to Hector in *ER*, eds. Stuart and Burnett, 2:566, 617, describe him as "medico."

141 See Bannerman, *The Beatons*, 59–62: The Beaton family served as physicians to Scottish kings over several generations, including David's father, Robert I, and then the Stewart kings. The Beatons perhaps had connections to Latin medical texts too: Bannerman notes that the *Lilium medicinae* by Bernard of Gordon was translated into Gaelic, *The Beatons*, 89–90.

142 During David's captivity: *Rot. Scot.*, ed. Illingworth et al., 1:751, 754–55. After 1357, and David's return to Scotland: *ER*, eds. Stuart and Burnett, 2:562, 566, 617.

autumn of 1357, David had a visit from Hector Beaton and was also attended by Edward III's physician, Jordan of Canterbury; the London apothecary, John Adam, also supplied an "electuario condayl" for the Scottish king in the same year.[143] Once the king returned to Scotland, Hector Beaton continued to serve David for at least the next two years. Unlike the period 1346–1357, Beaton's attention was seemingly not enough, and two additional physicians were paid for care between 1357–1360.[144] The exchequer accounts mention payment to two other *medici* for 1364, Donald Bannerman and John of Newcastle.[145] Meanwhile, in 1370, Thomas de Hall, *medico,* was paid for his service.[146]

This care from physicians, clustered around 1358–1359, the early 1360s, and then 1370 coincides with the years that David's childlessness was particularly integral to his political agenda. He was hoping to revive the succession deal with Edward III in 1359; he also proposed a new iteration of the succession peace deal to the Scottish council in 1364.[147] By 1370, he was trying to end his marriage to Margaret Logie and take a new wife to produce

---

143 I cannot find any contemporary description of this electuary or its ingredients. It could be related to "condyle," part of a joint, or "knuckle," so perhaps a remedy for arthritis or gout. Arthritis and gout seem unusual issues for a thirty-three-year-old, though. John Adam was paid in 1357: *Issues of the Exchequer*, ed. Devon, 166; Matthews, *Royal Apothecaries*, 12. For Jordan of Canterbury: Balfour-Melville, "Papers Relating to the Captivity," 32–33, contains a document with David's expenses in the final weeks of his captivity, recorded by William Trussel. Scots were banned from accessing David without leave while he was kept at Odiham, but Hector Beaton and a "Patrick of Aberdeen" were both allowed to see him in 1357: Balfour-Melville, "Papers Relating to the Captivity," 4, 32–34.

144 Hector Beaton served David on four occasions, between 1358–1359: *ER*, eds. Stuart and Burnett, 2:562 (1358), 566 (1359), 617 (1359); *ER*, eds. Stuart and Burnett, 2:6 (1359). Additionally, in 1359, John, "medici de Anglia" was summoned to Edinburgh for seven weeks. At the same time, both Hector Beaton and Master Nicolas, "medico," were also paid for their service: *ER*, eds. Stuart and Burnett, 1:616–17. Then in 1360, Master Nicholas, *medicus* of Flanders, was paid, perhaps the same Master Nicholas who had been mentioned with Hector and John of England the year before. In 1361 there was another new character, Thomas leche, although he is not specifically described as master or physician, *ER*, eds. Stuart and Burnett, 2:79. Thomas is never described as *magister* or *medicus* in the account, but neither is Hector Beaton, so he may still have been a physician. Thomas was paid two more times after the first mention: *ER*, eds. Stuart and Burnett, 2:88, 116.

145 *ER*, eds. Stuart and Burnett, 2:138 ("Douenaldo"). *ER*, eds. Stuart and Burnett, 2:178 (John).

146 *ER*, eds. Stuart and Burnett, 2:357; Talbot and Hammond, *Medical Practitioners*, 346. At this time, Thomas was paid £16. 13s. 4d. and granted 10 marks a year.

147 Penman, *David II*, 222–27, esp. 224 (1359 plans); 308–22 (1364 proposal).

a biological heir. David needed the Scottish magnates to agree to accept Edward III's son as his heir in order to resolve the substantial annual payment owed to the English for his ransom (conveniently also disinheriting his difficult nephew and heir presumptive, Robert the Steward). Without confirmation that David could produce his own child to ultimately override the agreement placing an English prince on the Scottish throne, the Scots were unwilling to accept the plan that would replace Robert the Steward with an English king if David died childless. Plausibly, David sought medical attention around 1358, 1364, and 1370 to gain support for his succession-peace deals in those years; either by finally siring a child to prove his fertility (ideally after the treaty was signed, so he might still fix the ransom problem), or, at least, to signal to the Scottish magnates that he was not *actually* planning to die without producing his own heir.[148] The increased employment of physicians in these years is significant, in part, because David could be *seen* by those who opposed his succession deal to be doing something about childlessness.

Of course, while the increased medical attention is clear, it can be interpreted in different ways. In his detailed study of David II, Penman states that the reason for the king's increased medical care after 1357 was unclear but he still relates it to the battle wounds from 1346 throughout his analysis.[149] Perhaps David did suffer for decades with a troublesome wound that required ongoing care; it is possible that an arrow barb had not been completely removed from his head.[150] If he still needed care, though, it seems

148 For another example of political messaging and being seen to invite fertility, see Mistry, "Ermentrude's Consecration (866)," 567–88.

149 Penman, *David II*, 139, 189. Penman also suggests that David's demand for medical care after 1357 was because of fear about the plague: Penman, "The Bruce Dynasty," 361. An anecdotal detail does suggest that the king took precautions against contracting the illness: Walter Bower, describing the murder of David's mistress Katherine Mortimer in 1360, notes that the deed took place when David, Katherine and much of the Scottish elite were on their way north because of "the sight and stories of many illnesses and deaths, the infections and impurities of the air, and the fear and dread of the plague then assailing the southern parts of the kingdom," quoted from Ormrod, "Katherine Mortimer's Death at Soutra," 111. The Scottish court might have been worried about plague, but the timing of the plague outbreaks in 1349/50 and then 1362 in Scotland does not quite explain the distinct increase in David's medical care from 1357, seven years after the first outbreak and five years before the second. Very little work has been done on the Black Death in Scotland though.

150 In his text of surgery, Henri de Mondeville gives detailed advice about how to clean wounds and remove something like an arrow lodged in a bone, and properly

strange that it only became a significant problem a decade later and suddenly needed regular treatment. Also, given that Edward III had sent the highest calibre of medical practitioners to David when he was first wounded in 1346, presumably David could have received additional care between 1346–1357 if he had needed it, but there is no sign that the wound was an issue after his initial treatments in 1346–1357 at Bamburgh and the Tower of London.

The only contemporary suggestion that David suffered continued grief from his head injury comes from the chronicler Jean Froissart. Froissart claimed that David II founded a church to St. Monan because the saint helped to relieve his headaches by removing the arrow barb from his head at the full moon.[151] In the fifteenth century, Walter Bower attributed David's interest in St. Monan to the miraculous removal of the arrow from the king's head after he prayed to the saint. In contrast though, another legend attributes David's interest in St. Monan to the saint's rescue of the king from a shipwreck while he was crossing the Forth.[152] Penman mentions these different narratives and perhaps undermines his own explanation for David's medical care by declaring that the shipwreck narrative is a "much more credible foundation legend" for St. Monan's.[153] The contradictory evidence of the three narratives, and Penman's interpretation of the chronicles, leaves space for another explanation of David's devotional behaviours coupled with regular medical care after 1357: they were responses to childlessness.

It must be considered whether David's need for more medical care in the last fourteen years of his life was because of the demands of age. David

---

removing debris from wounds was known by medieval surgeons to be important. Furthermore, face and head wounds in battle were not uncommon, even for medieval kings/elite: in the fifteenth century Henry V of England was wounded in the face in battle at Shrewsbury, and after being treated by surgeons, he made a full recovery. Livingston, "The Depth of Six Inches." Another fifteenth-century and Scottish example of the commonness of face/head wounds from battle: in John Barbour's *The Bruce*, when English soldiers meet the infamous Scottish warrior, James "the Black" Douglas in Spain, they cannot believe that it is him because no good knight could have such an unscarred face. John Barbour, *The Bruce*, 760, vv. 373–90. Finally, Penman, *David II*, 133 states that David's battle injury was identical to the one received by Philip VI at Crécy in 1346. An arrow barb lodged in Philip's jawbone.

151 *Chroniques de Jean Froissart*, ed. Luce, 1346–1356, 4:xi. In Bower: *Chron. Bower*, ed. Watt, 7:261n464. Penman cites this passage from Bower to justify David's medical care in the 1360s, Penman, *David II*, 139.

152 Discussed above in Chapter 4. The legend is mentioned by Watt, *Chron. Bower*, 7:261n464.

153 Penman, *David II*, 261.

died of unknown but seemingly natural cause when he was forty-six, though, and the increase in medical attention began when he was just thirty-three. Thirty-three and forty-six were not considered old or end-of-life ages according to medieval ideas of the life course and aging. Indeed, Alexander III's death at forty-four, a century earlier, was considered premature and caught the Scottish kingdom off-guard.[154] Equally, David seems to have thought he would live for much longer, as he was trying to end his marriage to Margaret Logie and hoping to make Agnes Dunbar his third queen around 1370–1371. His age and actions do not seem like those of an ill man who was suffering from either chronic illness or slipping into a frail existence and required regular medical attention from multiple physicians.

There is also a parallel between the timing of David II's medical care and the point when he began pursuing new spiritual support. It is not possible to pinpoint any specific fertility medicine in the annual payment to physicians but, from the point when David began to go on pilgrimages and found new churches and altars to saints, continued childlessness and personal frustration with his heir-presumptive had become a significant, politicized situation. Showing that he was working to invite fertility might have bolstered Scottish support for his succession deal with Edward III. Based on the political significance of David's childlessness by the 1350s and the timing of his new devotional practices and increased employment of physicians, it is plausible that he was working to maximize his health and fertility with the help of his physicians.

Gardens and the Lived Environment

A core part of medieval healthcare was balancing the body's humours by regulating the non-naturals, including air, food and drink, sleep and emotions. As such, external factors like one's surrounding environment and lifestyle habits had a significant effect on health and were an important part of medieval medicine. Indeed, the lived environment could be managed and manipulated for health. Traces of Henry III and Eleanor of Provence's decisions about their physical surroundings, particularly the gardens and decoration of their living spaces, suggest an awareness of humoral medical

154 *Wyntoun*, ed. Laing, 3:264–65 describes Scotland's grief; *Chron. Fordun*, ed. Skene, 309–10; *Liber Pluscardensis*, ed. Skene, 80–81. As insight into contemporary perceptions of "old," Matthew Paris considered Alexander II's death in 1241, when he was fifty, to be premature and the result of angering St. Columba: *The Illustrated Chronicles of Matthew Paris*, ed. Vaughan, 119–20.

theory and practice, and the impact of external factors like sight and smell on healthful balance and general wellbeing. As Henry III reached the peak age of masculine maturity, his health-seeking efforts involved behavioural adjustments that promoted humoral balance, moderation, and self-control which were not only key attributes of masculine maturity, but also necessary for fertility, according to medieval medical theories.

Medieval herb gardens were commonly built within the walls of castles and royal residences, beneath windows, in corners and between chambers.[155] In 1260, Albertus Magnus described small herb, or pleasure, gardens as spaces for growing medicinal and aromatic herbs, "but also for smell and sight, open air for health."[156] Herb gardens were theoretically "created principally to delight the senses of smell and sight and, thus, to promote health and contentment."[157] A herb garden was not simply a place to grow the ingredients for herbal medicines, but a therapeutic tool for effecting bodily balance in its own right, with beautiful scenes of plants and flowers and fragrant scented air. Walking through a garden also provided exercise and relaxation, both important for maintaining or restoring health.[158] Pleasant scenes and scents, in particular, were thought to be beneficial for restoring humoral balance within the body, and so gardens were often an initial port of call for those who felt sick.[159] Additionally, herb gardens and garden scenes were considered to be particularly beneficial for pregnant women who were thought to be especially susceptible to both good and bad sights, and frightening images could imprint on the developing fetus and cause deformities.[160] Gardens provided calm, pleasing views that benefited both mother and her unborn child.[161]

---

155 Landsberg, *The Medieval Garden*, 16; Colvin, "Royal Gardens in Medieval England," 7–22; McLean, *Medieval English Gardens*; Malcolm, "Gardens of the Castle," 111. David II had a garden at Edinburgh Castle, but the only surviving evidence is the appointment of a gardener in 1363. Alexander III also had a gardener in the 1260s at Forfar Castle, one of the royal residences frequently used by the thirteenth-century royal family: *ER*, eds. Stuart and Burnett, 1:li, 8.

156 Albertus Magnus, *De vegetabilibus libri VII*, ed. Meyer, 638. Cited and translated in Rawcliffe, "'Delectable Sightes and Fragrant Smelles,'" 12.

157 Rawcliffe, "'Delectable Sightes and Fragrant Smelles,'" 4.

158 Bartholomaeus Anglicus, *On the Properties of Things*, ed. Seymour, 1:562; 2:1299–1300. Cited by Rawcliffe, "'Delectable Sightes and Fragrant Smelles,'" 9.

159 Rawcliffe, "'Delectable Sightes and Fragrant Smelles,'" 9.

160 Rawcliffe, "'Delectable Sightes and Fragrant Smelles,'" 11.

161 Rawcliffe, "'Delectable Sightes and Fragrant Smelles,'" 11.

Henry III and Eleanor of Provence had several new herb gardens installed in the early years of their marriage, when there were concerns about their fertility. Between 1237–1239 new herb gardens were made between the king and queen's chapels at Winchester, between Eleanor's chamber and chapel at Windsor, and below the king's chambers at Everswell.[162] In 1238, there was a new door and set of stairs made from the queen's chamber so that she could more easily reach her herb garden at Kenyngton.[163] In the 1240s, when Eleanor was frequently pregnant and gave birth to four of the couple's five children, herb gardens were created by her chambers at Kenyngton, Woodstock and Clarendon.[164] In contrast, in the later 1250s to 1270s orders relating to gardens appear only occasionally in the administrative accounts.[165] This slump in plans for new gardens later in the reign might be because all desired additions and improvements had been completed earlier and anything else was unnecessary by the 1250s. Indeed, this correlation does not equal causation, yet the fact that the most significant plans and alterations for gardens occurred when Henry and Eleanor were first married and then having children, rather than in the 1220s, for instance, at the beginning of Henry III's majority rule, is worth noting.

The therapeutic value of gardens for pregnancy and birth could also be harnessed by depicting gardens inside birthing chambers on hanging tapestries and paintings.[166] Perhaps it was some of these images that were added to Eleanor of Provence's chambers for her confinement and the birth of Edward in June 1239. There is a payment on June 15, 1239, the day of Edward's birth, "for colours and paintings done in the queen's chamber from the octaves of the Holy Trinity until St. Barnabas [June 11]."[167] Floral scenes were also painted in some of Eleanor's rooms when she was pregnant: there is an order for her chamber at the Tower of London to be painted with

162 *CLR*, 1:319, 365, 405, 412.

163 *CLR*, 1:342.

164 *CLR*, 2:48, 307; *CLR*, 4:109.

165 There is an order for an herb garden to be installed at Westminster in the 1260s: "a small enclosed *herbarium* next to the pentice, or covered passageway, between the king's chamber and the neighbouring abbey, in which six pear trees were to be planted in 1262." *CCR* (1261–1264), 29; Colvin, "Royal Gardens," 13.

166 Rawcliffe, "'Delectable Sightes and Fragrant Smelles,'" 11. There is also evidence that gardens were used for their healthful effects by Edward I's second queen, Margaret. When she went to Winchester in 1306 when she was pregnant, the king had a new garden made there for her: Colvin, *The History of the King's Works*, 2:862.

167 *CLR*, 1:393.

flowers in 1238, and then in 1240 it was to be wainscoted and painted with roses.[168] While they do not correspond specifically to Eleanor's confinements, other wall paintings discovered at Windsor Castle have been dated to Henry III's reign, probably from the early years of Eleanor and Henry's marriage, or at least before the construction of the new royal apartments in 1240.[169] In the lower chamber of Windsor, spandrels are filled "by delicate stylized foliage set against a green background."[170] Florals and foliage were common decorative details, often included in medieval manuscript margins, for instance, so their inclusion at Windsor is not, in and of itself, clinching evidence. But such decorative details nonetheless fit with the emerging picture of a couple who valued gardens and reproduced their therapeutic scenes inside castle and palace walls in the years when there were concerns about their fertility, initially when they were childless but also during subsequent pregnancies and births.

The healthful effects of gardens were brought inside in another way too, when windows were installed in Eleanor or Provence's chambers, specifically so that she could look out at her herb gardens. At Windsor, part of the refurbishment of the queen's chambers in 1236–1237 included instructions for windows to be installed for looking onto the herb garden in the cloister below.[171] It was specified that these windows were to be made to open and shut, presumably to allow the pleasant smells of the garden to rise up into the queen's chamber. Around the same time (when Eleanor was pregnant), a herb garden was added between Eleanor's chapel and chamber at Rochester in February 1239, with a window installed in that chamber too.[172] In 1247 a new herb garden was made for Eleanor at Clarendon, and then in 1250 there are instructions that her chambers there be paved and fitted with a window overlooking her herb garden.[173] In addition to their desire for herb gardens around chambers and chapels, and efforts to bring flowers and foliage inside with painted decoration, the detailed instructions for windows gives an impression that Henry and Eleanor were thinking about the therapeutic effects of pleasant sights and smells.

---

168 *CLR*, 1:352, 444, 453; Colvin, *King's Works*, 2:714.

169 Park and Pender, "Henry III's Wall Paintings," 126.

170 Park and Pender, "Henry III's Wall Paintings," 126.

171 Colvin, *King's Works*, 2:867: cites Pipe Roll 20 H III, rot 1d. Also enrolled as E101/530/1, no. 23. Jansen, "Henry III's Windsor," 101.

172 *CLR*, 1:365.

173 *CLR*, 3:109, 296–97.

Some specific features of Henry and Eleanor's gardens also suggest that they planned (at least in part) their physical surroundings according to principles of humoral health. The design of some of the royal gardens seems to reflect the instructions for an ideal herb garden by thirteenth-century contemporary, Albertus Magnus:

> it should stand open to the North and East, since those winds bring health and cleanliness. To the opposite winds, namely the South and West, it should, however, be closed because of their turbulence and impurity and disease. Although the North wind delays the fruit, yet it greatly conserves the spirit and guards the health. Pleasure should be sought in the wind and not the fruit.[174]

Albertus also advised that the small pleasure garden should contain sweet-smelling herbs such as sage and flowers such as violets and roses. There should be seating, trees and vines to provide some shade if the sun gets too hot, fruit-bearing trees should be sweet ones like pears and apples and, if possible, there should be a stone fountain in the middle.[175] In 1237–1238, Henry had his herb garden at Nottingham Castle enclosed by a wall, and at Woodstock in 1240, the walls around his garden were repaired—perhaps to block winds from the south and west—and the stone fountain was restored.[176] A trellis was installed to support rose bushes, in what was possibly an enclosed rose garden.[177] In 1239 at Everswell—an idyllic royal residence renowned by the thirteenth century for its gardens—Henry had a new herb garden made around one of the pools and another in 1251–1252.[178] At Clarendon, a bench was fitted around the wall of the king's garden in 1250 and he specified that another garden was to be made to the north, under his chamber.[179] This evidence is only suggestive, but it hints that Henry and Eleanor used their lived environment as part of their healthcare, especially when read alongside the new herb gardens planted in the first years of their marriage, the installation of fragrant roses and fruit trees, seats and fountains, and careful attention to garden orientation during the decades when Eleanor was frequently pregnant and their children were born.

174 Translation from Rawcliffe, "'Delectable Sightes and Fragrant Smelles,'" 4–5.

175 Translation from Landsberg, *The Medieval Garden*, 13.

176 Colvin, *King's Works*, 2:758; McLean, *Medieval English Gardens*, 100. There was a herb garden created at Winchester in 1239, on the southern side of the hall, and a protective wall was to be installed around it: *CLR*, 2:405.

177 McLean, *Medieval English Gardens*, 100.

178 *CLR*, 1:412. Colvin, "Royal Gardens," 19; Colvin, *King's Works*, 2:1013–15. He also had one hundred pear trees planted here in 1264.

179 *CLR*, 3:296–97.

In addition to gardens, there was a recurring colour in Henry III and Eleanor's living spaces which had significance in medical theories about health and fertility because of its influence on the internal balance of the body's humours. Henry's chancery accounts contain multiple references to the painting and decoration of royal chambers, including many orders to paint various chambers green (frequently with gold stars).[180] These orders were for both Henry and Eleanor's chambers: for instance, in 1236 the queen's chamber at Woodstock was painted green around her bed and made to look like a curtain and orders for Henry's chamber at Westminster call for the same painted green curtain.[181] There were three separate orders in 1237–1238 alone for green painted chambers.[182] The instructions slow down in the following years but do not stop altogether: Henry's bed at Westminster was painted green and decorated in 1244 with "spangled gold, matching the prevailing colour scheme of the chamber in the 1230s."[183] In 1251, he also had his chamber and three chapels at Geddington painted green with gold stars, and chambers at Guildford painted green.[184] The chapel near Henry's

180 The first instance of this seems to be from 1231–1232, when the king's chamber, door, and window shutters at Woodstock were painted green, *CLR*, 1:194; 289; *CLR*, 4:272. From 1235 there are instructions for a chamber at Winchester to be painted green, and in 1237–1238 Henry's chamber there was to be a wainscoted and painted green with gold stars, and the ground-floor chamber and the queen's chambers were also to be painted green with gold stars in 1237–1238: *CLR*, 3:63 (ground floor); Colvin, *King's Works*, 2:914 (queen's chamber); Park and Pender, "Henry III's Wall Paintings," 126; Colvin, *King's Works*, 2:861. At the same time, Eleanor's chambers at Windsor were wainscoted and painted green with gold stars, Colvin, *King's Works*, 1:129; Janson, "Henry III's Windsor," 105.

181 *CLR*, 1:344. Colvin, *King's Works*, 2:1012; Binski, *Westminster Abbey*, 16.

182 Henry's chamber at Winchester was to be a wainscoted and painted green with gold stars, and the ground-floor chamber and the queen's chambers were also to be painted green with gold stars in 1237–1238: *CLR*, 3:63 (ground floor); Colvin, *King's Works*, 2:914 (queen's chamber); Park and Pender, "Henry III's Wall Paintings," 126; Colvin, *King's Works*, 2:861. At the same time, Eleanor's chambers at Windsor were wainscoted and painted green with gold stars, Colvin, *King's Works*, 1:129; Janson, "Henry III's Windsor," 105.

183 *CCR* (1242–1247), 169; quote from Binski, *Westminster Abbey*, 17.

184 Colvin, *King's Works*, 2:944, 951. After a fire at Guildford in 1254, the king's chambers and great hall were rebuilt and also painted green with gold stars: Colvin, *King's Works*, 2:951. The queen's chamber at Winchester was painted with the signature green walls and gold stars at the same time in 1251–1252, and Eleanor's chamber at Woodstock was painted green with a red border in 1252–1253. *CLR*, 4:3 (Woodstock), 95 (Winchester).

chamber at Clarendon was also tiled with green and yellow tiles arranged in concentric circles between 1234–1237.[185]

The colour green had meaning in thirteenth-century medical thought. According to theory from the medical school of Salerno, white and black were at two opposing ends of the colour spectrum, with green the mid-point between them.[186] In humoral theory the fundamental principle of health was balance and, based on this Salernitan understanding of colour, green was the representation of balance. Bartholomaeus Anglicus describes green as the most pleasing colour and he argued that gazing at it could restore health to the eyes and soothe the sense of sight because of its perfect balance.[187] Also, according to Bartholomaeus, colours were produced by different qualities: black and red were produced by heat, white by cold and green was the product of heat and moisture, as seen in leaves, fruit and grass.[188] The association of colour with qualities, particularly moisture, relates green to the medical ideas about fertility and sterility that were discussed above: Bernard of Gordon explained fertility as the combination of "warmth, windiness and moisture," and "so a deficiency causes sterility."[189] An anonymous fourteenth-century text on infertility from Montpellier, the *Treatise on the Sterility of Women* by Pseudo-Bernard, describes "sterility" as a complexional imbalance: either too much heat, cold, humidity or dryness in both men and women.[190] Therefore, a fertile body was both moist and warm and complexionally balanced, a description identical to that of the colour green.

185 *CLR*, 2:224; *CLR*, 3:362.

186 Woolgar, *Senses*, 156. Woolgar notes that this particular theory was known in England by ca. 1200. In the spectrum of colours, green was in the middle, with red between white and green, and blue between green and black.

187 Bartholomaeus Anglicus, *On the Properties of Things*, ed. Seymour, 2:1290–91. Cited in Rawcliffe, "'Delectable Sightes and Fragrant Smelles,'" 11n55. Bartholomaeus also explained that the therapeutic effect of vineyards came from the restorative effects of the colour green, discussed in Landsberg, *Medieval Garden*, 26. See also Landsberg, *Medieval Garden*, 37: Christine de Pizan wrote about grass at a nunnery in Poissy that was never allowed to go brown, and a twelfth-century French cleric Hugh of Fouilloy explained that green lawns were kept in the middle of monasteries in order to sooth and refresh eyes tired from studying, for "it is truly the nature of the colour green that it nourishes the eyes and preserves their vision."

188 Bartholomaus Anglicus, *On the Properties of Things*, ed. Seymour, 2:1284–90. Woolgar, *Senses*, 156.

189 See n115 above.

190 *Tractatus de sterilitate mulierum*, ed. Cartelle, 130–59. Monica Green discusses this: *Making Women's Medicine Masculine*, 88.

Scholars have recognized Henry III's penchant for green decoration in his residences. Paul Binski mentions that Henry had part of the St. Stephen chapel at Westminster painted green in 1236 and declares that it was a "decorative rather than figurative [design]," resembling the "considerable number of orders for purely decorative work involving green throughout Henry's residences."[191] Virginia Janson muses that "green seems to have been Henry's favourite colour."[192] This might have been the case but for a king who deeply believed in the power of imagery—for instance, he also filled his residences with meaningful Biblical scenes and carefully chosen images of certain saints—his recurrent desire to have his and his queen's daily living spaces painted green should at least be scrutinized for significance beyond an aesthetic taste for the colour and desire for decoration. Like the choices about gardens and painted floral scenes, the prevalence of green in the royal couple's homes was plausibly part of their health-promoting behaviour, and a conscious effort to encourage humoral balance and boost fertility, particularly in the late 1230s when there was concern about their childlessness.

When childlessness became concerning for Henry III and David II at the critical age of male physical perfection and social maturity, we can see traces of health-seeking behaviours by both kings which suggest that they were encouraging fertility by applying humoral medical principles. Significantly, both the medical therapies *and* the concern about childlessness are connected to the kings' behaviours. Henry was perhaps actively promoting royal health, and ultimately fertility, by controlling the non-naturals and regulating complexional balance through his lifestyle and physical surroundings. Moreover, without any suggestion that David II was ill in contemporary sources, it is unlikely that he was being treated by his physicians throughout the 1360s for a chronic illness. His employment of physicians looks more like an effort to promote overall health from the point when attention to his childlessness increased. This chapter suggested that David was hoping to maximize his fertility with the regular oversight of his physicians and the supervised application of humoral principles of balance like those set out by *regimen* guides to health. Although only from traces of evidence about their medical care, both Henry and David can be seen actively *doing* something to invite health and fertility, rather than receiving remedies for a bodily illness. By implementing preventative, *regimen*-style humoral medicine, a king

191 Binski, *Westminster Abbey*, 16. He cites the same evidence from the liberate rolls just described above, primarily that at Clarendon, Windsor and Winchester.

192 Janson, "Henry III's Windsor," 109n79.

could demonstrate specific behaviours, like self-control and balance, that were also associated with maturity and masculinity, and crucially, not physical failing or weakness.

* * *

Geaman has argued that Anne of Bohemia and Richard II both shared the burden of childlessness, but she focused on Queen Anne's search for treatment and commitment to finding a remedy.[193] More generally, there is an imbalance in the scholarly interest in female versus male experiences and responses to infertility.[194] As a result, we have skewed understandings of how couples managed problems with fertility.[195] What queens did to promote fertility and conception has received more attention from scholars because of the perceived importance of motherhood for queenship and, therefore, remedying infertility, the assumption runs, was primarily the queen's responsibility too. Modern historiography's fixation on how queens negotiated childlessness has resulted in a limited view of the ways that royal couples, and their extended familial groups, shared responsibility for and participated in the medical management of fertility and reproduction.

This chapter has nuanced understanding of the queen's role in royal healthcare. Using evidence like the letter from Margaret of France's physician to Edward I and the involvement of Henry III and Eleanor of Provence in decisions about their adolescent daughter Margaret's marriage, we can see how other people took an interest in and led the management of healthcare for queens. In fertility medicine specifically, the queen's body disproportionately bore the brunt of the reproductive labour and, as a result, was the recipient of medical treatments for reproduction, as indicated by the apothecary list for Isabella of France.

Yet, considering the practitioners who served in royal couples' households and the medical texts and knowledge which circulated in royal networks shed light on the queen's authority over medical care too. It is impossible to definitively discern who the recipients of medical treatments were from only payments to medical practitioners, but the queen's influence *is*

193 Geaman, "Anne of Bohemia and Her Struggle to Conceive," 224–44.

194 Noted in Rider, "Men and Infertility," 248.

195 Joan Cadden, for instance, argues that in practice, women were treated for fertility conditions/infertility far more than men, but Rider observes that we might have a distorted view of this because of the focus of modern scholars on women's experience of infertility, for instance, childless queens. See Cadden, *The Meanings of Sex Difference*, 228–58.

evident in the connections between royal practitioners and the queens' natal lands. The above discussion also located specific medical texts, like Aldobrandino's *regimen,* in the proximity of royal couples via queens and their familial networks. This sort of influence affected the medical treatment available to the royal couple, and it highlights how the personal relationships and trust of the queen were pivotal in shaping the royal medical entourage and ultimately the fertility medicine that could be administered to a royal couple. If the king or royal parents made decisions about healthcare and the queen's body, the treatment was carried out by *her* chosen physicians. The claim that Isabella of France owned practical medical texts provides yet another indication of the queen's active role in shaping royal medicine. The fact that this attribution was made so naturally suggests how readily contemporaries acknowledged and took for granted the queen's active role in determining royal healthcare.

Above all, this chapter demonstrated that both the king and queen were involved in the medical management of royal health and fertility, albeit in different ways. The importance of the king's behaviour for medieval perceptions of royal fertility problems has hitherto been overlooked; the queen's influential role in attracting medical practitioners and acquiring texts must not obscure the fact that kings were patients of fertility medicine too. As discussed above, the king's age in relation to his social maturity prompted attention to a couple's childlessness; the status of a king's social body was tied to the condition of his physical body. Any medical treatments received by Henry III and David II from the points of heightened concern about childlessness when they reached the peak male physical age are difficult to piece together from the surviving sources: there are no traces of specific treatments for any illness or infertility. The only healthcare that is visible for these kings is in their behavioural practices, whether David's regular employment of physicians or Henry's decisions about his and Eleanor's environment. Henry III, in particular, made choices about physical surroundings which suggest his awareness of the theory for promoting health according to humoral principles. Notably, there is no admission of physical weakness or illness in this kind of healthcare; controlling lifestyle factors to ensure health relied on some of the same key functions as the achievement of medieval masculinity, like demonstrating self-control and balance, which was undermined by remaining childless.

Chapter 6

REPRODUCTIVE POLITICS

RELIGIOUS PATRONAGE AND SPIRITUAL SUPPORT FOR ROYAL FERTILITY

MEDIEVAL REPRODUCTIVE SUCCESSES and failures existed in a religious framework and spiritual practices were an integral part of treatment and support for reproduction. Spiritual aids for fertility, like medieval devotional practices for illness generally, included appeals for saintly intercession at shrines, protective prayers inscribed on objects for use during birth, and rituals involving holy communion and holy water.[1]

We have considered the devotional habits of Henry III, Alexander II, and David II and Chapter 4 argued that the shifts in their pious practices were related to being childless around thirty, the peak age of masculine adulthood. This present chapter looks more closely at what royal couples did to support their fertility with spiritual practices. There is evidence that medieval royal couples prayed to saints, offered gold coins to shrines and used saints' clothing for help during childbirth. However, this chapter is not simply a catalogue of the things couples did to boost their fertility with spiritual support. Rather, it argues that the spiritual aids for fertility also had important political significance because royal piety and patronage were conspicuous, often intentionally so. Demonstrating devotion to saints and supporting religious institutions around the kingdom was a necessary part of English kingship and a potent means for solidifying power.[2] The king served as "the supreme patron" in his kingdom, and by making offerings "on the altar of St. Alban or St. Edmund, St. Thomas, or St. Wulfstan, he was not merely doing what was expected of him and enlisting the goodwill of the saints, but he was also setting a good example to his subjects great and small."[3] As royal patrons, the king and queen set pious examples, while their behaviour was also shaped by the expectations of their role.

The spiritual remedies that royal couples pursued for fertility problems were shaped by the fundamentally public nature of royal reproduction. Within scholarship on medieval women's practice of pilgrimage, Susan

1 Jones and Olsan, "Performative Rituals for Conception and Childbirth in England," 406–33; Oren-Magidor, *Infertility in Early Modern England*, 124–25.

2 Blick, "King and Cleric," 186; Blick, "Votives, Images, Interaction," 52.

3 Webb, *Pilgrimage in Medieval England*, 112.

Morrison argued that matters related to reproduction and motherhood were the primary motivation for medieval women to undertake pilgrimage.[4] However, a problem with fertility was "never the private business of the woman suffering it," and so neither were the spiritual remedies for reproductive conditions.[5] Scholarship on early modern infertility has also shown that the successes and failures of fertility were witnessed and discussed in relation to a woman's body by her family and community, and such social attention and expectation influenced women's experiences of and attempts to cure childlessness.[6] This interest was not out of concern for the woman, but because of the social significance of the body, illness and reproduction in early modern society.[7] More so than for other medieval couples, royal reproduction attracted particular attention from contemporaries. Whether the king and queen were childless or not was a matter of public knowledge, and the royal body, illness and fertility had implications for the political stability of the realm.

The conspicuousness of both royal reproduction and piety created a platform where royal actions mutually "conditioned and [were] conditioned by" the public view.[8] On a practical level, royal couples' spiritual remedies for fertility were witnessed by those around them, including members of their households, courtiers, advisors, the political elite, and all those associated with the institutions that housed the saints' relics and received royal patronage. Royal pilgrimages were particularly conspicuous endeavours because kings and queens travelled to various parts of the kingdom (or beyond) with large retinues and supplies, making their movements highly visible.

The expenses from these practices were enrolled in the court chancery documents and they were also frequently recorded by chroniclers, who were often individuals linked to the monastic and religious institutions involved. However, other chronicles offered different perspectives; for instance, the French chronicler Jean Froissart, who spent time with David II's court, also mentioned one of the king's pilgrimages in his history.[9] Some sources for royal pious practices, such as orders in the court liberate rolls for offerings following a birth, can be read as deliberate political communication by the

4 Morrison, *Women Pilgrims*, 3, for an outline, but it is a central argument of the book.

5 Morrison, *Women Pilgrims*, 3.

6 Smith, "La raillerie des femmes?," 205.

7 Smith, "La raillerie des femmes?," 205.

8 Morrison, *Women Pilgrims*, 4.

9 Penman, *David II*, 340–43.

king and queen, while others, like the chronicles, indicate broader interest in royal fertility. As the following chapter will demonstrate, the role of royal religious patronage and the conspicuousness of royal piety allowed for a king and queen to shape, or at least attempt to shape, perceptions of their fertility.

This chapter considers the devotional practices of the eight royal couples together, thereby mutually illuminating patterns which could not otherwise be associated with fertility support if the couples were studied in isolation. This methodology is crucial because it uncovers attention to saints like Thomas Becket who were not particularly associated with fertility, rather than only cataloguing devotion to recognized "patron saints" of fertility. This comparative approach is also important because it guards against interpreting everything in relation to a couple's fertility while simultaneously revealing spiritual strategies that couples employed to aid reproduction. Uncovering common spiritual practices among couples who suffered from reproductive anxiety is key for examining with precision the relationship between the management of royal fertility and devotional practices.

The chapter demonstrates that royal couples communicated messages about their fertility through their spiritual practices. The first section argues that kings and queens demonstrated their efforts for fertility by visiting sites and calling on saints with recognizable links to remedying fertility problems. The second section examines how couples used their established royal patronage networks to seek fertility support, strengthening existing ties with religious institutions and their saints. Finally, the last section investigates royal attention to saints with no preexisting royal connections or contemporary associations with fertility, arguing that such devotional choices allowed couples to forge new spiritual relationships that conveyed politically advantageous messages—such as a Scottish couple demonstrating Anglo-Scottish unity through devotion to a shared English saint.

The spiritual practices for fertility were gendered, much like the medical management of royal reproduction. This chapter suggests that the spiritual aids for fertility were exclusively focused on treating the queen's body, while the king called for prayers, made offerings and appealed to saints to give him a son or to help the queen during pregnancy. These kinds of spiritual practices for fertility by-passed the king's reproductive body and presented reproduction and fatherhood as a divinely determined decision without any suggestion of bodily weakness or involuntary failing on the king's part. Ultimately, this chapter argues that spiritual therapy for royal fertility constituted powerful political action and communication because of the conspicuousness of royal fertility *and* piety.

Fertility Saints and Sites

During the Middle Ages, several saints were believed to aid fertility and assist with reproduction. One such "fertility saint" was St. Margaret of Antioch, who was thought to protect mothers and infants during childbirth.[10] Particular sites, like the shrine of Our Lady of Walsingham in Norfolk, also developed reputations for helping with fertility-related issues and were visited by medieval women and men who had reproductive concerns.[11] Some of the pious practices of the royal couples included attention to St. Margaret and Our Lady of Walsingham, as will be discussed below. Crucially, this devotion was witnessed by many different people in various ways; royal pilgrimages included the king or queen's attendants and were observed by other pilgrims, locals and the religious community which housed the saintly relics. In other words, royal couples were *seen* to be doing things that were socially recognizable as fertility remedies.

This is significant because, by performing spiritual practices associated with promoting fertility, the royal couple actively demonstrated their attention to treating fertility concerns. Elizabeth L'Estrange suggested that religious images meant particular things to a medieval audience because of their specific cognitive habits and "situational eye": the idea that there were conditioned understandings of saints and images.[12] Cognitive habits and the situational eye meant that men and women seeing imagery of saints like St. Margaret and St. Anne (another popular fertility saint) understood them to be related to childbirth and fertility. It is significant that the fertility saints and sites called on by the royal couples were particularly associated with treating female reproductive issues: St. Margaret of Antioch was associated with help in childbirth, while the shrine of Our Lady of Walsingham in Norfolk, with its relics and imagery of breastmilk, was a particularly gendered site for supporting fertility. Henry III, Eleanor of Provence, and David II all had connections to St. Katherine of Alexandria, so this section will also discuss the miracles of St. Katherine as they show that this saint was specifically called on by elite husbands to cure their wives' sterility.

---

10 Wogan-Browne, *Saints' Lives and Women's Literary Culture*, 126.

11 Morrison, *Women Pilgrims*, 10–35.

12 L'Estrange, *Holy Motherhood*, 44–75, esp. 61–68.

St. Margaret of Antioch

St. Margaret of Antioch was perhaps the "official and most intensely culted helper of women in childbirth" from at least the late twelfth century.[13] A virgin martyr who defended her Christian faith in the face of torture, she was also swallowed by a dragon (Satan disguised) but burst forth from its stomach unharmed.[14] Derived from the narrative of her *vita*, St. Margaret's torture associated her with both the mother and infant in childbirth; the suffering of parturient women is paralleled in Margaret's endurance of pain while being tortured, while in the conflict with the dragon, St. Margaret is likened to the newborn when she bursts forth from the dragon's belly unscathed.[15] Extant thirteenth-century manuscript versions of her *vita* make Margaret's association with childbirth even more explicit.[16] In the final prayers of her passion, she promises to ensure the delivery of a healthy child, with the method for asking for her help varying by manuscript: labouring mothers could read or hear the saint's *vita*, call her name during birth, or have a copy of her *vita* placed on them.[17]

One thirteenth-century, Anglo-Norman version of St. Margaret's *vita*, in BL, MS Sloane 1611, promises that simply "faith on the part of the pregnant

---

13 Wogan-Browne, *Saints' Lives and Women's Literary Culture*, 126. See also Dresvina, *A Maid with a Dragon*; Alberts, "Suffering and Protection in Childbirth," 289–314; Larson, "Who Is the Master of This Narrative? Maternal Patronage and the Cult of St. Margaret," 94–104; Heyes, *Margaret's Monsters*; Donohoe, "'Unbynde Her Anoone,'" 139–56; Lewis, "The Life of St. Margaret of Antioch," 129–42.

14 Hill, *Women and Religion in Late Medieval Norwich*, 61. St. Margaret was commonly depicted in medieval psalters and Books of Hours with the dragon, demonstrating her primary association with childbirth: Wogan-Browne, "Women's Literary Culture in Twelfth- and Thirteenth-Century England," 125n9.

15 Alberts, "Spiritual Suffering," 297–300. Alberts's focus is on the *South English Legendary* versions of St. Margaret's *vita*, specifically. Juliana Dresvina suggests that St. Margaret's association with childbirth came from a link between exorcism and childbirth: Dresvina, "The Significance of the Demonic Episode in the Legend of St. Margaret of Antioch," 189–209. For a study of late medieval readings of St. Margaret's life and torture, see Lewis, "'Lete Me Suffre,'" 69–82.

16 The *Legenda aurea* does not have the prayer for childbirth, but it is included in Middle English versions of St. Margaret's life, including the Katherine Group and the *South English Legendary*; Alberts, "Spiritual Suffering," 292.

17 Wogan-Browne, "The Apple's Message," 51–52; Wogan-Browne, "Women's Literary Culture," 125; Alberts, "Spiritual Suffering," 291–93; Donohoe, '"Unbynde Her Anoone,'" 147–56. For a broader discussion of the spiritual practices used to support childbirth in the Middle Ages, see Harris Stoertz, "Suffering and Survival in Medieval English Childbirth," 101–13.

woman" would be enough to guarantee a safe delivery and a healthy child.[18] Significantly, St. Margaret's *vita* was bound together in this particular manuscript with Aldobrandino of Siena's *Régime du Corps*, the text composed at the request of Eleanor of Provence's mother.[19] The volume also contains a collection of medical remedies, featuring "recipes and invocations for women in labour."[20] Notably, all three texts were originally bound together.[21] The manuscript also has an inserted *curriculum vitae* for St. Anne, mother of the Virgin Mary, who was associated with miraculous fertility.[22] Likely all three texts were intended to be used together and indicate the reader's interest in childbirth.[23] While there is no internal evidence that this volume belonged to Eleanor of Provence, it embodies the contemporary therapeutic pluralism by which people might draw on both medical remedies and spiritual aids for fertility and childbirth.

While it is not possible to connect the Sloane manuscript to Henry III or Eleanor of Provence, there is some evidence that Eleanor of Provence called on St. Margaret for help. Henry III gave orders for a new timber chapel to be built at Rochester Castle and dedicated to St. Margaret in 1244, just before Eleanor's fourth pregnancy and when the couple was hoping for another son.[24] St. Margaret's life was also painted in the king's Upper Chamber at Clarendon in 1246.[25] This installation was perhaps in recognition of the saint's help after the birth of their second son, Edmund, in 1245. Images of saints functioned as a kind of stand-in for a saint's relics and were understood as capable of healing miracles in their own right.[26] Thus, the dedication and

---

18 Wogan-Browne, "The Apple's Message," 47.

19 See discussion of Aldobrandino's *regime* in Chapter 5. Meyer, "Notice du MS Sloan 1611 du Musée Britannique," 531–58, contains a description of the contents of the manuscript and transcription of the text of St. Margaret's *vita*. Monica Green mentions BL, MS Sloane 1611 in Green, "The Possibilities of Literacy," 26–27, and notes that the insertion of St. Anne's *curriculum vitae* was made after the chapter in the *Régime du corps* that describes remedies for obstetrical issues and discusses the nature of breastmilk.

20 Wogan-Browne, "The Apple's Message," 52.

21 Wogan-Browne, "The Apple's Message," 52.

22 Carole Hill, *Women and Religion*, 19–23.

23 Wogan-Browne, "The Apple's Message," 52.

24 *CLR*, 3:42; Colvin, *King's Works*, 2:808. The couple's desire for another son will be discussed below on pages 184–85.

25 *CLR*, 3:63.

26 Vauchez, *Sainthood in the Middle Ages*, trans. Birrell, 448–53. Morrison, *Women*

images of St. Margaret in Henry and Eleanor's residences indicate a desire for the healing/protective properties of the saint.[27]

Significantly, the images of St. Margaret painted in 1246 were strategically positioned to communicate the royal couple's fertility efforts to their court and household. The installation of these images in the king's chambers at Clarendon, rather than the queen's private apartments, demonstrates their communicative purpose; Henry III's apartments were more permeable and closer to the public spaces of the palace than Eleanor's rooms, which were situated deeper within the complex and farthest from public access routes.[28] By placing devotional images of St. Margaret—a saint associated with protection in childbirth—in the king's upper chamber where members of their court, households and visitors would observe them, the royal couple ensured that their spiritual efforts for fertility were conspicuously displayed to all who engaged with them. This strategic placement exemplifies how a royal couple used their devotional practices to communicate messages about their reproductive endeavours.

There is also other evidence that Eleanor of Provence appealed to St. Margaret for help in childbirth. Reflecting the practice of invoking the saint's name during labour, prescribed in thirteenth-century versions of St. Margaret's *vita*, Matthew Paris claimed that Henry and Eleanor's second child was named for St. Margaret because Eleanor called on her during the difficult birth in 1240.[29] It is significant that Paris knew about this detail in the first place (or at least claimed so), and also that he decided it was worth recording. By nature, chronicles preserved what happened in the past as a way to instruct the present; they actively "[shaped] both past and present."[30] In this light, Paris's decision to mention that the queen called on the patron saint of childbirth when she had a difficult labour cannot be dismissed as a meaningless detail. Paris's Eleanor demonstrated model piety when she appealed to St. Margaret during labour and the saint's favour is indicated by the birth of a healthy daughter, who was named Margaret to show the king and queen's gratitude. Eleanor's behaviour is an example of the power of the

---

Pilgrims, 14, states that by the high Middle Ages, saints were "not linked only to where their relics lay, but also to where their images were."

27 Lewis, "Pilgrimage and the Cult of St. Katherine," 46.

28 Richardson, "Gender and Space in English Royal Palaces," 132, 140.

29 *Chronica majora*, ed. Luard, 4:48: "Et quia in discrimine puerperii sanctam invocavit Margaretam" (And because of a crisis in childbirth she called on St. Margaret).

30 Galloway, "Writing History in England," 255; Weiler, "Matthew Paris and the Writing of History," 277.

saints, prayer, and divine reward in Paris's history. Paris is the only source to mention that Eleanor called on St. Margaret, but it is a reasonable claim, given the other evidence for the royal couple's interest in the saint and the naming of their daughter, Margaret. It is plausible that Paris recorded a contemporary narrative about the birth, publicized by Henry and Eleanor, which declared that the queen's appeal for help had been answered by the patron saint of childbirth.

The moment in Eleanor's labour when she invoked St. Margaret might also be read in the context of a broader shift in devotional practice in England. Beginning in the twelfth century, instead of making the journey to the saint's shrine when help was needed, one could make an appeal anywhere and promise future devotion if the saint delivered the desired outcome.[31] This practice of "invocation from afar" benefitted women in particular because they could travel to the shrine to give thanks after giving birth, when they would not or could not have travelled during pregnancy or labour.[32] The whole dynamic was shifted towards "thanksgiving as opposed to one of supplication" at shrines.[33] Henry and Eleanor's behaviour, the queen's supposed appeal to the saint during labour, and the paintings of St. Margaret in the king's chamber modelled contemporary spiritual practices for reproduction and fertility. When their children, Margaret and Edmund, were born in 1240 and 1245, respectively, their exemplary piety appeared to have been rewarded with divine favour.

Our Lady of Walsingham, Norfolk

Dedicated to the Virgin Mary, the shrine of Our Lady of Walsingham was not exclusively associated with fertility in the Middle Ages.[34] However, Susan Morrison argues that the shrine and the pilgrimage route leading to it were tailored specifically to female pilgrims seeking miracles related to fertility and motherhood because the route to the shrine was dominated by saints associated with milk, and culminated with the relic of the Virgin's breastmilk at Our Lady of Walsingham.[35] Mary's milk was connected in medieval

---

31 Vauchez, *Sainthood*, 453. Lewis, "Pilgrimage and the Cult of St. Katherine," 46.

32 Powell, "The Miracle of Childbirth," 797.

33 Powell, "The Miracle of Childbirth," 797.

34 There is no surviving chronicle from Our Lady of Walsingham. A study of material relating to the medieval shrine has been published: Dickinson, *The Shrine of Our Lady of Walsingham*.

35 Morrison, *Women Pilgrims*, 10, 16. See also Anne E. Bailey's work on female

thought to Christ's blood, her breasts a parallel to his wounds, and related to the image of Christ as lactating mother.[36] Morrison suggests that, to a medieval viewer, "milk signified not only femaleness, but motherhood and fertility, both symbolic and literal."[37] The shrine of Our Lady of Walsingham, and the path of smaller chapels and shrines that pilgrims passed through on the way to Walsingham, resonated with female pilgrims especially, many of whom were "on pilgrimage due to their experiences as mothers, [and] would have seen and identified with the saints depicted in churches on the way to Walsingham whose legends refer to milk and/or motherhood."[38]

Before Henry III, there is no sign of royal interest in Our Lady of Walsingham.[39] Royal pious activity included devotion to saints based on individual inclinations as much as sustaining support for preexisting connections to saints' cults and for religious institutions.[40] By the later Middle Ages, the shrine at Walsingham was a regular recipient of English royal devotion. J. C. Dickinson claims that it was Henry's influence which inspired his successors' attention to Our Lady of Walsingham; Diana Webb further suggests that Henry's attention to the shrine was either a response to contemporary trends or the creation of one, as Walsingham became a relatively popular pilgrimage destination in the late Middle Ages.[41] Although Henry's attention to the shrine seems to have inspired the spiritual practices of future kings and queens, the reason for his novel support for Our Lady of Walsingham appears to have been motivated by the shrine's contemporary reputation for fertility miracles.

Henry III's attention to Walsingham coincided with his hopes for fertility and the births of his and Eleanor's children. Beginning in the 1230s, the king visited the shrine at Our Lady of Walsingham semi-regularly until

pilgrims: Bailey, "Wives, Mothers and Widows on Pilgrimage," 197–219; Bailey, "'Flights of Distance," 292–309; Bailey, "'The Rich and the Poor,'" 9–29.

36 For the spiritual significance of milk and the comparison to Christ's blood, see: Morrison, *Women Pilgrims*, 32–33. Walker Bynum, *Jesus as Mother*; Walker Bynum, "The Body of Christ in the Later Middle Ages," 399–439; Olson, "Blood, Sweat, Tears, and Milk," 11–30.

37 Morrison, *Women Pilgrims*, 32. See also: Williamson, "The Virgin *lactans* as Second Eve," 105–38; Corrington, "The Milk of Salvation," 393–420; Phillips, "The Breasts of Virgins," 1–19.

38 Morrison, *Women Pilgrims*, 16.

39 Webb, *Pilgrimage in Medieval England*, 117; Dickinson, *The Shrine of Our Lady of Walsingham*, 17.

40 Webb, *Pilgrimage*, 116.

41 Dickinson, *The Shrine of Our Lady of Walsingham*, 17; Webb, *Pilgrimage*, 116.

1256 but after that he did not return again until just before his death in 1272.[42] The years 1236 to 1256 span exactly Henry's marriage to Eleanor of Provence, the births of their five children, and the illness, gradual decline and death of their youngest daughter in 1256 or 1257. Henry made a pilgrimage to Walsingham in June 1238, when he and Eleanor were still childless and just after this, Eleanor went on pilgrimage to Thomas Becket's tomb in Canterbury.[43] Then, two weeks after the birth of their first child, Edward, in June 1239, the couple offered a 4 lb (just under 2 kg) wax taper —generally, orders for tapers were about ½ lb (just over 220 g) of wax— "in the Church of St. Mary Walsingham to burn before the altar of St. Mary in her honour."[44] In November 1240, after Margaret's birth and Eleanor's purification, Henry ordered 1,000 lbs (just over 453 kg) of wax: half of which was to be used to make one thousand tapers for the shrine of St. Edmund, and the other half was for "the sacristan of Walsingham...to make 1000 tapers and place them in the chapel of St. Mary of Walsingham at the feast of her conception."[45] Other equally substantial gifts of wax were offered to Walsingham in 1241, 1242, and 1244; Eleanor was pregnant with the couple's third child in 1241, she gave birth to Beatrice in 1242, and they were praying for another son in 1244.[46] Henry only seems to have made this specific kind of offering to Walsingham around the births of his children.[47]

Henry's attention to Walsingham was new, but royal interest in the site became standard during the reigns of his successors; Dickinson remarks that Our Lady of Walsingham had become a shrine "of national importance"

42 Dickinson, *The Shrine of Our Lady of Walsingham*, 19.

43 Dickinson, *The Shrine of Our Lady of Walsingham*, 18.

44 *CLR*, 1:398.

45 *CLR*, 2:9.

46 *CLR*, 1:398; *CLR*, 2:9, 66, 114, 143, 245. These prayers for a son were requested from monastic men throughout the kingdom and will be discussed in the section in St. Thomas Becket, later in this chapter.

47 There was one other time when Henry made substantial offerings at Our Lady of Walsingham, when Edward was seriously ill in 1246. In January of that year, Henry ordered a golden crown for St. Mary's image at Walsingham (*CLR*, 3:18). In March, a chaplain was paid to celebrate divine service daily in the queen's chapel at Windsor (*CLR*, 3:30), cloth for St. Mary at Kaversham, the same to Fontevraud Abbey, and two copes to Westminster (*CLR*, 3:36). At same time, there was another offering to Walsingham of embroidered cloth (*CLR*, 3:37). Additionally, divine service and *salvus populi* was to be sung to "preserve the king and his household from sudden death" (*CLR*, 3:54), and tapers were to continually be burning in the chapel of Dover Castle. Finally, electuaries for king, queen and their children (*CLR*, 3:56).

by the end of the fourteenth century.[48] While Henry's practice of making offerings following the births of his children looks like thanksgiving to the shrine after praying for reproductive success, there is no sign that Edward I's patronage and pilgrimages to the shrine were motivated by fertility concerns. Rather, Edward likely supported the shrine because it had been established in royal devotional practice by his father, Henry III.[49]

Edward II and Isabella of France first visited the shrine in 1308/9, shortly after they were married, and in 1309 the Walsingham monks were granted the right to collect rents worth £40 at Queen Isabella's insistence.[50] The couple did not visit again until October 1315, at which time Isabella "seems to have outdone the king in the generosity of her oblations" to the shrine.[51] There is no further evidence of Edward and Isabella's interest in the site after 1315.[52] This early interest is notable, though. The couple's brief attention seems driven by Isabella and perhaps happened at moments when she felt pressure or concern about fertility. Isabella and Edward had been married for roughly a year by 1308/9 but Edward was focused on Piers Gaveston and neglecting Isabella and his reproductive duty as a result. Then, after having a son in 1312, Isabella probably suffered a miscarriage or stillbirth in 1313, and John was not born until August 1316, after the couple's final visit to Walsingham in 1315. English royal attention to Our Lady of Walsingham after Henry III cannot be assumed to be related to fertility. However, while it had become a normative part of royal devotion by the fourteenth century, the sporadic interest of Isabella of France does coincide in time with anxiety about the couple's fertility, experience of pregnancy loss and the period immediately preceding the conception of their second child.

There was no comparative tradition of royal patronage to Our Lady of Walsingham in fourteenth-century Scotland, making David II's two pilgrimages to the English shrine even more remarkable. The chronicler Jean Froissart spent time in Scotland with David's court and he recorded that David went on pilgrimage to Walsingham in 1363.[53] In the following year, Edward III

---

48 Dickinson, *The Shrine of Our Lady of Walsingham*, 24.

49 Webb, *Pilgrimage in Medieval England*, 122–23.

50 *CPR 1307–1313*, 156 (£40 of rents); Dickinson, *The Shrine of Our Lady of Walsingham*, 24.

51 Dickinson, *The Shrine of Our Lady of Walsingham*, 24. Quote from Webb, *Pilgrimage in Medieval England*, 130.

52 Dickinson, *The Shrine of Our Lady of Walsingham*, 24.

53 Froissart, *Chronicles of England, France, Spain*, ed. Johnes, 1:306. The point of Froissart's entry is not David's pilgrimage; the Scottish king was at Walsingham

granted David safe-conduct to make the journey to Our Lady of Walsingham again.[54] Penman suggests that David undertook these pilgrimages to Walsingham "out of genuine faith" but also as a diplomatic tool to help the negotiations with Edward III over the ransom.[55] If David's pilgrimages were intended to impress Edward and pave the way for negotiations, Walsingham is not the most obvious choice. Edward III visited Walsingham regularly in the first years of his reign, during the late 1320s and 1330s.[56] But, after 1343—still twenty years before David's first pilgrimage to Walsingham—there is no evidence of any further visits to the shrine in the remaining thirty-four years of Edward III's reign.[57] If David was hoping to appeal to Edward III by venerating his favourite saints and sites in the late 1350s and 1360s, Walsingham would have been an odd choice after 1343.

It also seems counterintuitive that David would go on pilgrimages to a shrine with targeted imagery of breastmilk, making it popular with mothers and pilgrims looking for fertility miracles, to help negotiate an agreement that depended on his dying without a biological heir. There is another explanation: David paid attention to the shrine of Our Lady of Walsingham, not to win over Edward III, as Penman suggests, but to sway the Scottish magnates. David had proposed versions of a succession-peace deal to the Scottish council at least twice by 1364, with no success, which suggests that there was real concern that he would never produce a biological heir and Scotland would one day have an English prince as their king if the deal was agreed with Edward III.[58] The sources suggest how the Scottish magnates would have known about these pilgrimages: Edward III granted safe-conduct to roughly fifty Scots (and their retinues) in 1363, around the same time that Froissart says David II was in Walsingham.[59] Travel between England and Scotland was also granted for clerics and for Scottish university students. Penman describes the men granted safe-conduct to travel to England as

---

when he apparently heard of a meeting happening in London between Peter I of Cyprus and the kings of England, France, and Denmark discussing recruitment of men for crusade.

54 *Rot. Scot.*, ed. Illingworth et al., 1:881; *Foedera*, ed. Rymer, 3.2:723; Dickson, *The Shrine of Our Lady of Walsingham*, 25; Penman, *David II*, 303, suggests that the safe-conduct in 1364 went unused.

55 Penman, "Christian Days and Knights," 256.

56 Dickinson, *The Shrine of Our Lady of Walsingham*, 24–25.

57 Dickinson, *The Shrine of Our Lady of Walsingham*, 25.

58 Penman, *David II*, 162–66.

59 *Rot. Scot.*, ed. Illingworth et al., 1:876–77.

"strong crown supporters and the core of David's chivalric cadre," as well as many of the men who the king was hoping to win over.[60] Essentially, most of David's court was granted leave to travel to England at the same time that he went on pilgrimage, and therefore would have been aware of, and perhaps even present to witness, the king's devotional activity. Making pilgrimages to Our Lady of Walsingham was an astute political move by David because it communicated to the Scottish political realm that the king was not actually happy to accept his childlessness and acknowledge an English heir by showing that he was actively seeking a remedy for fertility. His pilgrimage to the popular healing shrine, which had associations with fertility, can be interpreted, in part, as a demonstration of his commitment to remedying childlessness.

St. Katherine of Alexandria

The royals who venerated the shrine at Walsingham—David II, Henry III, and Eleanor of Provence—also showed interest in St. Katherine of Alexandria, one of the most popular and widely venerated saints in the medieval world.[61] St. Katherine had diverse roles that derived from elements of her *vita*, such as patron of scholars, as well as other associations which developed from the additions and versions of her *vita*; for instance, as a marriage-broker.[62] Generally, the versions of St. Katherine's life which circulated in the British Isles in the thirteenth and fourteenth centuries were based on the *Legenda aurea*, and the *Legenda aurea*'s source for St. Katherine's life was derived from a text that originated in Rouen, the centre of her cult in Europe, in the eleventh century.[63] The unexpanded narrative of St. Katherine's life in the *Legenda aurea* describes how, as a young queen, she defended her Christian faith against the emperor Maxentius. He arranged a debate between Katherine and fifty philosophers, and she managed to defeat and convert them. The empress and Porphirius, captain of the guard, were also inspired to convert to Christianity because of Katherine's example and they were martyred. Katherine was to be tortured

60 Penman, *David II*, 304.

61 Lewis, *The Cult of St. Katherine*, 1–2.

62 Lewis, *The Cult of St. Katherine*, 11–14; 58–60, 73. More recently, Lewis has also argued that the prose *Life* of St. Katherine contains ideologies of ideal masculinity and it appealed to medieval men in positions of authority: Lewis, "A King, Not a Servant," 397–416.

63 Lewis, *The Cult of St. Katherine*, 9.

on four nail-spiked wheels, but angels instantly destroyed the device in response to her prayers. The legend ends with St. Katherine's beheading, when milk poured from her neck instead of blood, and her body was translated to Mount Sinai.[64]

While she did have multiple associations as a patron saint, St. Katherine was not known as a saint of fertility or childbirth. St. Katherine's wide appeal likely came from her "non-specific nature" and the approach here is not to assume or push any fertility associations on the evidence.[65] However, fertility miracles were an element of St. Katherine's circulating reputation in the thirteenth and fourteenth centuries. Christine Walsh argues that St. Katherine came to have fertility associations because of the milk that flowed from her neck when she was beheaded.[66] As discussed, Morrison described the pilgrim route to Our Lady of Walsingham as the "milky way," and she notes that images of St. Katherine featured in some of the smaller chapels along the way to the relic of the Virgin's breastmilk at the shrine in Walsingham.[67] For a medieval audience, the milk in St. Katherine's *vita* conceivably led to an association with motherhood and fertility.

Furthermore, sterility miracles do appear to be part of St. Katherine's circulating image by the thirteenth century. Her cult grew in medieval Western Europe as a result of the focused promotion by the monks of Holy Trinity in Rouen, who had acquired some of her relics around 1046/7.[68] Walsh argues that the acquisition of the saint's relics was a calculated plan to fund the abbey by promoting it as a pilgrimage destination (a substantial revenue source for an abbey).[69] A text describing St. Katherine's translation and miracles was produced at the abbey in Rouen in the second half of the eleventh century and it survives in two later manuscripts.[70] This *miracula* text, which Walsh calls the Norman miracles because of its connection

64 Jacobus de Voragine, *The Golden Legend*, ed. Ryan, 720–25.

65 Lewis, *The Cult of St. Katherine*, 79.

66 Walsh, "The Role of the Normans," 27.

67 Morrison, *Women Pilgrims*, 27.

68 Walsh, "The Role of the Normans," 81.

69 Walsh, "The Role of the Normans," 27.

70 Walsh, *The Cult of St. Katherine of Alexandria*, 79. Both manuscripts are slightly different copies of an earlier text; one is from the twelfth and the other from the thirteenth century. Given the early date of the original *miracula* collection and the extant later copies which feature the same twenty-two miracles, Walsh argues that the Rouen *miracula* text of St. Katherine was relatively popular.

to Rouen, describes how St. Katherine cured several cases of sterility.[71] Walsh examined twelve other contemporary Norman miracle collections of different saints and found the *miracula* of St. Katherine to contain the highest proportion of sterility miracles, with four of the twenty-two miracles related to remedying childlessness.[72] The only other saint whose relics come close to producing cures for sterility on the scale of Katherine in Walsh's study is Vulfran, who performed just one sterility miracle.[73]

The author(s) of the Norman *miracula* had a vested interest in reporting miracles that would appeal to a lay audience, if St. Katherine's relics were to encourage interest in the abbey as a pilgrimage destination.[74] Significantly, the sterility miracles described in the Norman miracle text were all granted after the appeals of husbands. Nineteen of the total twenty-two petitioners mentioned in the text were adult men and the sterility miracles are presented "from the male point of view."[75] In the four sterility miracles, husbands seek aid from St. Katherine for their wives' childlessness, and while all four seem committed to finding a remedy and maintain hope for an heir, it is treated as if the sterility ultimately resided in their wives.[76] It is also notable that the majority of supplicants in all twenty-two miracles—when it is possible to determine—were wealthy and/or of high social status.[77] The Norman *miracula* texts shows that not only were sterility miracles part of

71 Walsh, *Cult of St. Katherine*, 79: The Norman miracles survive in Saint-Omer, BM, MS 27 (twelfth century) and Rouen, BM, MS U.22 (thirteenth century), "both contain the same basic text of Katherine's *Passio* followed by a description of the translation of relics of Katherine to Rouen (the *Translatio*) and a collection of miracles performed by her Rouen relics (the *Miracula*)." Walsh uses Rouen, BM, MS U.22 as her primary text.

72 Walsh, "The Role of the Normans," 27. For the other Norman miracle collections, see: Gonthier and Le Bas, "Analyse socio-économique," 3–36.

73 Walsh, "The Role of the Normans," 27.

74 Walsh, "The Role of the Normans," 27.

75 Walsh, *Cult of St. Katherine*, 93.

76 Walsh, *Cult of St. Katherine*, Appendix C, Miracles 3–6, pp. 175–76. See Finucane, *Miracles and Pilgrims*, for more examples of the blame for infertility being assigned to wives.

77 Walsh, *Cult of St. Katherine*, 93. See also Finucane, *Miracles and Pilgrims*, 148. Finucane identified that non-healing miracle cures recorded in miracle collections were most often for upper-class men. He also argued that medieval English women primarily visited local shrines, while it was mostly men (particularly upper-class men) who travelled further afield.

St. Katherine's reputation by the high Middle Ages, but the cures for sterility were specifically sought by elite men for their wives.[78]

Henry III and Eleanor of Provence cultivated devotion to St. Katherine from the beginning of their marriage. In 1236, the chapel near the queen's apartments at Clarendon was dedicated to St. Katherine and scenes of the saint's life were added to the walls.[79] In 1240, images of St. Katherine were installed in the church of St. Peter in the Tower of London.[80] The chapels at both Guildford and Nottingham Castle were also dedicated to St. Katherine and, in 1251, the story of St. Katherine was painted in the chapel at Guildford and on a tablet for the chapel at Nottingham Castle in 1252.[81] Notably, this work was commissioned after Henry and Eleanor experienced six to seven years of diminished fertility, with no births or evidence that they had conceived between 1245 and 1252. After installing images of St. Katherine's life in 1251 and 1252, Henry and Eleanor's fifth and final child was conceived and born in 1253 and named Katherine. The dedications and imagery of St. Katherine from the 1230s to 1250s were still there in the 1250s to 1270s, and Henry and Eleanor's devotion to St. Katherine continued after the births of

78 Walsh, "The Role of the Normans," 27, argues that because the Norman miracle collection was intended to promote the power of St. Katherine's relics, conveniently held in Rouen, "the author would have wanted to include [miracles] that would catch lay interest, [so] the collection can arguable be said to reflect lay attitudes towards Katherine's cult." The higher-than-average proportion of sterility miracles in the Norman miracles suggests that the Norman version of St. Katherine's cult propagated by the monks of Holy Trinity in Rouen was associated with sterility cures.

79 Colvin, *King's Works*, 914. There was work on the king's and queen's chambers and queen's chapel at Clarendon in 149–50: *CLR*, 3:67, 239, 296–97.

80 Borenius, "The Cycle of Images in the Palaces and Castles of Henry III," 49; Lewis, *The Cult of St. Katherine*, 64, mentions the dedications to St. Katherine in 1240 and 1252 and she suggests that the saint appealed to the couple because of her royal/noble status. I am not convinced that this fully explains the dedications, as there were some English royal saints who might have made good intercessors/patrons for Queen Eleanor. For instance, St. Edith of Wilton, who Henry did support. He sent a cloth to her shrine in 1239, for himself, Queen Eleanor and their son, Edward who was a few weeks old: *CLR*, 1:418. The images of St. Katherine from 1240 were installed alongside panels of St. Christopher, who had associations with protection against pestilence and sudden death and was often depicted with a child on his shoulder, and St. Nicholas, who was thought to protect children. This gives the sense that Henry and Eleanor were perhaps worried about the health of Prince Edward, born in 1239. Orme, *Medieval Children*, 233; Fredell, "The Three Clerks and St. Nicholas in Medieval England," 181.

81 Colvin, *King's Works*, 2:759 (Nottingham), 952 (Guildford); *Royal and Other Historical Letters*, ed. Waddington-Shirley, 67.

their children. However, the timing of the new images and dedications and the naming of their youngest daughter, after eight years of no births, suggests that Henry and Eleanor might have turned to St. Katherine for help with fertility.

There are also signs that David II venerated St. Katherine when he was concerned about childlessness. The mercat cross outside St. Giles Cathedral in Edinburgh was dedicated to St. Katherine and, in 1358, the king and Roger Hogg, an Edinburgh burgess, dedicated an altar to St. Katherine within St. Giles.[82] Penman suggests that David was also behind several other dedications to St. Katherine around the same time, including at the Dominican friary in Ayr, an altar in Holyrood, a chapel, hospital and altar in Dunfermline, an altar in Cambuskenneth, a house of the Blackfriars in Edinburgh, and the priory of Beauly.[83] There is no explicit evidence which connects David to these dedications, but his illegitimate nephew was prior of Beauly, and Dunfermline and Holyrood had long-standing royal significance and favour from Scottish medieval rulers.[84]

David II's veneration of St. Katherine seems related to remedying infertility particularly because of his connection to Rouen, the hub of St. Katherine's cult in Europe and where the *miracula* text featuring cures for sterility originated. In the 1330s, David and Joan spent seven years as guests of Philip IV at Château Gaillard in Normandy, forty kilometres from Rouen. During this time, "David seems to have found an ally in the archbishop of Rouen, Pierre Roger," later Pope Clement VI.[85] Whether David encountered the *miracula* of St. Katherine in Rouen or not, his teenage years in Normandy and his ties to the prominent Benedictine cleric Pierre Roger likely familiarized him with the St. Katherine stories told by the Benedictine monks of Holy Trinity.

Royal interest in St. Katherine fits the demographic profile of the supplicants represented in the Norman miracle collection—elite husbands seeking cures for their wives' infertility. Accepting that the timing of Henry III and Eleanor and David II's attention to St. Katherine happened at moments when they experienced concern or pressure for fertility, their interest in St. Katherine reveals a gendered approach to fertility concerns, in which the

---

82 *RRS*, ed. Webster, 6:no. 204. *CPL*, ed. McGurk, 300.

83 Penman, "Christian Days and Knights," 261n34; MacKinlay, *Ancient Church Dedications in Scotland*, 2:418 (Cambuskenneth and Dunfermline), 420 (Beauly), 424 (Holyrood and Blackfriars).

84 Penman, "Christian Days and Knights," 261.

85 Penman, "Christian Days and Knights," 253.

kings appealed to a saint who specifically cured infertile wives at the request of wealthy husbands.

This gendered dynamic extended to other "fertility saints" discussed in this section. St. Margaret supported labouring women who called on her for help and, according to Matthew Paris, Eleanor of Provence followed this practice and was duly rewarded. Pilgrimage to Our Lady of Walsingham was popular with female pilgrims praying for fertility or help for their children but, as an interesting inversion from the typical Walsingham pilgrim, it was David II and perhaps Henry III who venerated the shrine more visibly than their queens. Read together, the spiritual practices involving St. Margaret, St. Katherine, and Our Lady of Walsingham were designed to aid the queen's reproductive body and fertility problems. The king took an active role in seeking remedies and giving thanks, but crucially, these practices allowed him to address fertility concerns without admitting any bodily failing on his part.

Furthermore, David II and Henry III and Eleanor used the fertility associations of the saints and shrine discussed to control perceptions of their fertility, while also making use of the context of reproduction to communicate broader political messages. Henry III's offerings to Walsingham, with its links to female fertility and motherhood, and Eleanor of Provence's invocation of St. Margaret's name during labour displayed the couple's piety and demonstrated their divine favour through the successful births of their children. Appealing to saints like St. Margaret and making offerings at Our Lady of Walsingham also helped Henry and Eleanor control perceptions of their fertility by showing that royal reproduction was something determined by the divine and managed with pious practices. In David II's case, his pilgrimages to the shrine of Our Lady of Walsingham and interest in St. Katherine demonstrated to the political elites of Scotland that he was still intent on producing his own biological heir regardless of any succession deal he might make with Edward III.

Calling on Old Friends: Established Royal Patronage and Management of Fertility

While cultivating new relationships with institutions like Our Lady of Walsingham was usual for kings and queens, maintaining established relationships with religious institutions was also important to the practice of monarchy.[86] Being *seen* to seek saintly support was important, and who and

86 Webb, *Pilgrimage in Medieval England*, 112, 116; Blick, "King and Cleric," 187.

how you asked mattered. Pre-conquest English saints, particularly royal ones, were appealing figures for legitimizing and reinforcing dynasty and kingship in the Middle Ages, and all thirteenth- and fourteenth-century English royal couples showed their devotion by carrying out regular pilgrimages and making substantial offerings to institutions like Bury St. Edmunds, which housed the relics of St. Edmund of Anglia.[87] Another saint, St. Thomas Becket, initially posed an opportunity for anti-monarchical sentiment in the twelfth century, but was quickly co-opted as one of the preeminent royal allies and his shrine in Canterbury became a primary focus for English royal devotion.[88] It makes sense that royal couples would utilize their relationships to these saintly figures and their associated institutions when seeking spiritual support for reproduction.

Appealing to saints like St. Thomas and St. Edmund for fertility issues displayed a couple's veneration of the saints and institutions that were most politically significant to their dynasty and kingdom—an expected practice—and confirmed the favour, close relationship and power of those key saints and institutions when their prayers were answered. Due to the conspicuousness of both royal reproduction and royal devotion, this section argues that couples strategically promoted their relationships with chosen saints and institutions through their spiritual management of fertility. At the same time, as "supreme patrons" in their realms, being seen to enlist the favour of the foremost dynastic and national saints and their associated institutions when a royal couple needed assistance was an important and expected practice of monarchy.

St. Thomas Becket and Canterbury

Almost all the kings and queens discussed in this book—English and Scottish—showed devotion to St. Thomas Becket, some particularly when they were childless or looking for help with fertility. Eleanor of Provence went on a pilgrimage to Canterbury in 1237, just before Matthew Paris reported fears about her fertility after two years of childless marriage.[89] She was joined by another childless queen and her sister-in-law, Joan Plantagenet, queen of Scotland.[90] Margaret Howell declares that "there can

87 Webb, *Pilgrimage in Medieval England*, 120–21.

88 Webb, *Pilgrimage in Medieval England*, 115; Blick, "King and Cleric," 185.

89 *Chronica de Mailros*, ed. Stevenson, 148: "regina Scotiae cum regina Anglie causa orationis Cantuariam adiit" (the queen of Scotland with the queen of England went to Canterbury to pray).

90 *Chronica de Mailros*, ed. Stevenson, 148.

be little doubt as to the likely purpose of their prayers."[91] There is no contemporary explanation of the queens' purpose but the *Chronicle of Melrose* recorded that they went to Canterbury to pray and so perhaps the reason was implied by both women's childlessness.

Some couples also sent offerings to Becket's tomb and publicly called for prayers for help with fertility. With a son and two daughters, Eleanor of Provence and Henry III felt some pressure to have a second son.[92] Henry made this clear, as Matthew Paris wrote that the king requested prayers from "religious men" (not exclusively those of Canterbury) for a son in 1244.[93] Henry also ordered 1,000 ½ lb wax tapers—the same quantity that he sent to Walsingham after the births of his children—to be placed at St. Thomas's shrine at Canterbury and the same at the church of St. Augustine of Canterbury in November, "for the preservation of the health and delivery of the queen, who is with child."[94] Offerings of gold coins were sent to the churches of the Holy Trinity and St. Augustine in Canterbury at the same time too.[95] The prayers were apparently answered when Edmund was born in January 1245.

---

91 Howell, "Royal Women," 169.

92 Howell, *Eleanor of Provence*, 44. After Edward's birth in 1239, there was an order for tapers to be offered in the chapel of Caversham and in the chapel of Dover Castle (*CLR*, 1:398). The chapel at Caversham was dedicated to St. Anne, with a shrine of Our Lady. One chapel at Dover Castle was dedicated to Thomas Becket and the other to Mary. St. Anne and Mary had fertility associations, so the inclusion of St. Thomas in this instance strengthens the impression that he was also called on to support royal fertility.

93 *Historia Anglorum*, ed. Madden, 2:499. The entry is titled "The king asked for prayers that God would send him a son" (*Rex petiit orari pro eo, ut Deus sibi prolem mitteret masculinam*). In the passage, Paris says that Henry, "the lord king, most Christian of kings, requested prayers from religious men, so that God...might grant a child for the strength of the kingdom; relying on the prayers and the alms, which he had never ceased to pay" (*dominus rex, utpote regum Christianissimus, postulavit a viris religiosis orations, ut Dominus noster...prolem sibi ad regni robur conferre dignaretur; confisus orations et, quas non cessavit erogare, elemosinis*). The next chapter is titled "A son is born to the lord king, and called Edmund" (*Natus est domino regi filius, et vocatus est Edmundus*), demonstrating Paris's approval of Henry's piety, and highlighting that his prayers had been answered.

94 *CLR*, 2:275. Eleanor gave birth to Edmund in January 1245.

95 *CLR*, 2:275. Henry also ordered a golden garland to be placed at the head of St. Thomas's shrine in Canterbury in 1244. It is unclear if this reflects a specific request for help, or, as the order directs that the garland was to be placed over the altar-table "where there is a defect," a glimpse at Henry's general support of the shrine (in this case, when it required some maintenance).

In another instance, Henry sent gold coins to St. Thomas's shrine in 1251.[96] Eleanor is not known to have been pregnant in 1251, but the offering does coincide with their installation of images of St. Katherine's life in 1251 and 1252, just before the conception and birth of their last child in 1253, after eight years without any known pregnancies or successful births. Perhaps the gift of gold coins to Becket's shrine in 1251 was a plea for divine intervention in the couple's fertility.

Edward I's second queen, Margaret of France, called on St. Thomas for help during her difficult labour in 1300 and offered thanks to his Canterbury shrine after the successful birth.[97] Webb suggests that the gold coins sent by Margaret to Canterbury in gratitude following the birth had been placed on her belly as an aid during labour.[98] Edward II and Isabella of France also appealed to St. Thomas before the birth of their first child in 1312. Edward requested prayers from "our brothers, monks and priests" to the Blessed Virgin, the Holy Spirit and St. Thomas for the protection of "the queen, who is pregnant."[99]

A royal couple's offerings and requests for prayers communicated concerns about reproduction because they were witnessed by their attendants, courtiers and the religious communities who were asked to pray. Who and how the couples asked for help is particularly significant. Sarah Blick argues that English royal patronage of St. Thomas's tomb, "with the aid of the Canterbury monks, made Becket their champion and source of legitimacy."[100] Following Becket's violent martyrdom at the hands of Henry II's knights in 1170, Henry II quickly co-opted his former opponent's memory, transforming the archbishop into one of the preeminent royal allies. From this point in the twelfth century through to the Reformation, no king of England missed "the importance of as close an appreciative relationship with St. Thomas's

96 *CLR*, 3:385.

97 *Willelmi Rishanger*, ed. Riley, 438.

98 Webb, *Pilgrimage in Medieval England*, 129; Blick, "Votives, Images," 49.

99 *Concilia magnae Britanniae et Hiberniae*, ed. Wilkins, 2:421: "Edwardi, Dei gratia…ac statum dominae Isabellae reginae, quam in utero gravidam…quingentas missas concedimus celebrari per confratres nostros, et commonachos et sacerdotes; viz. centum et sexaginta missas de Spiritu Sancto, et centum et sexaginta de B. virgine, et centum et octoginta de B. Thoma martyre glorioso" (Edward, by the grace of God…for the condition of Lady Isabella, the queen, who is pregnant…we request our brothers, monks and priests to celebrate 500 masses; that is 160 masses for the Holy Spirt, 160 for the Blessed Virgin, and 180 for the glorious Blessed martyr St. Thomas).

100 Blick, "King and Cleric," 186.

community as his other commitments allowed."[101] The calls for St. Thomas's help with pregnancies and births shows how royal couples enlisted and were *seen* to enlist the support of the saints and communities whose favour was integral to the workings and identity of the medieval English monarchy. Becket's political significance, his widespread popularity in England and further afield, and the tradition of royal patronage to his shrine meant that royal couples faced some expectation to support and seek assistance from Becket and the Canterbury monks when they needed help. At the same time, appealing to St. Thomas and the Canterbury monks shared the management of royal fertility with the religious community and emphasized the spiritual nature of royal reproduction, making it a matter between anointed royals, their spiritual champion and his institution. Ultimately, when Henry III requested prayers for a successful birth, like in 1244/1245, and they were answered, it demonstrated the power and favour of both St. Thomas and his Canterbury cult.

Scottish royal interest in St. Thomas's tomb in Canterbury differed from the attention English royal couples paid to the shrine, because having St. Thomas and the monks of Canterbury onside was not fundamental to the Scottish monarchy. Nonetheless, there was a connection between the Scottish crown and St. Thomas by the thirteenth century. William the Lion had founded and dedicated Arbroath Abbey to St. Thomas in the twelfth century, and Becket's resistance against the English king, Henry II, made him an appealing figure in Scotland, particularly in the fourteenth century.[102] Canterbury was also the most popular English destination for Scottish pilgrims in the fourteenth century and fairly large numbers of Scottish pilgrims were granted safe-conduct to visit the shrine between 1357 and the late 1360s, although numbers diminished in the 1370s.[103] Alexander II had made the journey to Canterbury in 1223, two years after marrying Joan Plantagenet.[104]

101 Dobson, "The Monks of Canterbury Cathedral in the Later Middle Ages," 142.

102 Webb, *Pilgrims and Pilgrimage in the Medieval West*, 215. For Penman's analysis of Scottish interest in St. Thomas's tomb in Canterbury in the fourteenth century, and his suggestion of possible motivations for veneration: Penman, "Bruce Dynasty," 346–70.

103 Webb, *Pilgrims and Pilgrimage in the Medieval West*, 214–15. Penman, "Bruce Dynasty," 347, suggests that the increased number of Scots travelling to Canterbury in David II's reign was a reflection of the more peaceful relations between England and Scotland cultivated by David and Edward III.

104 *CDS*, ed. Bain, 1:nos. 831, 855; *CPR 1216–1225*, 338. Penman, "Bruce Dynasty," 351 asserts this was motivated by illness or fears about infertility, but he does not

And discussed above, Joan Plantagenet went on pilgrimage to Canterbury too, with Eleanor of Provence in 1237.

At the critical turning point for concerns about his childlessness, David II made his first pilgrimage to Canterbury in 1357 and gave 30*d.* in alms.[105] Over the next decade and a half, Edward III granted his requests to travel to Canterbury in July 1358, April 1363, February and November 1364, March and October 1366, January 1369 and February 1370.[106] David married Margaret Logie in 1363, and in 1366, she was granted safe-conduct in her own right to visit St. Thomas's tomb, while the royal couple was also issued a joint safe-conduct by Edward III to travel to Canterbury in 1366.[107] David's interest in St. Thomas's shrine marks the shift in his devotional behaviour at thirty-three that lasted for the rest of his life. Penman suggests that David's interest in Becket, like his visits to Our Lady of Walsingham, was an attempt to win favour with Edward III, by showing interest in one of the English king's principal saints, at a time when the Scottish king's release was being negotiated.[108] Yet this does not explain David's continuing desire for pilgrimages to Canterbury after his release was agreed in 1357.

Rather, David's new and sustained interest in Becket—precisely during the period when producing an heir was critical—suggests that the Scottish king undertook pilgrimage to remedy infertility. Becket's tomb straddled divisions: it was a shrine that "was at one and the same time the scene of great public occasions, the receptacle of opulent benefactions from the

---

explain this interpretation, nor why Alexander might have been worried about infertility so early in the marriage.

105 David II made the trip to Canterbury in September 1357, just before his return to Scotland; Balfour-Melville, *Papers Relating to the Captivity*, 21–29. David might also have gone on a pilgrimage to Canterbury in January 1357. See Penman, *David II*, 189, and accounts from David's captivity: BL, Additional MS 24512, fols. 4–6; Additional MS 24511, fols. 83–87.

106 *Rot. Scot.*, ed. Illingworth et al., 1:828, 872, 881, 887, 900, 917, 928. *Foedera*, ed. Rymer, 3.2:787. It is difficult to confirm how many of these safe conducts David actually used. Penman, *David II*, 328, 371, suggests that joint grants for David and Queen Margaret to visit Canterbury in 1364 and again in 1368 went unused. However, Penman, "The Bruce Dynasty," 363 also posits that the king went to Canterbury in February 1370 (a trip not previously noticed by historians) because he identified a gap in royal grants issued by the king during this time which suggests that David was not in Scotland. Ultimately, it is hard to trace exactly how many of the grants David (and Margaret) actually made use of but it is still significant that they made the requests.

107 *Rot. Scot.*, ed. Illingworth et al., 1:899a, 900.

108 Penman, "Christian Days and Knights," 256.

great, and a healing shrine and object of popular pilgrimage."[109] More specifically, while his shrine in Canterbury was not *primarily* a fertility shrine, pilgrims did call on Becket for help with fertility problems. In the *Miracles of St. Thomas*, recorded by William of Canterbury, women were treated for issues related to pregnancy and childbirth and cured of sterility.[110] Indeed, the comparative evidence that the English royal couples called on the saint for support for conception, pregnancy and childbirth indicates that Becket's intercession for royal fertility was already established practice by the fourteenth century.

David's repeated trips to Becket's tomb—sometimes joined by Queen Margaret—would have been witnessed or at least known by his Scottish court, many of whom shared his interest and desire for pilgrimage to Canterbury.[111] Penman's suggestion that David's attention to Becket was a political manoeuvre is apt. However, there is a more nuanced interpretation: by making annual pilgrimages to a popular and potent healing shrine, David was communicating to the Scottish council that he was *indeed* concerned about his and Margaret's childlessness and was not content to accept his apparent infertility and take an English prince as heir. This means that Becket was perhaps partly a "fertility saint" for David, but the preexisting popularity of pilgrimage to Canterbury in fourteenth-century Scotland, and the earlier royal devotion demonstrated by William the Lion, also means that David's interest was informed by preexisting connections and expectations of royal devotion that were meaningful to a Scottish audience.

St. Edmund of East Anglia and Bury St. Edmunds

Like the successes and failures of royal fertility, the spiritual practices of a royal couple were witnessed by their entourages and the religious communities involved. Sarah Blick argues that requests for prayers for the royal family's health, success in war, and remembrance of their dead served to inform "England's population ...of the initiatives of the royalty, whether military, political, or personal such as their safe travel."[112] This can be applied to royal fertility too. In spiritual efforts for royal fertility, "the point of view of the monarchy" was put before the religious communities of the

109 Webb, *Medieval European Pilgrimage*, xi.

110 *Materials for the History of Thomas Becket*, ed. Robertson, 1:264–65, 383, 469–70.

111 Webb, *Pilgrims*, 214–15.

112 Blick, "King and Cleric," 193.

realm with, for instance, Henry III's request for prayers for a son or Edward II's calls for prayers for Isabella when she was pregnant.[113] Royal couples framed their reproductive successes, failures and hopes as a spiritual matter negotiated by special saintly intercessors and the institutions associated with those saints.

One such important relationship between royalty, saint and institution was that between Henry III, St. Edmund of Anglia and his cult at Bury St. Edmunds. According to early medieval accounts, Edmund was a ninth-century king who was killed by Danish invaders. The narrative of Edmund's life was developed in the tenth century in a hagiographical account by Abbo of Fleury, which formed the basic version of Edmund's *vita* and martyrdom.[114] Although his martyrdom did not happen at Bury St. Edmunds, the saint's incorrupt body was moved from its original location to Bury St. Edmunds sometime around the early tenth century.[115] Promoted by the monks of Bury St. Edmunds and venerated as an ideal king and model Christian, St. Edmund was a versatile saint and his relics in Bury St. Edmunds became one of the most popular pilgrimage destinations in medieval England by the twelfth century.[116] A model of ideal kingship who was connected to the wealthy, East Anglian Benedictine abbey, St. Edmund was popular with medieval English royalty too; Henry II and John, Henry III's grandfather and father, had both venerated St. Edmund and shown their support for the Abbey of Bury St. Edmunds.[117]

Before the development of his devotion to St. Edward the Confessor in the mid- to late 1230s, Henry III seems to have seen St. Edmund of East Anglia as his special patron, and he continued to promote this relationship alongside the development of his veneration of the Confessor and connection to Westminster.[118] It is therefore not surprising that in 1245 Henry III and Eleanor of Provence named their second son Edmund, after the ninth-century

113 Blick, "King and Cleric," 193.

114 Bale, *St. Edmund*, 2–3.

115 Bale, *St. Edmund*, 3; Gransden, "The Cult of St. Mary"; Pinner, *The Cult of St. Edmund in Medieval East Anglia*.

116 Bale, *St. Edmund*, 4.

117 Webb, *Pilgrimage in Medieval England*, 115–19. See also, Webster, "The Cult of St. Edmund, King and Martyr, and the Medieval Kings of England," 636–51. Late medieval kings venerated St. Edmund too, particularly Richard II and Henry VI: see Geaman, "Childless Queens and Child-like Kings," 155–61; Lewis, "Edmund of East Anglia, Henry VI and Ideals of Kingly Masculinity," 158–73.

118 Webb, *Pilgrimage in Medieval England*, 118.

English king and martyr. This act of royal thanks and devotion to the saint of Bury St. Edmunds was recorded in the Abbey's institutional chronicle, and Henry III wrote to the monastery to declare the good news himself and acknowledge the saint's help. The *Bury St. Edmunds* chronicler wrote that a son was born to the king and queen and named Edmund, "after the glorious king and martyr Edmund; King Henry, in a letter...instructed Henry, abbot of Bury St. Edmunds, to announce this to his monks."[119] In this letter, written two days after Edmund's birth, Henry claimed that "our consort Queen Eleanor was labouring in distress, and was delivered of her sorrow by the playing of the antiphon of St. Edmund."[120] He also wrote: "and you know that just as you asked us, if memory recalls, we have named our son Edmund."[121] Henry's letter attests to St. Edmund's potency as intercessor and his favour for Henry and Eleanor, while demonstrating his and Eleanor's faith in and relationship with the monks of Bury St. Edmunds, one of the richest and most influential medieval English abbeys. The *Bury* chronicler's mention of the letter decisively confirms that it was *their* saint who had aided the royal birth, which reinforced the mutually beneficial relationship between Bury St. Edmunds and the monarchy.

Henry's letter of declaration to the abbey that it was St. Edmund who had aided the birth indicates that he meant this to be known by the Bury St. Edmunds community and probably more widely through the religious houses of England; the *Bury St. Edmunds* chronicler even mentions that Henry asked the abbot to share the news with the other monks (perhaps knowing the news would soon trickle through to other institutions?). Henry's letter and its preservation in the chronicle indicate how the context of a royal birth allowed a royal couple to demonstrate their piety and show that *they* had special saintly favour on their side, while simultaneously fulfilling the expectations of their role as supreme religious patrons in the realm. The pressure of this relationship meant that the royal couple acknowledged and reaffirmed their support and relationship with Bury St. Edmunds and St. Edmund through the spiritual thanksgiving for the conception and successful birth of their longed-for second son.

---

119 *Chronicle of Bury St. Edmunds*, ed. Gransden, 13.

120 The letter (dated January 18, 1245) is printed in Arnold, *Memorials of St. Edmunds Abbey*, 3:28: "laborante dilecta consorte nostra Æ[lianora] regina nostra tristitia pariendi, fecimus pro ea psallere antiphonam de sancto Edmundo."

121 Arnold, *Memorials of St. Edmunds Abbey*, 3:28: "Et sciatis quod sicut nos ipsi rogastis, si memoriter retinetis, faciemus ad ipsum filium nostrum, Edmundum nuncupari."

Royal couples confirmed their relationships with important dynastic saints and displayed their support for certain religious institutions by turning to these entities to support fertility. This communicated a powerful message about the special relationship between royals and the divine when they had a child, as well as exhibiting the power of their chosen saint and bolstering the standing of the institutions that managed the saints' cults. Scottish royal devotion to St. Thomas Becket seems to have been influenced by contemporary devotional practices, given the veneration of Becket in Scotland and the popularity of his Canterbury shrine with Scottish pilgrims in the thirteenth and fourteenth centuries. The evidence for appeals to St. Thomas and the monks of Canterbury by English royal couples suggests that royal devotional practices for reproduction were shaped by contemporary expectations of royal patronage too. In England, kings and queens seeking spiritual intercession enlisted (or at least were seen to enlist) the support of Becket, St. Edmund, and their associated institutions because of their political significance and preeminence in existing royal devotional practices. Notably, the evidence of English queens' devotion to important saints for help in the reproductive process highlights the political communication inherent in the spiritual management of royal fertility. As a new queen, Margaret of France's appeal to St. Thomas Becket for support during the birth of her first child with Edward I was a clear display of her commitment to her new marital land and role, as she embraced (and was seen to receive the favour) of such a critically important and popular English saint.

Building Connections: New Saints for Royal Fertility

Royal couples sometimes turned to saints and institutions with no established royal connections nor contemporary fertility associations, yet these devotional practices can still be interpreted as part of their spiritual management of reproduction. Indeed, it was Henry III's newfound interest in St. Edward the Confessor in the mid-1230s that suggested the connection between the king's age, behaviours, and concern about childlessness.[122] Here, the following discussion argues that Henry III and Eleanor of Provence called on Edward the Confessor and another new saintly interest, Edmund of Abingdon, as part of their spiritual management of fertility, while some Scottish royal interest in St. Edward and St. Edmund can also be interpreted as spiritual support for fertility. More than just practices for boosting

122 See Chapter 4.

fertility, though, royal couples negotiated perceptions of their fertility with these devotional practices and, ultimately, they used this management of reproduction as political communication.

St. Edward the Confessor and St. Joseph

Henry III's devotion was the origin point for English royal patronage of St. Edward the Confessor and his cult based at Westminster. The beginning of Henry's focused promotion of St. Edward's cult between 1235 and 1238 coincided with the first years of his marriage to Eleanor of Provence and the concerns about the couple's childlessness, suggesting that Henry was looking to the Confessor to help support fertility. However, the Confessor was not a "fertility saint" so to speak; he seems like a paradoxical choice for encouraging Henry III's fertility, as a king whose reputedly chaste marriage and resulting childlessness led to his sanctity and canonization.[123] Henry's devotion to St. Edward and his longstanding support for the cult based at Westminster also cannot be interpreted as spiritual therapy for fertility in every instance; Henry's veneration of the Confessor lasted throughout his reign. Yet, Henry's behaviour in the mid-1230s hints at a connection between his veneration of St. Edward and his childlessness at that point. The evidence suggests that St. Edward was something more complex for Henry than a mere spiritual intercessor for fertility. Rather, the Confessor also provided an alternative model of kingship for Henry III, one without biological fatherhood, if his new royal marriage proved infertile.[124]

From 1236, there was an interesting pairing of images of St. Edward and St. Katherine of Alexandria in Henry and Eleanor's royal residences and chapels.[125] When St. Edward was painted in the chapel of All Souls at Clarendon in 1236, St. Katherine was painted in Eleanor's private chapel there, too.[126] In 1251, an image of St. Edward was painted in the chapel of St. Katherine at Guildford, at the same time that the scenes of Katherine's life were added

123 Wogan-Browne, "The Apple's Message," 40–41, writes that Edward was "a saint particularly associated with cures of blindness." Huntington, "Edward the Celibate, Edward the Saint," 119–39.

124 See Katherine Lewis's argument about Richard II's devotion to Edward the Confessor: Lewis, "Becoming a Virgin King," 86–100.

125 Lewis, *The Cult of St. Katherine of Alexandria*, 65: There was a connection made between the two saints, as the Confessor was supposed to have brought back a relic of St. Katherine (oil from her thumb) to Westminster Abbey during his reign.

126 Colvin, *King's works*, 2:914. For more details on the queen's chapel, *CLR*, 3:67, 239, 296–97.

around the altar.[127] When the story of St. Katherine was added in the chapel of St. Katherine in Nottingham Castle in 1252, the story of St. Edward was painted in the king's chapel there.[128] These pairings happened at two significant points for Henry and Eleanor's fertility. In 1236 they were concerned about childlessness and, by 1251–1252, despite producing four children by 1245, they had not conceived a child in six or seven years. If, when Henry and Eleanor were childless, St. Edward was a figure for Henry to identify with, an alternative model for his own rule if the royal marriage did turn out to be infertile, perhaps the pairing of St. Katherine with the Confessor in the late 1230s was a similar cultivation of an alternative royal model for Queen Eleanor, should she need it. From the evidence of the images and royal chapel dedications to St. Katherine, Lewis has argued that the saint, royal herself, was considered a fitting patron and a figure for young Queen Eleanor to identify with.[129] Not only royal, St. Katherine was also associated with milk, a symbol of motherhood and fertility. Henry's promoted connections to St. Edward and St. Katherine look like a response to concerns about childlessness because both saints supplied the royal couple with alternatives to biological reproduction that could be used to ennoble their childlessness.

Henry III looked to another saintly alternative to biological fatherhood too. In February 1238, he had the history of St. Joseph painted on the back of his seat in the small chapel at Westminster.[130] In the same period as the pairing of St. Edward and St. Katherine's images, Henry had St. Joseph depicted again in the new chapel at Winchester in 1250.[131] St. Joseph became associated with fatherhood and masculinity in the later Middle Ages but his cult did not yet have a devotional focal point in the thirteenth century and veneration of Christ's adopted father was not common.[132] Despite this devotional ambiguity, the depiction of the saint on Henry III's chair is interesting and seems distinctly designed to be seen. Westminster was a central hub of Henry's court and government so the image would be widely and regularly viewed, while the choice of its placement on his seat makes the association

127 Colvin, *King's Works*, 2:759.

128 Borenius, "The Cycle of Images," 48–49.

129 Lewis, *The Cult of St. Katherine*, 63–64.

130 Borenius, "The Cycle of Images," 43.

131 *CLR*, 3:325.

132 Sheingorn, "Constructing the Patriarchal Parent," 171–72; Dzon, "Joseph and the Amazing Christ-Child,"135–57; Payan, "Paternité de Joseph et filiation du Christ," 383–92.

between the king and Joseph strikingly personal, particularly when the king sat on his chair.[133] Perhaps Henry was reminding his court—and himself—that childlessness was not always permanent or, depending on the associations attached to St. Joseph, he may have been cultivating another model of masculinity that did not rely on producing biological children.

Like the Scottish royal devotion to St. Thomas, royal attention to St. Edward the Confessor had a different meaning in Scotland. Rather than offering an alternative to royal reproduction, St. Edward emphasized the royal lineage of Alexander II and Joan Plantagenet's future children. The dedication of Balmerino Abbey to St. Edward by Alexander II and his mother, Ermengarde, in the late 1220s was unusual.[134] Matthew Hammond argued that despite Alexander II's official involvement, Balmerino was really his mother's institution, and she chose to dedicate the abbey to St. Edward to emphasize the significance of Alexander and Joan's marriage and to encourage their fertility with St. Edward's support.[135] Edward the Confessor was the last king of England from the ancient line of Alfred and, after his death, the bloodline was preserved through his great-niece, Margaret.[136] Margaret became queen of Scotland after marrying Malcolm III, and so her descendants—including Alexander II—had royal Anglo-Saxon ancestry.[137] Association with the saint-queen, Margaret, would have highlighted the Scottish kings' lineage and their claim to the English throne (and intimated that the Norman kings of England were usurpers). When considering Balmerino's dedication St. Edward, it is important to note that St. Margaret of Scotland was not canonized until 1250 and so she was not an official option for dedication in the 1230s when Balmerino was founded.[138]

The dedication of the new Cistercian abbey of Balmerino to St. Edward distinctly emphasized the re-joining of a branch with the trunk of the

133 Richardson, "Gender and Space," 155, suggests that images on seats indicated a personal identification with that saint.

134 Discussed earlier, in Chapter 1 and Chapter 3. Hammond, "Queen Ermengarde," 9, 15.

135 Hammond, "Royal and Aristocratic Attitudes," 76–77; Oram, *Alexander II*, 134, agrees with Hammond.

136 Hammond, "Queen Ermengarde," 5.

137 Hammond, "Queen Ermengarde," 5. The prophesy of the branches being reunited with the tree in Aelred of Rievaulx's *vita* of the Confessor had already been realized once, by the thirteenth century, when St/Queen Margaret's daughter Matilda married Henry I of England.

138 Hammond, "Queen Ermengarde," 3.

ancient royal Alfredic line. The choice of St. Edward communicated the dynastic significance of Alexander and Joan's future children, who would link the Scottish and English royal families, and highlighted the significance of the royal couple's fertility and the noble lineage of their future children. The Scottish royal devotion to St. Edward in the thirteenth century communicated the standing and royal prestige of Alexander II and Joan's offspring, the next kings of Scotland, rather than specifically trying to remedy a fertility problem. Indeed, this aligns with Alexander II's efforts in the 1220s–1230s to elevate the office of Scottish kingship; for instance, his attempt to secure papal approval for the anointment of Scottish kings in the coronation ceremony, akin to the English and French rites. Ultimately, the Scottish dedication to St. Edward intimates a focus on progeny, the future, and dynasty in the 1220s–1230s.

St. Edmund of Abingdon

When Eleanor of Provence gave birth to Edmund in 1245, and Henry III sent the letter of thanks to Bury St. Edmunds to acknowledge St. Edmund of East Anglia's help and favour, he also gave £10 to "two sisters who brought the pall of St. Edmund to Westminster against the queen's delivery."[139] Another St. Edmund, not the king and martyr of East Anglia, but an archbishop of Canterbury, Edmund of Abingdon had died in Pontigny in 1240 and his relics very quickly developed a reputation for healing miracles.[140] After his death, Edmund's pall, or perhaps cloak, was sent to his two sisters, nuns at Catesby Priory, and it is seemingly this other St. Edmund's cloth that is referred to in the liberate rolls and brought to Eleanor of Provence in 1245.[141] In contrast to the narrative portrayed by Henry's letter, which reinforced the importance of Bury St. Edmunds and its relationship with the monarchy, the chancery accounts suggest that it was the pall of St. Edmund of Abingdon that had helped the queen in labour. The importance of reinforcing existing royal connections to saints and institutions as a part of royal patronage explains Henry's letter to Bury St. Edmunds, but why would the queen call for Edmund of Abingdon's cloak to aid childbirth?

The nature of St. Edmund of Abingdon's sainthood and popularity is the key to understanding why his cloak was used during Eleanor's labour.

139 *CLR*, 2:284. The order is dated January 14, 1245, two days before Edmund's birth.

140 Creamer, "St. Edmund of Abingdon and Henry III," 129–30.

141 Creamer, "Edmund of Abingdon and Henry III," 130.

Edmund, as archbishop of Canterbury, had married Henry and Eleanor in 1236. However, relations between the king and archbishop soured when Edmund criticized royal power and opposed Henry's involvement in church affairs and interference in episcopal elections, and they were still at odds when Edmund died in 1240.[142] After Edmund's death, his royal opposition became foundational in the narrative of his sanctity. Versions of his *vita* composed in the 1240s modelled him after St. Thomas Becket, both in his conflict with the king, and his death at Pontigny.[143] Joseph Creamer argued that St. Edmund's resemblance to Becket was due to the efforts of English bishops who weaponized his image to oppose the king's power in disputes with Henry III in the early 1240s.[144] In fact, contrary to the hagiographical narrative, Edmund was not exiled by Henry III in 1240.[145] However, the narrative of royal opposition served the bishops in the 1240s when they made claims that the king had violated the terms of *magna carta*.[146]

Edmund was not canonized until 1246, but there were reports of miracles at his tomb as early as 1241.[147] Indeed, Matthew Paris described how Eleanor and Henry's own physician, Nicholas of Farnham, was finally cured from an illness in 1244 (before Edmund was canonized) after drinking holy water containing preserved trimmings from Edmund's beard.[148] Furthermore, Paris also wrote a *vita* of St. Edmund around 1247–1253, and he includes the bequest of Edmund's cloak to Catesby Priory.[149] Paris's *vita* mentions that Edmund's relics at Catesby developed a reputation for miracles.[150] With the growing reputation for miracles and sanctity associated with Edmund of Abingdon by the mid-1240s, Henry III likely feared a threat to his kingship similar to that posed by Becket to Henry II in the twelfth century.[151]

---

142 Howell, *Eleanor of Provence*, 1.

143 Creamer, "Edmund of Abingdon and Henry III,"136. For discussion of the *vitae*, see Lawrence, *St. Edmund of Abingdon*, 30–104.

144 Creamer, "Edmund of Abingdon and Henry III," 133; 136.

145 Lawrence, St. *Edmund of Abingdon*, 168–82; Creamer, "Edmund of Abingdon and Henry III," 132.

146 Creamer, "Edmund of Abingdon and Henry III,"134–39.

147 *Chronica de Mailros*, ed. Stevenson, 151; *Chron. Bower*, ed. Watt, 5:189–91; *Chronica majora*, ed. Luard, 4:103, 324; Lawrence, *St. Edmund of Abingdon*, 270, 279.

148 *Chronica majora*, ed. Luard, 4:330.

149 Lawrence, *St. Edmund of Abingdon*, 70–100, esp. 99–100.

150 Lawrence, *St. Edmund of Abingdon*, 270 and 278.

151 Creamer, "St. Edmund of Abingdon and Henry III," 138–39.

Like the letter to Bury St. Edmunds, Edmund of Abingdon's assistance in Eleanor's labour was still clearly intended to be witnessed: the evidence comes from a substantial £10 gift of thanks sent by the king to the two sisters who delivered St. Edmund's cloak to the queen and the order was enrolled in the official account of court expenses. As mentioned, Paris's *vita* of St. Edmund mentions the bequest of the cloak to Catesby, so an association between St. Edmund's cloak and Catesby Priory existed by at least the late 1240s or early 1250s. It is plausible that the royal use of the cloak in 1245 was the beginning of a trend and conditioned Paris's *vita* of St. Edmund written a few years later. The miracle-working of St. Edmund's cloak at Catesby was at least part of the saint's contemporary circulating image when Paris composed the *vita*. Most significantly and indicated by Paris's text, the Catesby connection would have been known to the bishops and churchmen who promoted the saint's cult in the early 1240s and used his image to oppose the king's power. Significantly, they would have recognized the significance of the king and queen's devotional behaviour when Eleanor had the cloak delivered to her in 1245.

The pregnancy in 1245, on the eve of St. Edmund's canonization in 1246, presented Henry and Eleanor with an opportunity to co-opt a new and problematic saint as a spiritual supporter.[152] Showing that Eleanor had used Edmund's cloak to aid in labour demonstrated both royal devotion and saintly favour and limited the opportunity for Edmund of Abingdon to be venerated as an opponent to the English crown, becoming a second Becket in both his martyrdom *and* royal devotion. In this instance, childbirth and the name of the infant enabled the king to control the narrative and declare his relationship with St. Edmund of Abingdon, while at the same time conveniently still confirming the favour of the royal saint and institution of Bury St. Edmunds too.

Queen Margaret, Henry and Eleanor's daughter, and her husband, Alexander III of Scotland, also venerated relics of St. Edmund of Abingdon. A late thirteenth-century inventory from Edinburgh Castle and Holyrood includes, among several valuable objects, a "box of silver-gilt and gems containing part of the Holy Cross and many small relics of the confessor St. Edmund, in a burse bearing the arms of the kings of France, with other relics which that king sent to Alexander king of Scotland."[153] Penman suggests that Louis

152 In 1249, Henry ordered an image of "St. Edmund of Pontigny" to be added in his chapels at both Cliff and Guildford: *CLR*, 3:248; Colvin, *King's Works*, 2:969; Creamer, "St. Edmund and Henry III," 130.

153 *CDS*, ed. Bain, 5:no. 494: the other objects were a "papal golden rose, the 'Blak

IX perhaps sent relics of St. Edmund of Abingdon to Alexander II in 1247, after the saint was canonized in 1246 and his remains translated to Pontigny Abbey in 1247.[154] Or, alternatively, the relics might have been gifted by Louis IX at a later date, perhaps after peace talks with Henry III in 1259–1260.[155] Penman proposes that the Scottish royal interest in St. Edmund stemmed from the overlap of St. Edmund's feast days with the festivals of St. Margaret of Scotland.[156] St. Margaret's feasts were June 10 or 19, and November 16, while St. Edmund's were June 9 and November 16.[157] This overlap, while convenient, does not explain Alexander III and Margaret's interest in St. Edmund entirely. St. Margaret was canonized in 1250 and so her feast days were marked by the Scottish monarchy from at least that point.[158]

There is another explanation for Scottish interest in St. Edmund of Abingdon: it was inspired by Henry III and Eleanor of Provence's devotion in 1245. If relics were in Scotland by 1247, they would have been sent to Alexander II. Yet, his interest in the contemporary English saint seems less likely, especially since he had remarried after Joan's death in 1238 to a French noblewoman, Marie de Coucy. Penman also reasons that it was almost certainly Alexander III and Margaret who were the owners and chief devotees

---

Rude' of St. Margaret and another bejewelled 'crux Sancte Elene de Scoc.'" Also noticed by Penman, "Royal Piety," 24.

154 Penman, "Royal Piety," 24.

155 Penman, "Royal Piety," 25.

156 Penman, "Royal Piety," 25.

157 Penman, "Royal Piety," 25.

158 Penman, "Royal Piety," 25. St. Margaret (along with "devout and respectable women") is also credited with delivering a woman's long-dead fetus, so there is some association with reproduction in her *miracula*: see Barlett, *The Miracles of St. Æbbe of Coldingham and St. Margaret of Scotland*, 80–83. Intriguingly, Barlett, *The Miracles of St. Æbbe of Coldingham and St. Margaret of Scotland*, 87–89 (no. 7), notes that possibly around 1263 St. Margaret of Scotland's "serk began to be used as a birthing shirt for Scottish queens in labour." I have not found any other evidence for this, but the suggestion indicates that St. Margaret was venerated in her own right (to aid royal reproduction/fertility!) by that point. By the fifteenth century, Scottish queens associated St. Margaret of Scotland with protection in childbirth, perhaps conflating her with her namesake, St. Margaret of Antioch. Both Mary of Guelders and Margaret Tudor used her shirt, or "serk" as an aid during labour. In 1566, Mary, Queen of Scots requested that relics of St. Margaret be taken from Dunfermline Abbey to Edinburgh, to assist her during the birth of her son: see Lee, "The Miracles and Cult of St. Margaret," 3. Lee also notes that late medieval Scottish queens (Elizabeth de Burgh and Annabella Drummond) gave birth at Dunfermline, perhaps indicating their desire to be close to the saint's relics and tomb for protection during labour.

of St. Edmund's relics.[159] The later arrival date of 1259–1260 also connects Henry III to the relics, if they came to Scotland via his meeting with Louis IX. Perhaps it was his influence that caused the relics to be sent to his daughter and son-in-law. It is tempting to relate the gift of the relics—given Eleanor of Provence's use of St. Edmund's cloak in childbirth—to Alexander III and Margaret's fertility because the queen would have been pregnant with the couple's first child (born in early 1261), or perhaps hoping to conceive, when the relics arrived in Scotland. It is possible that after Henry III and Eleanor's use of St. Edmund's cloak in 1245, their daughter was sent the same saint's relics for support during her pregnancy and childbirth.

Margaret and Alexander III's possession of St. Edmund's relics also displayed a significant political message. Beginning with their wedding in 1251, their marriage forged peace between England and Scotland. Penman argues that "the convergence of observation" of the Scottish veneration of St. Margaret and the English interest in Edmund of Abingdon "probably provided strong common ground for the Scottish and English monarchies."[160] Alexander and Margaret certainly promoted a closer relationship with the English court, and the Scottish king and queen made more regular visits to England than other Scottish royal couples.[161] On these visits, Alexander III witnessed and participated in Henry III's devotional practices and almsgiving on several occasions, and was perhaps inspired by Henry's influence and example of piety.[162] More than just a convenient overlap with their observance of St. Margaret's feast days, Alexander III and Margaret's veneration of St. Edmund of Abingdon, perhaps an effort to aid fertility, was also an expression of the closer ties with the English monarchy and Margaret's parents, Henry III and Eleanor of Provence.

* * *

Royal devotional activity was a powerful platform through which, as Blick puts it, "the point of view of the monarchy was repeatedly put before the populace," with religious images, pilgrimages to sites and requests for prayers from religious communities.[163] This conspicuousness was significant; royal couples communicated their initiatives, both personal and political, with

159 Penman, "Royal Piety," 24.

160 Penman, "Royal Piety," 25.

161 Penman, "Royal Piety," 23.

162 Penman, "Royal Piety," 23.

163 Blick, "King and Cleric," 193.

their devotional practices. Equally conspicuous was a royal couple's production of children. The mixed evidence of royal spiritual practices for fertility—attention to fertility saints, as well as saints and institutions with longstanding royal connections, and those without preexisting royal *or* fertility associations—suggests that royal couples used the context of reproduction to reinforce important messages.

Through their spiritual practices, royal couples also controlled how their fertility was perceived. Showing attention to saints and institutions with preexisting royal connections to aid fertility framed royal childlessness and fertility concerns as spiritual issues with spiritual cures. Compared to the evidence for royal medical care, the spiritual practices for aiding reproduction, because of the nature of royal religious patronage and piety, were more visible to greater numbers of the population (and, therefore, also to modern historians); they were, at least, visible to the institutions who received the offerings, said the prayers or were visited by the kings and queens on pilgrimage. Notably, the spiritual practices seem to distance royal reproduction from the biological process and portray it as a matter between the royal couple, important religious institutions and their saints, which ultimately reinforced the unique (and elevated) relationship between anointed rulers and the divine.

Royal spiritual practices for fertility highlight the nature of another relationship, between rulers, religious institutions and the wider population. The requests for prayers for reproductive success or for the queen and infant's health gave others a role in managing royal fertility too. In work on an early modern French king, Henri III, Penny Roberts argues that Henri and Queen Louise's public processions, masses, and requests for prayers for a son and heir "simultaneously spread the responsibility for resolving the monarch's infertility, and underlined that this was a public issue."[164] In a similar way, requesting prayers for a son (as Henry III did) or asking the whole religious community of the realm to pray for the health of a pregnant queen (as Edward II did for Isabella) assigned a task in the management of royal fertility to the monks and whoever heard and participated in their prayers. This placed the success of royal fertility on the behaviours of others and not just on the royal couple.

The spiritual practices for supporting royal fertility were also gendered. The finding about the queens' influence over medical care in royal households operates in the inverse way in this chapter; the queens do not seem to

164 Roberts, "Sterility and Sovereignty," 161.

have determined which saints were called on for help with fertility. Eleanor of Provence, Eleanor of Castile, Isabella of France, and Margaret of France were not English and, with the exception of Margaret Logie, the queens of Scotland were either English or French princesses. There is no sign that the queens of England promoted any saints from their natal lands. In fact, Webb argues that English queens' "homage to the saints of their adoptive kingdom" was politically crucial, particularly because many English queens were French by birth and relations between England and France were often strained in the thirteenth and fourteenth centuries.[165] Margaret of France, Edward I's second wife, offers a good example of this dynamic when she called on St. Thomas Becket for support during childbirth. This does not seem to have been because of any preexisting personal devotion to Becket, and she had been in England for less than a year when her first child was born, making it unlikely that she developed that devotion in such a short time. Margaret's appeal to Becket, like other English queens' adoption of the devotional practices and saintly intercessors of their marital land in support of reproduction and fertility, highlights how both royal reproduction and spiritual practices were politically charged undertakings. It also underlines how a new queen could communicate politically significant messages about her identity and loyalties through her choice of spiritual intercessors for fertility.

Some of the queens of Scotland, on the other hand, seem to have inspired or at least maintained some devotion to the saints of their homeland. Joan Plantagenet, Margaret of England, and Joan of the Tower were all English princesses. Joan Plantagenet travelled to Canterbury on pilgrimage, Margaret had relics of St. Edmund of Abingdon, and Balmerino Abbey was dedicated to St. Edward the Confessor, a distinctly English royal saint, when Alexander II was married to Joan Plantagenet. This attention to English saints can be explained by the nature of the relationship between England and Scotland. In England, there was particular criticism of foreign queens, and it was dangerous for a queen to seem more foreign—particularly French—than English when France was often at political odds with England in the thirteenth and fourteenth centuries. However, devotion to English saints by Scottish royalty helped to forge closer ties with the English monarchy, already linked by familial bonds, and promoted more peaceful relations between the two kingdoms. This benefited the political aims of Alexander II, Alexander III, and David II, all of whom pursued peaceful initiatives with

165 Webb, *Pilgrimage in Medieval England*, 129.

the English (at least for a time), including their marriages to daughters and sisters of English kings.

The gendering of the spiritual practices for fertility is also apparent in how the king and the queen were involved in the therapies. Like the traces of medical treatment, the focus is squarely on treating the queen's body; the king's body is never the object nor explicit recipient of spiritual aid for fertility. The requests for prayers for the pregnant queen's health, the calls for saintly intercession during labour, and seeking support from "fertility saints" like St. Margaret were all efforts directed at the queen's body, whether the king or queen initiated the action. It was also the queen's body where the successes and failure of royal reproduction were observed, where the prayers for a son were answered and which needed help from St. Margaret and St. Edmund during labour. Morrison states that the production of family was centred on the woman's fertile body, and "if this body could not function properly—if it were sterile, if the child it carried miscarried, if the child it carried died or was sickly, if the body could not heal after birth, if the body could not produce milk to feed the child—then the body...needed to be cured."[166] Morrison asserts that to treat and heal a woman's body was to heal the family, and so a woman's body symbolized "the state of her family's health."[167] In the same way, to manage royal fertility was to treat the queen's body, and the queen's body symbolized not just her family's health but the stability of the realm.

The locus of reproduction might be the female body, but both husband and wife, king and queen, felt the impact of childlessness. In the early modern English context, Daphna Oren-Magidor describes how a wife's "barren" body caused social shame for the husband too, as it showed that he was also being punished by God.[168] Or, a husband could be punished for his sinful behaviour by his wife's body being made infertile.[169] Of the cases discussed in this chapter, Henry III's spiritual practices related to fertility do suggest

166 Morrison, *Women Pilgrims*, 3.

167 Morrison, *Women Pilgrims*, 3.

168 Oren-Magidor, *Infertility in Early Modern England*, 86.

169 Oren-Magidor, *Infertility in Early Modern England*, 86. There is an early medieval example of this too: Pope Nicholas I, in a letter to Lothar II and Theutberga in the ninth century, wrote that Theutberga's supposed sterility was caused by Lothar's wickedness rather than any "infertility of the body." See Mistry, "Ermentrude's Consecration (866)," 577; Airlie, "Private Bodies and the Body Politic in the Divorce Case of Lothar II," 3–38; Stone and West, *The Divorce of King Lothar and Queen Theutberga*, 1–80; esp 6–7, 78.

that he shared the social burden of reproductive pressure with Eleanor, but it was still her body where reproduction happened, fertility was witnessed, and cures took place. Moreover, Henry's interest in St. Joseph and Edward the Confessor skirted around any issue with *his* reproductive body and presented royal childlessness and fatherhood as a divine decision and even a reflection of sanctity. This distinction aligns with broader societal understanding and practices which associated fertility, or the creation of "family," with the female body.

REPRODUCTIVE OUTCOMES

CONCLUSIONS ABOUT THE PRESSURE FOR ROYAL FERTILITY

THE FERTILITY CONCERNS and reproductive difficulties faced by the royal couples examined in this book have remained largely unstudied, in part because their experiences do not fit within the narrow definition of "infertility" as the inability to conceive. This study has highlighted the diversity of reproductive difficulties beyond childlessness and argued that such difficulties were more commonly experienced by medieval royal couples than has previously been recognized. By taking a more expansive approach to studying fertility and reproduction in history, the chapters asked what raised contemporary concerns about a royal couple's fertility? How, when and why did royal couples experience pressure to be fertile? How did couples react to pressure and concerns about their fertility? Were the practices for managing reproduction gendered? The indications that all of the royal couples considered here encountered some kind of reproductive concern, whether mentioned by their contemporaries or pieced together from the patterns and evidence of their lives, suggest that managing fertility was an intrinsic part of medieval rulership and integral to perceptions of kingship and queenship.

While the evidence showed that kings *and* queens shouldered the responsibility for remedying and encouraging fertility, attention to royal fertility was certainly gendered in the narrative sources. Medieval chroniclers concentrated explicitly on the queen when writing about royal reproduction. The most striking example was Matthew Paris's report of fears that Eleanor of Provence was barren at the age of fourteen, while the accusations by two different chroniclers that Yolande de Dreux and Margaret Logie had pretended to be pregnant in order to secure their futures hinged on the perceived importance of fertility for queens, and showed, ultimately, how infertility might be weaponized against them. The importance of fertility and risk of infertility communicated in these accounts was also highly gendered; the chroniclers carefully passed over implicating the kings in the queens' deception and spared them blame for the consequences of royal childlessness, whether the succession crisis of the early 1290s or the end of David II and Margaret's marriage. Crucially, a fake pregnancy was a gendered accusation used by chroniclers against queens, which shows how infertility could cost the queen her position but not the king his.

Yet, this is not the entire picture. By keeping the focus on royal couples, rather than queens in isolation, it was possible to uncover the gendered divisions in the management of fertility by medieval queens *and* kings. While the chronicles only really mentioned royal fertility in relation to queens and, in some cases, even reduced queens to their reproductive role, what they wrote about fertility was still shaped by their perceptions of the king. The way that the chronicles handled David II's adultery or described Edward II's favouritism of Piers Gaveston demonstrates that childlessness was certainly not seen as unilaterally the queen's fault. Chroniclers emphasized Isabella of France's fertility in the 1310s as a way to reconstruct her gendered image after her part in the deposition of her husband in 1326, but chroniclers' descriptions of Edward II's neglect of his wife and failure to secure the succession in the 1310s also indicated his poor kingship. Fertility or, at the very least, producing an heir, was a critical part of both good queenship and good kingship. Not only were chroniclers still thinking about kings while writing about queens' fertility, but it was the king's age, in relation to his masculine identity, which led to the problematization of a couple's childlessness, despite what the explicit comment on a queen's fertility by Matthew Paris might incline us to presume.

If the degree of scrutiny of the queen's fertility—recorded by Paris—was triggered by the king's age and need for an heir, queens nonetheless did have influence and agency in the management of royal health and fertility. The connections and origins of the medical practitioners who served royal households indicate that queens, such as Eleanor of Provence and Eleanor of Castile, chose practitioners from their natal lands to provide healthcare for the royal family. The queens' role in the transmission of medical texts should not be underestimated either; the analysis of Chapter 5 placed medical texts in the proximity of royal couples based on the queens' connections. Moreover, medieval understandings of the gestational period, and reproduction more generally, gave queens like Margaret Logie and Yolande de Dreux some influence as potential mothers of heirs in a time of "unpregnancy," before it was possible to know—for the queens themselves but also, for instance, the nobles waiting at Stirling for a royal birth in 1286—whether they were pregnant.

In a different way, the matter of public knowledge ran through royal couples' efforts to aid fertility. The spiritual practices for fertility entailed forms of powerful political communication because of the conspicuousness of royal fertility *and* piety. These communications both displayed concerns and sought to control perceptions of royal fertility, like David II's attention to the shrines in Walsingham and Canterbury. In David's case, his piety demonstrated to the Scottish magnates that he was still committed to producing his own biological heir. In other instances, like Eleanor of Provence's request for St. Edmund of Abingdon's cloak as an aid in childbirth, the context of the queen's labour was used to control the narrative around a figure with a growing reputation for sanctity and an image which was being deployed to oppose Henry III's kingship. These findings do not ignore that royal couples called on trusted saintly intercessors and institutions in genuine faith to remedy their fertility concerns. But the highly visible nature of royal pious practices (whether pilgrimages, gifts to shrines, requests for prayers from monks of a particular institution, or the installation of images in royal chapels and chambers) was also a critical aspect of the royal couples' spiritual practices for fertility.

A pivotal premise of this research has been to think about "infertility" as more than permanent childlessness. Taking into account the reproductive experiences of kings and queens who, in many cases, have not been conventionally considered infertile uncovered concerns about the fertility of couples who had, or went on to have, children. The contemporary anxieties about the childlessness of couples like Henry III and Eleanor of Provence, and Edward II and Isabella of France, stemmed from perceptions of the kings in the 1230s and 1310s, respectively. Crucially, (in)fertility had a considerable impact on perceptions of good kingship: an aspect of kingship that had received little scrutiny. This study has firmly demonstrated that chroniclers blamed royal couples' childlessness on the king when they wished to communicate the broader failings of that king. Approaching infertility as more than the inability to conceive children also brought into focus the experiences of miscarriage and stillbirth by queens who were already mothers, or who would become mothers. Because of these queens' motherhood, scholars of infertility had neglected to consider their reproductive labour and concerns over fertility because they successfully produced children.

This book also offers a solution to the dilemma of how to study men and masculinity without leaving out women in the history of infertility, and vice versa. An enduring objection from feminist scholars toward histories of men and masculinity is that, when the focus is placed on the male social hierarchy and the construction of masculine identities, which are often formed (and discussed) in relation to other men, women are, again, forgotten.[1] Toby Ditz reflected that, despite making significant contributions to our understanding of the complexities and social differences between men, the

1 Ditz, "The New Men's History," 7–9.

history of masculinity "leaves us with the queasy feeling that, cumulatively, it risks repeating the oppressive omissions of conventional history."[2] Men, once again, are at the centre of the historical narrative. At the same time, though, women's bodies and experiences tend to remain the focus in the history of infertility, to the detriment of studying men's role in management and experiences of infertility.[3] As Ditz suggested, masculinity can be studied more productively by asking what effect the construction of masculinity had on women too.[4]

The value of this methodology regarding masculinity has been demonstrated above: uncovering the pattern between the king's age and concerns about childlessness shows not only how infertility affected kings' masculine identity, but also, fundamentally, that the king's age was the switch that activated the intense scrutiny of the queen's fertility. The significance of fertility for a king's masculine maturity determined when and why the royal couple sought to manage their fertility with spiritual and medical therapies—remedies which were disproportionately directed at, and experienced by, the queen's body. It is both possible and necessary to include men without losing sight of women in the history of infertility, and equally to include women without excluding men.

Finally, there continues to be a divide in historiography on medieval England and Scotland and it is worth stating that it is possible to focus on English and Scottish royal couples in the same study, while appreciating the differences between the two regional contexts and not making one secondary to the other. The evidence that shed light on the English royal couples' experiences, particularly for Henry III and Eleanor of Provence, initially seemed richer than what survives for all of the Scottish couples in this study combined. However, it was the Scottish evidence that shaped the primary conclusions of this book, leading to both the discovery of the significance of the kings' age for the problematization of childlessness and the political communication in spiritual practices for fertility. How the Scottish kings

---

2 Ditz, "New Men's History," 7.

3 Mistry, "Review Essay: Infertility in History and the History of Reproduction," 661.

4 Ditz, "New Men's History," 9. Marcia Inhorn demonstrated the value of this approach in her work on infertility in modern Egypt. She considered how men's infertility affected their masculinity and impacted their wives. She argued that male infertility is a crisis of masculinity for Egyptian men and demonstrated that the consequences of this are experienced by their wives who continue to be blamed for the marriage's infertility and suffer threats of divorce and abandonment: Inhorn, "'The Worms Are Weak,'" 236–56.

responded to childlessness, and how chroniclers wrote about the Scottish queens' fertility, is not an afterthought or illustrative sideline to the English evidence but, rather, it has defined the key arguments of this book. It has also been worthwhile remembering that these kings and queens were not only English and Scottish royals, but also brothers-in-law, sisters, sons, and daughters from the same social and familial context. It is worthwhile uniting them in a gendered study of reproduction and (in)fertility.

BIBLIOGRAPHY

Manuscript and Archival Sources

Cambridge, Peterhouse, MS 222.
Cambridge, University of Cambridge Library, MS Ee.3. 59.
Kew, The National Archives (TNA)
Exchequer: E101 King's Remembrancer: Various Accounts.
Special Collections: SC 1 Ancient Correspondence.
London, British Library (BL)
MSS Additional 24511, 24512.
MS Sloane 1611.
London, The Wellcome Collection, MS 5262.

Digitized Primary Sources

Correspondence of Aldobrandino of Siena to Beatrice of Savoy, 1256. https://epistolae.ctl.columbia.edu/letter/501.html, accessed October 14, 2025.

Incipit antidotarium Nicholai (1471). https://www.loc.gov/item/2014659217/, accessed October 14, 2025.

Printed Primary Sources

Albertus Magnus. *De vegetabilibus libri VII*. Edited by E. F. H. Meyer. Berolini, 1867.

"Annales Londoniensis." In *Chronicles of the Reigns of Edward I and Edward II*. Edited by William Stubbs. *Rolls Series* 76, vol. 1, 1–251. Longman, 1882.

"Annales Paulini." *Chronicles of the Reigns of Edward I and Edward II*. Edited by William Stubbs. *Rolls Series* 76, vol. 1, 253–370. Longman, 1882.

Aristotle, *Rhetoric*. Edited by J. H. Freese, http://www.perseus.tufts.edu/hopper/text?doc=Perseus%3Atext%3A1999.01.0060%3Abook%3D2, accessed October 14, 2025.

Arnold, Thomas. *Memorials of St. Edmunds Abbey*. 3 vols. HMSO, 1890–1896.

Balfour-Melville, E. W. M, ed. "Papers Relating to the Captivity and Release of David II." In *Miscellany of the Scottish History Society, Ninth Volume*, 3–51. Constable, 1958.

Barbour, John. *The Bruce*. Canongate, 2007.

Bartholomaeus Anglicus. *On the Properties of Things: John Trevisa's Translation of Bartholomaeus Anglicus' De proprietatus rerum*. Edited by M. C. Seymour. 3 vols. Clarendon, 1975–1988.

Bond, E. A. "Notices of the Last Days of Isabella, Queen of Edward the Second, Drawn from an Account of the Expenses of her Household." *Archaeologia* 35 (1854): 453–69.

Bower, Walter. *Scotichronicon*. Edited by D. E. R. Watt. 9 vols. Aberdeen University Press, 1987–1998.

Bracton: On the Laws and Customs of England. Edited by George Woodbine and translated by Samuel E. Thorne. 4 vols. Belknap, 1968.

Calendar of Close Rolls Preserved in the Public Record Office of the Reign of Henry III. 14 vols. HMSO, 1902–1938.

Calendar of Documents Relating to Scotland. Edited by Joseph Bain. 5 vols. H. M. Public Record Office, 1881–1888.

Calendar of Entries in the Papal Registers Relating to Great Britain and Ireland: Petitions to the Pope. Vol. 1: 1198–1304. Edited by William H. Bliss. HMSO, 1896.

Calendar of Liberate Rolls Preserved in the Public Record Office of the Reign of Henry III. 6 vols. HMSO, 1916–1964.

Calendar of Papal Letters to Scotland of Benedict XIII of Avignon, 1394–1419. Edited by F. McGurk. Scottish History Society, 1976.

Calendar of Patent Rolls Preserved in the Public Record Office of the Reign of Edward II. 5 vols. HMSO, 1894–1904.

Chaplais, Pierre. *English Medieval Diplomatic Practice in the Middle Ages*. Black, 2003.

——. "Some Letters of Edward I." *English Historical Review* 77 (Jan 1962):79–86.

Charters of the Priory of Beauly. Edited by Edmund Chisholm Batten. Grampian Club, 1877.

The Chartularies of Balmerino and Lindores. Edited by William Turnbull. Abbotsford Club, 1841.

Chronica de Mailros. Edited by Joseph Stevenson. AMS, 1835.

The Chronicle of Bury St. Edmunds, 1212–1301. Edited by Antonia Gransden. Nelson, 1964.

The Chronicle of Lanercost 1272–1346. Edited and translated by Herbert Maxwell. Maclehose, 1913.

The Chronicle of Melrose: A Stratigraphic Edition. I: Introduction and Facsimile Edition. Edited by Dauvit Broun and Julian Harrison. Scottish History Society. Boydell, 2007.

Chronicles of the Reigns of Edward I and Edward II. Edited by William Stubbs. Longman, 1882–1883.

Chronicon de Lanercost. Edited by Joseph Stevenson. Bannatyne Club, 1839.

"Chronique John St. Victor." In *Recueil des historiens des Gaules et de la France*. Edited by Martin Bourquet. Palmé, 1840.

Chronique métrique de Godefroy de Paris. Edited by J. A. Buchon. Verdière, 1827.

Chroniques de Jean Froissart. Edited by Simeon Luce. 13 vols. Société de l'Histoire de France, 1869–1879.

Concilia magnae Britanniae et Hiberniae. Edited by David Wilkins. 4 vols. Gosling, 1737.

English Coronation Records. Edited by Leopold G. W. Legg. Constable, 1901.

Flores historiarum. Edited by Henry R. Luard. 3 vols. HMSO, 1890.

Froissart, Jean. *Chronicles of England, France, Spain, and the Adjoining Countries*. Edited and translated by Thomas Johnes. 2 vols. Smith, 1839.

Gordon, Bernard of. *Practica seu Lilium medicinae*. Naples, 1480. http://wellcomecollection.org/works/v8ssnagx/items?canvas=1, accessed October 14, 2025.

Gray, Sir Thomas. *Scalacronica*. Edited and translated by Andy King. Boydell, 2005.

The Historical Works of Gervase of Canterbury. Edited by William Stubbs. 2 vols. Longman, 1879–1880.

Isidore of Seville. *Etymologies*. Edited by Stephen A. Barney et al. Cambridge University Press, 2006.

Issues of the Exchequer: Being a Collection of Payments Made out of His Majesty's Revenue from King Henry III to King Henry VI. Edited by Frederick Devon. Murray, 1837.

Johannis de Fordun Chronica gentis Scotorum. Edited by W. F. Skene. Edmonston, 1871.

"Johannis de Trokelowe Annales." In *Johannis de Trokelowe et Henrici de Blaneforde chronica et annales*. Edited by Henry Thomas Riley. Longman, 1866.

Landouzy, Louis, and Roger Pépin, eds. *Le régime du corps de Maitre Aldebrandin de Sienne*. Champion, 1911.

Le Baker, Geoffrey. *Chronicon*. Edited by Edward Thompson. Clarendon, 1889.

Liber Pluscardensis. Edited by Frederick Skene. 2 vols. Paterson, 1877–1880.

Liber Sancte Marie de Melros. Edited by Cosmo Innes. Bannatyne Club, 1877.

Luard, Henry R., ed. *Annales monastici*. 5 vols. Longman, 1864.

——. *Lives of Edward the Confessor*. Longman, 1858.

Macer, Floridus. *De viribus herbarum*. Leopoldi Vossii, 1832.

Matthew Paris. *Chronica majora*. Edited by Henry R. Luard. 7 vols. Longman, 1872–1883.

——. *Historia Anglorum*. Edited by Frederic Madden. 3 vols. Longman, 1866–1868.

Miracles of Saint Æbbe of Coldingham and Saint Margaret of Scotland. Edited and translated by Robert Bartlett. Clarendon, 2003.

Pagel, Julius. "Raymundus de Moleriis und seine Schrift de Impedimentis Conceptionis." *Janus* 8 (1903): 530–37.

Platearius, Matthaeus. *Liber de simplici medicina* (1512). https://books.google.co.uk/books/about/Liber_de_simplici_medicina.html?id=wok8AAAAcAAJ&redir_esc=y, accessed October 14, 2025.

Pseudo-Arnald. *Tractatus de sterilitate: Anónimo de Montpellier (s. XIV) atribuido a A. de Vilanova, R. de Moleris y J. de Turre*. Edited and translated by E. M. Cartelle. Universidad de Valladolid, 1993.

Regesta regum Scottorum: The Acts of David II, 1329–71. Edited by Bruce Webster. Edinburgh University Press, 1982.

Regiam majestatem and quoniam attachiamenta. Edited and translated by Thomas Cooper. Stair Society, 1947.

Robertson, James C., ed. *Materials for the History of Thomas Becket Archbishop of Canterbury*. 7 vols. Longman, 1875.

Rôles gascons transcrits et publiés: Tome première 1242–1254. Edited by Francisque Michael. Imprimerie nationale, 1885.

Rotuli scaccarii regum Scotorum: The Exchequer Rolls of Scotland. Edited by John Stuart and George Burnett. 23 vols. H. M. General Register House, 1878.

Rotuli Scotiae in Turri Londensi et in domo capitulari Westmonasteriensi asservati. Edited by William Illingworth et al. 2 vols. Eyre, 1814–1819.

Royal and Other Historical Letters Illustrative of the Reign of Henry III from the Originals in the Public Record Office, Volume II: 1236–1272. Edited by Walter Waddington-Shirley. 2 vols. Longman, 1862–1866.

Rymer, Thomas, ed. *Foedera, conventiones, litterae, et cujuscunque generis acta publica, inter reges Angliae et alios quosvis impeatores, reges, pontifices, principes, vel communitates: Ab ingressu Gulielmi I. in Angliam, A.D. 1066, ad nostra usque tempora habita aut tractate*. 20 vols. 1816.

Scoular, J. M., ed. *Handlist of the Acts of Alexander II, 1214–1249*. Edinburgh University Press, 1959.

Sir Thomas Gray's Scalacronica. Edited by Herbert Maxwell. MacLehose, 1907.

Statuta capitulorum generalium ordinis Cisterciensis tomus II, 1221–1261. Edited by Joseph Marie Canivez. Bureaux de la Revue, 1934.

Tractatus de sterilitate mulierum. Edited by E. M. Cartelle. In *Tractatus de conceptu, Tractatus de sterilitate mulierum*. Edited and translated by Pedro Conde Parrado et al. Lingüistica y filología 37. Universidad de Valladolid, 1999.

The Trotula: A Medieval Compendium of Women's Medicine. Edited by Monica Green. University of Pennsylvania Press, 2001.

Vita Edwardi secundi. Edited by Wendy Childs and N. Denholm-Young. Clarendon, 2005.

Voragine, Jacobus de. *The Golden Legend: Readings on the Saints*. Edited by William Granger Ryan, with introduction by Eamon Duffy. Princeton University Press, 2012.

Wallis, Faith. *Medieval Medicine: A Reader*. University of Toronto Press, 2010.

Willelmi Rishanger, quondam Monachi S. Albani, et quoarundam Anonymorum: Chronica et annales, regnatibus Henrico tertio et Edwardo primo. Edited by Henry T. Riley. Longman, 1865.

Wyntoun, Andrew of. *The Orygynale Cronykil of Scotland*. Edited by David Laing. 3 vols. Edmonston, 1872–1879.

Secondary Works

Abrams, Lynn, and Elizabeth Ewan. *Nine Centuries of Man: Manhood and Masculinity in Scottish History*. Edinburgh University Press, 2017.

Adams, Tracy. "Anne de France and Gift-Giving: The Exercise of Female Power." In *Women, Power, and Authority at the French Court, 1483–1563*. Edited by Susan Broomhall, 65–84. Amsterdam University Press, 2018.

——. "'Make Me Chaste and Continent, but Not Yet': A Model for Clerical Masculinity?" In *Masculinities and Femininities in the Middle Ages and Renaissance*. Edited by Frederick Kiefer, 1–29. Arizona Studies in the Middle Ages and the Renaissance 23. Brepols, 2010.

Alberts, Allison A. "Suffering and Protection in Childbirth in the *South English Legendary*." *Journal of Medieval and Early Modern Studies* 46, no. 2 (2016): 289–314.

Amundsen, Darrel, and Carol J. Diers. "The Age of Menopause in Medieval Europe." *Human Biology* 45, no. 4 (December 1973): 605–12.

Aram, Bethany. "Authority and Maternity in Late-Medieval Castile: Four Queens Regnant." In *Aspects of Power and Authority in the Middle Ages*. Edited by B. Bolton and C. Meek, 121–29. Brepols, 2007.

Arnold, John. "Gender and Sexuality." In *A Companion to the Medieval World*. Edited by C. Lansing and E. D. English, 161–84. Wiley, 2009.

Bailey, Anne E. "Flights of Distance, Time and Fancy: Women Pilgrims and their Journeys in English Medieval Miracle Narratives." *Gender & History* 24, no. 2 (2012): 292–309.

——. "'The Rich and the Poor, the Lesser and the Great': Social Representations of Female Pilgrims in Medieval England." *Cultural and Social History* 11, no. 1 (2014): 9–29.

——. "Wives, Mothers and Widows on Pilgrimage: Categories of 'Woman' Recorded at English Healing Shrines in the High Middle Ages." *Journal of Medieval History* 39, no. 2 (2013): 197–219.

Bak, Janos. *Coronations: Medieval and Early Modern Monarchic Ritual*. University of California Press, 1990.

Bale, Anthony. St. *Edmund, King and Martyr: Changing Images of a Medieval Saint*. Cambridge: Cambridge University Press, 2009.

Bannerman, John. *The Beatons: A Medical Kindred in the Classical Gaelic Tradition*. Donald, 1986.

Barclay, Katie. *Love, Intimacy and Power: Marriage and Patriarchy in Scotland, 1650–1850*. Manchester University Press, 2011.

Barclay, Katie, et al. "The State of Scottish History: Gender." *Scottish Historical Review* 92, Supp., no. 234 (2013): 83–107.

Barefield, Laura D. *Gender History in Medieval Chronicle and Romance*. Lang, 2003.

Bartlett, Robert. *The Miracles of St. Æbbe of Coldingham and St. Margaret of Scotland*. Oxford University Press, 2003.

——. *Royal Blood: Dynastic Politics in Medieval Europe*. Cambridge University Press, 2020.

Beattie, Cordelia. "The Life Cycle: The Ages of Medieval Women." In *A Cultural History of Women: In the Middle Ages*. Edited by Kim Phillips, 15–38. Bloomsbury, 2013.

Bell, Susan Groag. "Medieval Women Book Owners: Arbiters of Piety and Ambassadors of Culture." *Signs* 7 (1982): 742–68.

Benz St. John, Lisa. "Queen Consort, Queen Mother: The Power and Authority of Fourteenth-Century Plantagenet Queens." PhD diss., University of York, 2009.

——. *Three Medieval Queens: Queenship and the Crown in Fourteenth-Century England*. Palgrave, 2012.

Berry, Helen, and Elizabeth A. Foyster. "Childless Men in Early Modern England." *The Family in Early Modern England*. Edited by Helen Berry and Elizabeth A. Foyster, 158–83. Cambridge University Press, 2007.

Biller, Peter. *The Measure of Multitude: Population in Medieval Thought*. Oxford University Press, 2003.

Binski, Paul. *Becket's Crown: Art and Imagination in Gothic England, 1170–1300*. Yale University Press, 2004.

——. "Reflections on *La estoire de Seint Aedwardi le Rei*: Hagiography and Kingship in Thirteenth-Century England." *Journal of Medieval History* 16, no. 4 (1990): 333–50.

——. *Westminster Abbey and the Plantagenets: Kingship and the Representation of Power, 1200–1400*. Yale University Press, 1995.

Blackley, F. D. "Adam, the Bastard Son of Edward II." *Bulletin of the Institute of Historical Research* 37, no. 95 (1964): 76–77.

Blick, Sarah. "King and Cleric: Richard II and the Iconography of St. Thomas Becket and St. Edward the Confessor at Our Lady of Undercroft, Canterbury Cathedral." In *Beyond Pilgrim Souvenirs and Secular Badges: Essays in Honour of Brian Spencer*. Edited by Sarah Blick, 182–200. Oxbow, 2007.

——. "Votives, Images, Interaction and Pilgrimage to the Tomb and Shrine of St. Thomas Becket, Canterbury Cathedral." In *Push Me, Pull You: Imaginative, Emotional, Physical, and Spatial Interaction in Late Medieval and Renaissance Art*. Edited by Sarah Blick and Laura Gelfand, 21–58. Brill, 2011.

Boardman, Stephen. "Chronicle Propaganda in Fourteenth-Century Scotland: Robert the Steward, John of Fordun and the 'Anonymous Chronicle.'" *The Scottish Historical Review* 76, no. 201, pt. 1 (April 1997): 23–43.

——. *The Early Stewart Kings: Robert II and Robert III, 1371–1406*. Tuckwell, 1996.

——. "A People Divided? Language, History and Anglo-Scottish Conflict in the World of Andrew of Wyntoun." In *Ireland and the English World in the Late Middle Ages*. Edited by Brendan Smith, 112–29. Palgrave, 2009.

Bologne, Jean Claude. *La naissance interdite: Stérilité, avortement, contraception au Moyen Âge*. Orban, 1988.

Borenius, Tancred. "The Cycle of Images in the Palaces and Castiles of Henry III." *Journal of the Warburg and Courtauld Institutes* 6 (1943): 40–50.

Borland, Jennifer. "Female Networks and the Circulation of a Late Medieval Illustrated Health Guide." In *Moving Women Moving Objects (400–1500)*. Edited by Tracy Chapman Hamilton and Mariah Proctor-Tiffany, 107–36. Brill, 2019.

Braekman, W. L. *Studies on Alchemy, Diet, Medecine [sic] and Prognostication in Middle English*. Omirel, 1986.

Broun, Dauvit. "Creating and Maintaining a Year-by-Year Chronicle: The Evidence of The Chronicle of Melrose." In *The Medieval Chronicle VI*. Edited by Erik Kooper, 141–52. Brill, 2009.

——. "A New Look at *Gesta annalia* Attributed to John of Fordun." In *Church, Chronicle and Learning in Medieval and Renaissance Scotland*. Edited by B. E. Crawford, 9–30. Birlinn, 1999.

Brown, Cynthia J. "Family Female Networking in Early Sixteenth-Century France: The Power of Text and Image." In *Women, Power, and Authority at the French Court, 1483–1563*. Edited by Susan Broomhall, 209–40. Amsterdam University Press, 2018.

Brown, Keith, and Roland J. Tanner, eds. *Parliament and Politics in Scotland, 1235–1560: The History of the Scottish Parliament*. Edinburgh University Press, 2004.

Bruso, Steven. "Bodies Hardened for War: Knighthood in Fifteenth-century England." *Journal of Medieval and Early Modern Studies* 47, no. 2 (2017): 255–77.

Buck, Rosemary. "Woman's Milk in Anglo-Saxon and Later Medieval Medical Texts." *Neophilologus* 96 (2012): 467–85.

Bullough, Vern. "On Being a Male in the Middle Ages." In *Medieval Masculinities: Regarding Men in the Middle Ages*. Edited by Clare A. Lees et al., 31–46. University of Minnesota Press, 1994.

Burrow, J. A. *The Ages of Man: A Study in Medieval Writing and Thought*. Oxford University Press, 1988.

Butler, Sara M. "More than Mothers: Juries of Matrons and Pleas of the Belly in Medieval England." *Law and History Review* 37, no. 2 (2019): 353–96.

Cadden, Joan. *The Meanings of Sex Difference in the Middle Ages: Medicine, Science, and Culture*. Cambridge University Press, 1993.

Carpenter, David. *Henry III: The Rise to Power and Personal Rule, vol. 1: (1207–1258*). Yale University Press, 2020.

——. "King Henry III and Saint Edward the Confessor: The Origin of the Cult." *English Historical Review* 122, no. 498 (2007): 865–91.

Cavanaugh, Susan. "Royal Books: King John to Richard II." *The Library* 5, no. 10 (1988): 304–16.

Chaplais, Pierre. *Piers Gaveston: Edward II's Adoptive Brother*. Oxford University Press, 1994.

Colvin, Howard. "Royal Gardens in Medieval England in Medieval Gardens." In *Dumbarton Oaks Colloquium on the History of Landscape Architecture* 9 (1986): 7–22.

——, et al. *The History of the King's Works*. 2 vols. HMSO, 1963.

Comba, M. "Methods of Queenship in Matrimonial Diplomacy: Fifteenth-Century Scottish Royal Women." *Constellations* 5, no. 2 (2014). https://doi.org/10.29173/cons22030.

Connell, R. W. *Masculinities*. 2nd ed. Polity, 2005.

Cooke, Jessica. "Nice Young Girls and Wicked Old Witches: The 'Rightful Age' of Women in Middle English Verse." In *The Court and Cultural Diversity: Selected Papers from the Eighth Triennial Congress of the International Courtly Literature Society, the Queen's University of Belfast, 26 July–1 August 1995*. Edited by Evelyn Mullally and John Thompson, 219–28. Boydell, 1997.

Corrington, Gail P. "The Milk of Salvation: Redemption by the Mother in Late Antiquity and Early Christianity." *The Harvard Theological Review* 82 (1989): 393–420.

Cowan, Ian B., and David E. Easson. *Medieval Religious Houses in Scotland*. Longman, 1976.

Creamer, Joseph. "St. Edmund of Abingdon and Henry III Under the Shadow of Thomas Becket." In *Thirteenth-Century England XIV: Proceedings of the Aberystwyth and Lampeter Conference, 2011*. Edited by Björn Weiler et al., 129–40. Boydell, 2013.

Crossley, Paul. "The Architecture of Queenship: Royal Saints, Female Dynasties and the Spread of Gothic Architecture in Central Europe." In *Queens and Queenship in Medieval Europe*. Edited by Anne J. Duggan, 263–300. Boydell, 1997.

Cullum, P. H. "Clergy, Masculinity and Transgression in Late Medieval England." In *Masculinity in Medieval Europe*. Edited by Dawn M. Hadley, 178–96. Longman, 1999.

D'Avray, David. *Papacy, Monarchy and Marriage 860–1600*. Cambridge University Press, 2015.

Davis, Angela. "Oral History and Women's Accounts of Infertility in Postwar England." In *The Palgrave Handbook of Infertility in History: Approaches, Contexts and Perspectives*. Edited by Gayle Davis and Tracy Loughran, 123–40. Palgrave, 2017.

Davis, Gayle, and Tracy Loughran. "Introduction." In *The Palgrave Handbook of Infertility in History: Approaches, Contexts and Perspectives*. Edited by Gayle Davis and Tracy Loughran, 1–25. Palgrave, 2017.

Davis, Isabel. *Writing Masculinity in the Later Middle Ages*. Cambridge University Press, 2007.

Davis, Rachel M. "Elite Women and Power in Late Medieval Scotland, 1296–1458." PhD diss., University of Edinburgh, 2020.

Dean, Lucinda. "Crowning the Child: Representing Authority in the Inaugurations and Coronations of Minors in Scotland, c. 1214 to c. 1567." In *The Image and Perception of Monarchy in Medieval and Early Modern Europe*. Edited by Sean McGlyn and Elena Woodacre, 254–80. Cambridge Scholars, 2014.

———. "Negotiating Youth, Old Age and Manhood: A Comparative Approach to Late Medieval Scottish Kingship." In *Gender in Scotland, 1200–1800: Place, Politics and Faith*. Edited by Janay Nugent et al., 193–209. Edinburgh University Press, 2024.

Demaitre, Luke. *Medieval Medicine: The Art of Healing, From Head to Toe*. Praeger, 2013.

DeWitte, Sharon, and Mary Lewis. "Medieval Menarche: Changes in Pubertal Timing Before and After the Black Death." *American Journal of Human Biology* 33, no. 2 (2020). https://doi.org/10.1002/ajhb.23439.

Dickinson, J. C. *The Shrine of Our Lady of Walsingham*. Cambridge University Press, 1956.

Dobson, Barrie. "The Monks of Canterbury Cathedral in the Later Middle Ages, 1220–1540." In *A History of Canterbury Cathedral*. Edited by Patrick Collinson et al., 69–153. Oxford University Press, 1995.

Donohoe, Róisín. "'Unbynde Her Anoone': The Lives of St. Margaret of Antioch and the Lying-In Space in Late Medieval England." In *Gender in Medieval Places, Spaces and Thresholds*. Edited by Victoria Blud et al., 139–56. Institute of Historical Research, 2019.

Doran, Susan. "Monarchy and Masculinity in Early Modern England." In *The Palgrave Handbook of Masculinity and Political Culture in Europe*. Edited by Christopher Fletcher et al., 201–23. Palgrave, 2018.

Dove, Mary. *The Perfect Age of Man's Life*. Cambridge University Press, 1986.

Downie, Fiona. "Queenship in Late Medieval Scotland." In *Scottish Kingship, 1306–1542: Essays in Honour of Norman MacDougall*. Edited by Michael Brown and Roland Tanner, 232–54. Donald, 2008.

——. *She is But a Women: Queenship in Scotland, 1424–1463*. Donald, 2006.

Dresvina, Juliana. *A Maid with a Dragon: The Cult of St. Margaret of Antioch in Medieval England*. Oxford University Press, 2016.

——. "The Significance of the Demonic Episode in the Legend of St. Margaret of Antioch." *Medium Ævum* 81, no. 2 (2012): 189–209.

——, and Nicholas Sparks, eds. *Authority and Gender in Medieval and Renaissance Chronicles*. Cambridge Scholars, 2012.

Drexler, Marjorie. "The Extant Abridgements of Walter Bower's 'Scotichronicon.'" *The Scottish Historical Review* 61, no. 171 (1982): 62–67.

Duncan, A. A. M. *The Kingship of the Scots, 842–1292: Succession and Independence*. Edinburgh University Press, 2002.

——. *The Kingship of the Scots, 842–1292: Succession and Independence*. 2nd ed. Edinburgh University Press, 2016.

——. "Sources and Uses of the *Chronicle of Melrose*, 1165–1297." In *Kings, Clerics and Chronicles in Scotland, 500–1297: Essays in Honour of Marjorie Ogilvie Anderson on the Occasion of her Ninetieth Birthday*. Edited by Simon Taylor, 146–85. Four Courts, 2000.

Dunn, Carolyn, and Elizabeth Carney, eds. *Royal Women and Dynastic Loyalty*. Palgrave, 2018.

Dzon, Mary. "Joseph and the Amazing Christ-child in Late Medieval Legend." In *Childhood in the Middle Ages and the Renaissance: The Results of a Paradigm Shift in the History of Mentality*. Edited by Albrecht Classen, 135–57. De Gruyter, 2005.

Earenfight, Theresa. *Queenship in Medieval Europe*. Palgrave, 2013.

——. "Trastámara Kings, Queens, and the Gender Dynamics of Monarchy." In *The Emergence of León-Castile, c. 1065–1500: Essays Presented to J. F. O'Callaghan*. Edited by James Todesca, 141–60. Ashgate, 2015.

——. "Without the Persona of the Prince: Kings, Queens and the Idea of Monarchy in Late Medieval Europe." *Gender & History* 19, no. 1 (April 2007): 1–21.

——, ed. *Royal and Elite Households in Medieval and Early Modern Europe: More than Just a Castle*. Brill, 2018.

Earenfight, Theresa, and Kristen Geaman. "Neither Heir Nor Spare: Childless Queens and the Practice of Monarchy in Pre-Modern Europe." In *The Routledge History of Monarchy*. Edited by Elena Woodacre et al., 518–33. Routledge, 2019.

Evans, Jennifer. "'They are Called Imperfect Men': Male Infertility and Sexual Health in Early Modern England." *Social History of Medicine* 29, no. 2 (2016): 311–32.

Evans, Michael R. *Inventing Eleanor: The Medieval and Post-Medieval Image of Eleanor of Aquitaine*. Bloomsbury, 2014.

Ewan, Elizabeth. "A History of Women in Scotland," History Scotland, Feb. 2018. https://www.historyscotland.com/history/scottish-history/a-history-of-women-in-scotland, accessed October 14, 2025.

——. "A New Trumpet? The History of Women in Scotland, 1300–1700." *History Compass* 7, no. 2 (2009): 431–46.

——. "Women's History in Scotland: Towards an Agenda." *The Innes Review* 46, no. 2 (1995): 155–64.

——, and M. Meikle, eds. *Women in Scotland, c .1100–c. 1750*. Tuckwell, 1999.

Facinger, Marion. "A Study of Medieval Queenship Capetian France, 987–1237." *Nebraska Studies in Medieval and Renaissance History* 5 (1968): 1–48.

Finucane, Ronald. *Miracles and Pilgrims: Popular Beliefs in Medieval England*. Rowman, 1977.

Fitch, Audrey-Beth. "Maternal Mediators: Saintly Ideals and Secular Realities in Late Medieval Scotland." *The Innes Review* 57, no. 1 (Spring 2006): 1–35.

Fleiner, Carey, and Elena Woodacre, eds. *Virtuous or Villainess? The Image of the Royal Mother from the Early Medieval to the Early Modern Era*. Palgrave, 2016.

Fletcher, Catherine. "The Ladies' Peace Revisited: Gender, Counsel and Diplomacy." In *Queenship and Counsel in Early Modern Europe*. Edited by Helen Matheson-Pollock et al., 111–33. Palgrave, 2018.

Fletcher, Christopher. "Manhood, Kingship and the Public in Late Medieval England." *Edad media: Revista de historia* 13 (2012): 123–42.

——. *Richard II: Manhood, Youth, and Politics 1377–99*. Oxford University Press, 2008.

——. "The Whig Interpretation of Masculinity? Honour and Sexuality in Late Medieval Manhood." In *What is Masculinity?: Historical Dynamics from Antiquity to the Contemporary World*. Edited by Sean Brady and John H. Arnold, 57–75. Palgrave, 2011.

Fredell, Joel. "The Three Clerks and St. Nicholas in Medieval England." *Studies in Philology* 92, no. 2 (1995): 181–202.

Galloway, Andrew. "Writing History in England." In *The Cambridge History of Medieval English Literature*. Edited by David Wallace, 255–83. Cambridge University Press, 1999.

Geaman, Kristen. "Anne of Bohemia and Her Struggle to Conceive." *Social History of Medicine* 29 (2016): 224–44.

——. "A Bastard and a Changeling? England's Edward of Westminster and Delayed Childbirth." In *Unexpected Heirs in Early Modern Europe: Potential Kings and Queens*. Edited by Valerie Schutte, 11–33. Palgrave, 2017.

——. "Beyond Good Queen Anne: Anne of Bohemia, Patronage, and Politics." In *Medieval Elite Women and the Exercise of Power, 1100–1400: Moving Beyond the Exceptionalist Debate*. Edited by Heather J. Tanner, 67–89. Palgrave, 2018.

——. "Childless Queens and Child-like Kings: Negotiating Royal Infertility in England, 1382–1471." PhD diss., University of Southern California, 2013.

Getz, Faye. "Medical Practitioners in Medieval England." *Social History of Medicine* 3, no. 2 (August 1990): 245–83.

——. *Medicine in the English Middle Ages*. Princeton University Press, 1998.

Gibson, Gail McMurray. "Blessings from Sun and Moon: Churchings as Women's Theatre." In *Bodies and Disciplines: Intersections of Literature and History in Fifteenth-Century England*. Edited by Barbara Hanawalt and David Wallace, 139–54. University of Minnesota Press, 1996.

Gilchrist, Roberta. *Medieval Life: Archaeology and the Life Course*. Boydell, 2012.

Given-Wilson, Chris. *Chronicles: The Writing of History in Medieval England*. Bloomsbury, 2007.

——. "Vita Edwardi secundi: Memoir or Journal?" In *Thirteenth Century England VI: Proceedings of the Durham Conference, 1995*. Edited by Michael Prestwich et al., 165–76. Boydell, 1997.

——, and Alice Curteis. *The Royal Bastards of Medieval England*. Routledge, 1984.

Gonthier, Dominique and Claire Le Bas. "Analyse socio-économique de quelques recueils de miracles dans la Normandie du XIe au XIIIe siècle." *Annales de Normandie* 24, no. 1 (1974): 3–36.

Grana Cid, Maria del Mar. "Catherine of Lancaster, the Order of Preachers, and Queenship: Monastic Policies." *Edad media: Revista de historia* 18 (2017): 75–100.

Gransden, Antonia. "The Cult of St. Mary at Beodricsworth and then in Bury St. Edmunds Abbey to c. 1150." *Journal of Ecclesiastical History* 55 (2004): 627–53.

——. *Historical Writing in England: c. 550 to c. 1307*. 2 vols. Routledge, 1974.

Grauer, Anne. "Life Patterns of Women from Medieval York." In *The Archaeology of Gender: Proceedings of the Twenty-Second Annual Conference of the Archaeological Association of the University of Calgary*. Edited by Dale Walde and Noreen D. Willows, 407–13. University of Calgary Archaeological Association, 1991.

Green, Monica. "Flowers, Poisons and Men: Menstruation in Medieval Western Europe." In *Menstruation: A Cultural History*. Edited by Andrew Shail and Gillian Howie, 51–64. Palgrave, 2005.

——. *Making Women's Medicine Masculine: The Rise of Male Authority in Pre-Modern Gynaecology*. Oxford University Press, 2008.

——. "The Possibilities of Literacy and the Limits of Reading: Women and the Gendering of Medical Literacy (Essay VII)." In *Women's Healthcare in the Medieval West*. Ashgate, 2000.

Haines, Roy. *King Edward II: Edward of Caernarfon, His Life, His Reign and its Aftermath, 1284–1330*. McGill-Queens University Press, 2003.

Hamilton, J. S. "Some Notes on Royal Medicine." In *Fourteenth Century England. Edited by* Chris Given-Wilson, 33–43. Vol. 2. Boydell, 2002.

Hamilton, Tracy Chapman, and Mariah Proctor-Tiffany, eds. *Moving Women Moving Objects (400–1500)*. Brill, 2019.

Hammond, Matthew. "Queen Ermengarde and the Abbey of St. Edward, Balmerino." *Cîteaux: Commentarii cisterciensis* 59 (2008): 1–27.

——. "Royal and Aristocratic Attitudes to Saints and the Virgin in Twelfth- and Thirteenth-Century Scotland." In *The Cult of Saints and the Virgin Mary in Medieval Scotland*. Edited by Steve Boardman and Eila Williamson, 61–85. Boydell, 2010.

Harrill, Claire Louise. "Politics and Sainthood: Literary Representations of St. Margaret of Scotland in England and Scotland from the Eleventh to the Fifteenth Century." PhD diss., University of Birmingham, 2017.

Harris-Stoerz, Fiona. "Pregnancy and Childbirth in Twelfth and Thirteenth-Century French and English Law." *Journal of the History of Sexuality* 21, no. 2 (May 2012): 263–81.

——. "Suffering and Survival in Medieval English Childbirth." In *Medieval Family Roles*. Edited by Cathy Jorgensen Itnyre, 101–20. Garland, 1996.

Hayes, Amy. "The Late Medieval Scottish Queen, c. 1371–c. 1513." PhD diss., University of Aberdeen, 2016.

Herrero, Maria del Carmen Garcia, and Angela Munoz Fernandez. "Queenship and Monastic Foundations in the Crowns of Castile and Aragon: An Approach to the Topic." *Edad media: Revista de historia* 18 (2017): 16–48.

Herrup, Cynthia. "The King's Two Genders." *Journal of British Studies* 45 (2006): 493–510.

Heyes, Michael E. *Margaret's Monsters: Women, Identity, and the Life of St. Margaret in Medieval England*. Routledge, 2019.

Hill, Carole. *Women and Religion in Late Medieval Norwich*. Boydell, 2010.

Hodgson, Natasha. "Normans and Competing Masculinities on Crusade." In *Crusading and Pilgrimage in the Norman World*. Edited by Kathryn Hurlock and Paul Oldfield, 195–213. Boydell, 2015.

Hollander, Melissa. "The Name of The Father: Baptism and The Social Construction of Fatherhood in Early Modern Edinburgh." In *Finding the Family in Medieval and Early Modern Scotland*. Edited by Elizabeth Ewan and Janay Nugent, 63–72. Routledge, 2008.

Hopwood, Nick, et al., eds. *Reproduction: Antiquity to the Present Day*. Cambridge University Press, 2018.

Howell, Margaret. "The Children of King Henry III and Eleanor of Provence." In *Thirteenth Century England IV: Proceedings of the Newcastle upon Tyne Conference 1991*. Edited by P. R. Coss and S. D. Lloyd, 57–72. Boydell, 1992.

——. *Eleanor of Provence: Queenship in Thirteenth-Century England*. Wiley, 2001.

——. "Royal Women of England and France in the Mid-Thirteenth Century: A Gendered Perspective." In *England and Europe in the Reign of Henry III*. Edited by Björn Weiler and L. W. Rowlands, 163–81. Ashgate, 2002.

Huneycutt, Lois. "The Idea of the Perfect Princess: The 'Life of St. Margaret' in the Reign of Matilda II (1100–1118)." *Anglo Norman Studies* 12 (1990): 81–98.

——. "Intercession and the High-Medieval Queen: The Esther Topos." In *Power of the Weak: Studies on Medieval Women*. Edited by Jennifer Carpenter and Sally-Beth MacLean, 126–46. University of Illinois Press, 1995.

——. *Matilda of Scotland: A Study of Medieval Queenship*. Boydell, 2003.

——. "'Proclaiming her Dignity Abroad': The Literary and Artistic Network of Matilda of Scotland, Queen of England 1100–1118." In *The Cultural Patronage of Medieval Women*. Edited by June Hall McCash, 155–74. University of Georgia Press, 1996.

——. "Public Lives, Private Ties: Royal Mothers in England and Scotland, 1070–1204)." In *Medieval Mothering*. Edited by John Carmi Parsons and Bonnie Wheeler, 295–311. Garland, 1996.

Huntington, Joanna. "Edward the Celibate, Edward the Saint." In *Medieval Virginities*. Edited by Anke Bernau et al., 119–39. University of Toronto Press, 2003.

Inhorn, Marcia. "'The Worms Are Weak': Male Infertility and Patriarchal Paradoxes in Egypt." *Men and Masculinities* 5, no. 3 (2003): 236–56.

Jacquart, Danielle. "Aristotelian Thought in Salerno." In *A History of Twelfth-Century Western Philosophy*. Edited by Peter Dronke, 407–28. Cambridge University Press, 1988.

Jansen, Virginia. "Henry III's Windsor: Castle-Building and Residences." In *Windsor: Medieval Archaeology, Art and Architecture of the Thames Valley*. Edited by Laurence Keen and Eileen Scarff, 95–109. British Archaeological Association, 2002.

Jones, Peter, and Lea Olsan. "Performative Rituals for Conception and Childbirth in England, 900–1500." *Bulletin of the History of Medicine* 89, no. 3 (2015): 406–33.

Jotischky, Andrew. "Saints' Cults and Devotions on the Norman Edge: The Case of St. Katherine of Alexandria." In *The Normans and the "Norman Edge": Peoples, Polities and Identities on the Frontiers of Medieval Europe*. Edited by Keith J. Stringer and Andrew Jotischky, 191–218. Routledge, 2019.

Kane, Bronach. *Impotence and Virginity in the Late Medieval Ecclesiastical Court of York, No. 114*. Borthwick, 2008.

Karras, Ruth M. *From Boys to Men: Formations of Masculinity in Late Medieval Europe*. University of Pennsylvania Press, 2003.

Kehnel, Annette. "The Narrative Tradition of the Medieval Franciscan Friars on the British Isles: Introduction to the Sources." *Franciscan Studies* 63 (2005): 461–530.

King, Andy. "Englishmen, Scots and Marchers: National and Local Identities in Thomas Gray's *Scalacronica*." *Northern History* 33, no. 2 (2000): 217–31.

——. "A Helm with a Crest of Gold: The Order of Chivalry in Thomas Gray's *Scalacronica*." In *Fourteenth-Century England*. Edited by Nigel Saul, 21–36. Boydell, 2000.

——. "Scaling the Ladder: The Rise and Rise of the Grays of Heaton, c. 1296–c. 1415." In *North-East England in the Later Middle Ages*. Edited by Christian D. Liddy and Richard H. Britnell, 57–73. Boydell, 2005.

Krause, Kathy M. "From Mothers to Daughters: Literary Patronage as Political Works in Ponthieu." In *Medieval Elite Women and the Exercise of Power, 1100–1400*. Edited by Heather J. Tanner, 113–33. Palgrave, 2019.

Lamb, Rory. "David II's Chapel Royal at St. Monans in the Context of Medieval Pilgrimage." *Innes Review* 68, no. 2 (2017): 117–31.

Landsberg, Sylvia. *The Medieval Garden*. University of Toronto Press, 2003.

Larson, Wendy. "Who Is the Master of This Narrative? Maternal Patronage and the Cult of St. Margaret." In *Gendering the Master Narrative*. Edited by Mary Erler and Maryanne Kowaleski, 94–104. Cornell University Press, 2003.

Lawrence, Clifford. St. *Edmund of Abingdon: A Study in Hagiography and History*. Clarendon Press, 1960.

Laynesmith, Joanna. "Fertility Rite or Authority Ritual? The Queen's Coronation in England, 1445–1487." In *Social Attitudes and Political Structures in the Fifteenth Century*. Edited by T. Thornton, 52–68. Sutton, 2000.

——. *The Last Medieval Queens: English Queenship, 1445–1503*. Oxford University Press, 2004.

L'Estrange, Elizabeth. *Holy Motherhood: Gender, Dynasty and Visual Culture in the Later Middle Ages*. Manchester University Press, 2008.

Lee, SangDong. "The Miracles and Cult of St. Margaret of Scotland." *The Scottish Historical Review* 97, no. 1 (2018): 1–11.

Lewis, Katherine J. "Becoming a Virgin King: Richard II and Edward the Confessor." In *Gender and Holiness: Men, Women and Saints in Late Medieval Europe*. Edited by S. E. J. Riches and S. Salih, 86–100. Routledge, 2002.

——. *The Cult of St. Katherine of Alexandria in Late Medieval England*. Boydell, 2000.

——. "Edmund of East Anglia, Henry VI and Ideals of Kingly Masculinity." In *Holiness and Masculinity in the Middle Ages*. Edited by P. H Cullum, and Katherine Lewis, 158–73. University of Wales, 2004.

——. "A King, Not a Servant: The Prose Life of St. Katherine of Alexandria and Ideologies of Masculinity in Late Medieval England." In *Hagiography and the History of Latin Christendom, 500–1500*. Edited by Samantha Kahn Herrick, 397–416. Brill, 2019.

——. *Kingship and Masculinity in Late Medieval England*. Routledge, 2013.

——. "'Lete Me Suffre': Reading the Torture of St. Margaret of Antioch in Late Medieval England." In *Medieval Women: Texts and Contexts in Late Medieval Britain. Essays for Felicity Riddy*. Edited by Jocelyn Wogan-Browne et al., 69–82. Brepols, 2000.

——. "The Life of St. Margaret of Antioch in Late Medieval England: A Gendered Reading." *Studies in Church History* 34 (1998): 129–42.

——. "Pilgrimage and the Cult of St. Katherine of Alexandria in Late Medieval England." In *St. Katherine of Alexandria: Texts and Contexts in Western Medieval Europe*. Edited by Katherine Lewis and Jacqueline Jenkins, 37–52. Brepols, 2003.

Lewis, Mary, F. Shapland, and R. Watts. "On the Threshold of Adulthood: A New Approach for the Use of Maturation Indicators to Assess puberty in Adolescents from Medieval England." *American Journal of Human Biology* 28 (2016): 48–56.

Lindgren, Amy. "The Wandering Womb and the Peripheral Penis: Gender and the Fertile Body in Late Medieval Infertility Treatises." PhD diss., University of California Davis, 2005.

Livingston, Michael. "The Depth of Six Inches: Prince Hal's Head Wound at the Battle of Shrewsbury." In *Wound and Wound Repair in Medieval Culture*. Edited by L. Tracy and K. DeVries, 215–31. Brill, 2015.

MacKinlay, James. *Ancient Church Dedications in Scotland*. 2 vols. Douglas, 1910–1914.

Malcolm, C. A. "Gardens of the Castle." In *The Book of the Edinburgh Club*, 101–200. Vol. 14. Edinburgh, 1925.

Mapstone, Sally. "Older Scots Literature and the Court." In *The Edinburgh History of Scottish Literature: From Columba to the Union (until 1707)*. Edited by Ian Brown et al., 273–85. Edinburgh University Press, 2007.

Martin, Russell E. "Introduction Part III: Dynasty and Succession." In *The Routledge History of Monarchy*. Edited by Elena Woodacre et al., 411–19. Routledge, 2019.

Matthews, Leslie. *The Royal Apothecaries*. Wellcome Historical Medical Library, 1967.

McCracken, Peggy. "The Body Politic and the Queen's Adulterous Body in French Romance." *Feminist Approaches to the Body in Medieval Literature*. Edited by Linda Lomperis and Sarah Stanbury, 38–64. University of Pennsylvania Press, 1993.

McGladdery, Christine. "Liber Pluscardensis." In *Encyclopedia of the Medieval Chronicle*. Edited by Graeme Dunphy and Cristian Bratu. Brill, 2010.

McLaughlin, Megan. "Secular and Spiritual Fatherhood in the Eleventh Century." In *Conflicted Identities and Multiple Masculinities: Men in the Medieval West*. Edited by Jacqueline Murray, 25–44. Routledge, 1999.

McLean, Teresa. *Medieval English Gardens*. Viking, 1981.

McQueen, Alison A. B. "Parliament, the Guardians and John Balliol, 1284–1296." In *Parliament and Politics in Scotland, 1235–1560*. Edited by Keith Brown and Roland J. Tanner, 29–49. Edinburgh University Press, 2004.

McQueen, Hector L. "'Regiam majestatem,' Scots Law, and National Identity." *Scottish Historical Review* 74, no. 197 (1995): 1–25.

Meale, Carol. "'…Alle the Bokes That I Haue of Latyn, Englisch, and Frensch': Laywomen and Their Books in Late Medieval England." In *Women and Literature in Britain 1150–1500*. Edited by Carol Meale, 128–58. 2nd ed. Cambridge University Press, 1996.

Meikle, Maureen. "The World of Women: Recent Medieval and Early Modern Publications." *The Innes Review* 45, no. 1 (1994): 71–77.

Menache, Sophia. "Chronicles and Historiography: The Interrelationship of Fact and Fiction." *Journal of Medieval History* 32, no. 4 (2006): 333–45.

——. "Isabella of France: A Postscript." *Revue belge de philologie et d'histoire* 90, no. 2 (2012): 493–512.

Meyer, Paul. "Notice du MS Sloan 1611 du Musée Britannique." *Romania* 40 (1911): 531–58.

Middlemass, Rachel, and Theresa Tyers. "Disabling Masculinity: Manhood and Infertility in the High Middle Ages." In *Social Dimensions of Medieval Disease and Disability*. Edited by Sally Crawford and Christina Lee, 47–58. Archaeopress, 2014.

Mielke, Christopher. "Doubly Crowned: The Public and Private Image of Two Fourteenth-Century Hungarian Queens." In *Ambiguous Women in Medieval Art*. Edited by Walker Vadillo and Monica Ann, 146–67. Trivent, 2019.

Miller, Peter. "The Mercat Cross of Edinburgh, from 1365 to 1617—Its Site and Form." *Proceedings of the Society of Antiquaries of Scotland* 20 (1886): 377–89.

Mistry, Zubin. "Ermentrude's Consecration (866): Queen-Making Rites and Biblical Templates for Carolingian Fertility." *Early Medieval Europe* 27, no. 4 (2019): 567–88.

Morrison, Susan. *Women Pilgrims in Late Medieval England: Private Piety as Public Performance*. Routledge, 2000.

Moss, Rachel E. *Fatherhood and Its Representations in Middle English Texts*. Boydell, 2013.

Neal, Derek. *The Masculine Self in Late Medieval England*. University of Chicago Press, 2008.

——. "What Can Historians Do with Clerical Masculinity? Lessons from Medieval Europe." In *Negotiating Clerical Identities: Priests, Monks and Masculinity in the Middle Ages*. Edited by Jennifer D. Thibodeaux, 16–36. Palgrave, 2010.

Nelson, Janet. "Early Medieval Rites of Queen-Making and the Shaping of Medieval Queenship." In *Queens and Queenship in Medieval Europe*. Edited by A. J. Duggan, 301–15. Boydell, 1997.

——. "Monks, Secular Men and Masculinity, c. 900." In *Masculinity in Medieval Europe. Edited by* D. M. Hadley, 121–42. Longman, 1999.

Nelson, Jessica. "Queens and Queenship in Scotland, circa 1067–1286." PhD diss., King's College University of London, 2006.

Neville, Cynthia J. "Making a Manly Impression: The image of Kingship on Scottish Royal Seals in the High Middle Ages." In *Nine Centuries of Man: Manhood and Masculinity in Scottish History*. Edited by Lynn Abrams and Elizabeth L. Ewan, 101–21. Edinburgh University Press, 2017.

Nutton, Vivian. "Medicine in the Greek World." In *The Western Medical Tradition: 800 BC to AD 1800*. Edited by Lawrence Conrad et al., 11–38. Cambridge University Press, 1995.

——. "Medieval Western Europe." In *The Western Medical Tradition: 800 BC to AD 1800*. Edited by Lawrence Conrad et al., 139–206. Cambridge University Press, 1995.

O'Boyle, Cornelius. *The Art of Medicine: Medical Teaching at the University of Paris, 1250–1400*. Brill, 1998.

Olson, Vibeke. "Blood, Sweat, Tears, and Milk: 'Fluid' Veneration, Sensory Contact, and Corporeal Presence in Medieval Devotional Art." In *Binding the Absent Body in Medieval and Modern Art: Abject, Virtual, and Alternate Bodies*. Edited by Emily Kelled, 11–30. Routledge, 2017.

Oram, Richard. *Alexander II: King of Scots, 1214–1249*. Birlinn, 2012.

——, ed. *The Kings and Queens of Scotland*. Stroud: Tempus, 2007.

Oren-Magidor, Daphna. *Infertility in Early Modern England*. Palgrave, 2017.

——. "Literate Laywomen, Male Medical Practitioners and the Treatment of Fertility Problems in Early Modern England." In *Infertility in Medieval and Early Modern Medicine*. Edited by Daphna Oren-Magidor and Catherine Rider. Special issue of *Social History of Medicine* 29, no. 2 (2016): 290–310.

——, and Catherine Rider eds. "Introduction: Infertility in Medieval and Early Modern Medicine." In "Infertility in Medieval and Early Modern Medicine," edited by Daphna Oren-Magidor and Catherine Rider, special issue *Social History of Medicine* 29, no. 2 (2016): 211–23.

Orme, Nicholas. *Medieval Children*. Yale University Press, 2003.

Ormrod, W. M. "Katherine Mortimer's Death at Soutra." In *SHARP Practice 4: Fourth Report on Researches into the Medieval Hospital at Soutra, Lothian/Borders Region, Scotland*. Edited by Brian Moffat, 110–20. Soutra Hospital Archaeoethnopharmacological Research Project, 1992.

——. "Monarchy, Martyrdom and Masculinity: England in the Later Middle Ages." In *Holiness and Masculinity in the Middle Ages*. Edited by P. H. Cullum and Katherine J. Lewis, 174–91. University of Wales Press, 2004.

——. "Personal Religion of Edward III." *Speculum* 64, no. 4 (October 1989): 849–77.

——. "The Sexualities of Edward II." In *The Reign of Edward II: New Perspectives*. Edited by Gwilym Dodd and Anthony Musson, 22–47. York Medieval, 2006.

Park, David and Robyn Pender. "Henry III's Wall Paintings of the Zodiac in the Lower Ward of Windsor Castle." In *Windsor: Medieval Archaeology, Art and Architecture of the Thames Valley*. Edited by Laurence Keen and Eileen Scarff, 125–31. British Archaeological Association, 2002.

Parsons, John Carmi. *Eleanor of Castile: Queen and Society in Thirteenth-Century England*. St. Martin's, 1995.

——. "Family, Sex and Power: The Rhythms of Medieval Queenship." In *Medieval Queenship*. Edited by John Carmi Parsons, 1–12. Palgrave, 1998.

——. "Intercessionary Patronage of Queen Margaret and Isabella of France." In *Thirteenth Century England VI: Proceedings of the Durham Conference, 1999*. Edited by Michael Prestwich et al., 81–97. Boydell, 1998.

——. "Mothers, Daughters, Marriage, Power: Some Plantagenet Evidence, 1150–1500." In *Medieval Queenship*. Edited by John Carmi Parsons, 63–78. Palgrave, 1998.

——. "The Pregnant Queen as Counsellor and the Medieval Construction of Motherhood." In *Medieval Mothering*. Edited by John Carmi Parsons and Bonnie Wheeler, 39–61. Garland, 1996.

——. "Ritual and Symbol in the English Medieval Queenship to 1500." In *Women and Sovereignty*. Edited by Louise O. Fradenburg, 60–77. Edinburgh University Press, 1992.

——. "The Year of Eleanor of Castile's Birth and Her Children by Edward I." *Medieval Studies* 46 (1984): 245–65.

Payan, Paul. "Paternité de Joseph et filiation du Christ: Variations autour d'un cas-limite (XIVe–début XVIe siècle)." In *Bâtards et bâtardises dans l'Europe médiévale et modern*. Edited by Carole Avignon, 383–92. Presses universitaires de Rennes, 2016.

Penman, Michael. "The Bruce Dynasty and Scottish Pilgrimage to Canterbury, c. 1178–c. 1404." *Journal of Medieval History* 32 (2006): 346–70.

——. "Christian Days and Knights: The Religious Devotions and Court of David II of Scotland, 1329–1371." *Historical Research* 75, no. 189 (August 2002): 249–71.

——. *David II, 1329–1371*. Tuckwell, 2004.

——. "Royal Piety in Thirteenth-Century Scotland: The Religion and Religiosity of Alexander II (1214–49) and Alexander III (1249–86)." In *Thirteenth-Century England XII: Proceedings of the Gregynog Conference, 2007*. Edited by Janet Burton et al., 13–30. Boydell, 2009.

Phillips, Kim. "The Breasts of Virgins: Sexual Reputation and Young Women's Bodies in Medieval Culture and Society." *Society, Culture and Social History* 15, no. 1 (2018): 1–19.

——. "Maidenhood as the Perfect Age of Woman's Life." In *Young Medieval Women*. Edited by Katherine J. Lewis et al., 1–24. St. Martin's, 1999.

——. *Medieval Maidens: Young Women and Gender in England, 1270–1540*. Manchester University Press, 2003.

Phillips, Seymour. *Edward II*. Yale University Press, 2010.

Pinner, Rebecca. *The Cult of St. Edmund in Medieval East Anglia*. Boydell, 2015.

Post, J. B. "Ages at Menarche and Menopause: Some Mediaeval Authorities." *Population Studies* 25, no. 1 (1971): 83–87.

Powell, Hilary. "The 'Miracle of Childbirth': The Portrayal of Parturient Women in Medieval Miracle Narratives." *Social History of Medicine* 25, no. 4 (2012): 795–811.

Prestwich, Michael. *Edward I, King of England*. Yale University Press, 1997.

Proctor-Tiffany, Mariah. "Transported as a Rare Object of Distinction: The Gift-Giving of Clémence of Hungary, Queen of France." *Journal of Medieval History* 41, no. 2 (2015): 1–21.

Rawcliffe, Carole. "'Delectable Sightes and Fragrant Smelles': Gardens and Health in Late Medieval and Early Modern England." *Garden History* 36, no. 1 (2008): 3–21.

——. *Medicine and Society in Later Medieval England*. Sutton, 1995.

Reid, Norman. *Alexander III, 1249–1286: First Among Equals*. John Donald, 2019.

——. "The Kingless Kingdom: The Scottish Guardianships of 1286–1306." *Scottish Historical Review* 61, no. 1 (1982): 105–29.

——, ed. *Scotland in the Reign of Alexander III 1249–1286*. John Donald, 1990.

——, and Michael Penman. "Guardian–Lieutenant–Governor: Absentee Monarchy and Proxy Power in Scotland's Long Fourteenth Century." In *Absentee Authority Across Medieval Europe*. Edited by Fréderique Lachaud and Michael Penman, 191–218. Boydell, 2017.

Richardson, Amanda. "Gender and Space in English Royal Palaces *c.* 1160–*c.* 1547: A Study in Access Analysis and Imagery." *Medieval Archaeology* 47 (2003): 131–65.

Rider, Catherine. "'A Defect of the Mind or Body': Impotence and Sexuality in Medieval Theology and Canon Law." In *The Ends of the Body*. Edited by Suzanne Conklin Akbari and Jill Ross, 193–210. University of Toronto Press, 2012.

——. "Gender, Old Age, and the Infertile Body in Medieval Medicine." In *Gender, Health, and Healing, 1250–1500*. Edited by Sara Ritchey and Sharon Strocchia, 267–88. Amsterdam University Press, 2020.

——. "Men and Infertility in Late Medieval English Medicine." *Social History of Medicine* 29, no. 2 (2016): 245–66.

——. "Men's Responses to Infertility in Late Medieval England." In *The Palgrave Handbook of Infertility in History*. Edited by Gayle Davis and Tracy Loughran, 273–90. Palgrave, 2017.

Roberts, Penny. "Sterility and Sovereignty: The Succession Crisis of the Late Valois Monarchy." In *The Palgrave Handbook of infertility in History*. Edited by Gayle Davis and Tracey Loughran, 151–69. Palgrave, 2017.

Rohr, Zita Eva. "Lessons for My Daughter: Self-Fashioning Stateswomanship in the Late Medieval Crown of Aragon." In *Self-Fashioning and Assumptions of Identity in Medieval and Early Modern Iberia*. Edited Laura Delbrugge, 46–78. Brill, 2014.

——, and Lisa Benz, eds. *Queenship, Gender, and Reputation in the Medieval and Early Modern West, 1060–1600*. Palgrave, 2016.

Romm, Aviva. "Pregnancy and Botanical Medicine: Use and Safety." In *Botanical Medicine for Women's Health*. Edited by Aviva Romm, 321–33. Churchill Livingstone, 2010.

Royan, Nicola. "Some Conspicuous Women in the *Original Chronicle, Scotichronicon* and *Scotorum Historia*." *Innes Review* 59, no. 2 (2008): 131–44.

Rubin, Miri. "A Decade of Studying Medieval Women, 1987–1997." *History Workshop Journal* 46 (1998): 213–39.

Sands, T. R. *The Company She Keeps: The Medieval Swedish Cult of Saint Katherine of Alexandria and Its Transformations*. Arizona Center for Medieval and Renaissance Studies, 2010.

Seabourne, Gwen. "'It is Necessary that the Issue Be Heard to Cry or Squall Within the Four [Walls]': Qualifying for Tenancy by the Curtesy of England in the Reign of Edward I." *The Journal of Legal History* 40, no. 1 (2019): 44–68.

Sears, Elizabeth. *The Ages of Man: Medieval Interpretations of the Life Cycle*. Princeton University Press, 1986.

Shahar, Shulamith. *Growing Old in the Middle Ages*. Routledge, 1997.

Sheingorn, Pamela. "Constructing the Patriarchal Parent: Fragments of the Biography of Joseph the Carpenter." In *Framing the Family: Narrative and Representation in the Medieval and Early Modern Periods*. Edited by Rosalynn Voaden and Diane Wolfthal, 161–80. Arizona Center for Medieval and Renaissance Studies, 2005.

Shenton, Caroline. "Phillippa of Hainault's Churchings: The Politics of Motherhood at the Court of Edward III." In *Family and Dynasty in Late Medieval England: Proceedings of the 1997 Harlaxton Symposium*. Edited by Richard Eales, 105–21. Tyas, 2003.

Simon, Anne. *The Cult of Saint Katherine of Alexandria in Late-Medieval Nuremberg: Saint and City*. Routledge, 2016.

Simpson, Andrew R. C. "The Scottish Common Law: Origins and Development, *c.* 1124–*c.* 1500." In *The Oxford Handbook of European Legal History*. Edited by Heikii Pihlajamäki et al., 451–74. Oxford University Press, 2018.

Slater, Laura. "Rumour and Reputation Management in Fourteenth-Century England: Isabella of France in Text and Image." *Journal of Medieval History* 47, no. 2 (2021): 257–92.

Smith, Julie Ann. "The Earliest Queen-Making Rites." *Church History* 66, no. 1 (1997): 18–35.

Smith, Kathryn A. *Art, Identity, and Devotion in Fourteenth-Century England: Three Women and Their Books of Hours*. University of Toronto Press, 2003.

Smith, Lisa. "La raillerie des femmes? Les femmes, la stérilité et la société en France à l'époque moderne." In *Femmes en fleurs: Santé, sexualité et génération du Moyen Âge aux Lumiéres*. Edited by Cathy McClive and Nicole Pellegrin, 203–20. Presses universitaires de Saint-Étienne, 2010.

Smith, Michelle Ann. "Assessing Gender in the Construction of Scottish Identity, *c.* 1286–*c.* 1586." PhD diss., University of Auckland, 2010.

Sotres, Pedro Gil. "The Regimens of Health." In *Western Medical Thought from Antiquity to the Middle Ages*. Edited by Mirko Grmek, 291–318. Harvard University Press, 1998.

Stafford, Pauline. "The King's Wife in Wessex 800–1066." *Past & Present* 91 (1981): 3–27.

——. "Powerful Women in the Early Middle Ages: Queens and Abbesses." In *The Medieval World*. Edited by Janet L. Nelson and P. Linehan, 398–415. Routledge, 2001.

——. *Queens, Concubines and Dowagers: The King's Wife in the Early Middle Ages*. University of Georgia Press, 1983.

——. *Queens, Concubines and Dowagers: The King's Wife in the Early Middle Ages*. 2nd ed. Leicester University Press, 1998.

Staniland, K. "The Nuptials of Alexander III of Scotland and Margaret Plantagenet." *Nottingham Medieval Studies* 30 (1986): 20–45.

Stephenson, Patricia. "Where a Cleric and Ælfgyva… ." In *The Bayeux Tapestry: New Approaches: Proceedings of a Conference at the British Museum*. Edited by Michael J. Lewis et al., 71–74. Oxbow, 2011.

Stringer, Keith J. "Kingship, Conflict and State-making in the Reign of Alexander: The Wars of 1215–17 and Their Context." In *The Reign of Alexander II*. Edited by Richard Oram, 99–156. Brill, 2005.

——. "The Scottish 'Political Community' in the Reign of Alexander II (1214–1249)." In *New Perspectives on Medieval Scotland, 1093–1286*. Edited by Matthew Hammond, 53–84. Boydell, 2013.

Strohm, Paul. *Hochon's Arrow: The Social Imagination of Fourteenth-Century Texts*. Princeton University Press, 1992.

Strohman, Anne-Marie. "'A More Natural Mother': Concepts of Maternity and Queenship in Early Modern England." PhD diss., University of Massachusetts, 2014.

Stuard, Susan Mosher, ed. *Women in Medieval History and Historiography*. University of Pennsylvania Press, 1987.

Swanson, R. N. "Angels Incarnate: Clergy and Masculinity from Gregorian Reform to Reformation." *Masculinity in Medieval Europe*. Edited by Dawn M. Hadley, 160–77. Longman, 1999.

Talbot, Charles H., and E. A Hammond. *The Medical Practitioners in Medieval England: A Biographical Register*. Wellcome Historical Medical Library, 1965.

Tanner, Heather J., et al. "Introduction." In *Medieval Elite Women and the Exercise of Power, 1100–1400: Moving Beyond the Exceptionalist Debate*. Edited by Heather J. Tanner, 1–18. Palgrave, 2019.

Taylor, Alice. *The Shape of the State in Medieval Scotland, 1124–1290*. Oxford University Press, 2016.

Tintinalli, Judith E., et al. *Tintinalli's Emergency Medicine: A Comprehensive Study Guide*. 9th ed. McGraw Hill, 2019.

Toepfer, Regina. *Infertility in Medieval and Early Modern Europe: Premodern Views on Childlessness.* Translated by Kate Sotejeff-Wilson. Palgrave, 2022.

———. *Negotiating Childlessness in the Middle Ages: Stories of Desired, Refused and Regretted Parenthood*. Translated by Kate Sotejeff-Wilson. Arc Humanities, 2025.

Toulalan, Sarah. "'Elderly Years Cause a Total Dispaire of Conception': Old Age, Sex and Infertility in Early Modern England." *Social History of Medicine* 29, no. 2 (2016): 333–59.

Trabut-Cussac, Jean-Paul. "Itinéraire d'Édouard I en France, 1286–1289." *Bulletin of the Institute of Historical Research* 25 (1952): 160–203.

Trease, G. E. "Spicers and Apothecaries of the Royal Household in the Reigns of Henry III, Edward I and Edward II." *Nottingham Medieval Studies* 3 (1959): 19–52.

Trivett, Emma. "'Because She Pretended to Be Pregnant and Was Not'" In *The Art of Illness: Malingering and Inventing Health Conditions*. Edited by Wendy J. Turner, 115–37. Routledge, 2023.

——. "Intercessor, Patron and Medical Authority?: Late Medieval Queenship and the Dietary of Queen Isabella." MSc thesis, University of Edinburgh, 2016.

Tyers, Theresa. "'In the Merry Month of May': Instructions for Ensuring Fertility in MS British Library, Lansdowne 380." *Social History of Medicine* 29, no. 2 (2016): 267–89.

——. "The Rebirth of Fertility: The Trotula and Her Travelling Companions c. 1200–1450." PhD diss., University of Nottingham, 2012.

Van Houts, Elisabeth. *Memory and Gender in Medieval Europe, 900–1200*. Palgrave, 1999.

Vauchez, Andre. *Sainthood in the Middle Ages*. Translated by Jean Birrell. Cambridge University Press, 1997.

Verskin, Sara. *Barren Women: Religion and Medicine in the Medieval Middle East*. De Gruyter, 2020.

Voigts, Linda E., and Ann Payne. "Medicine for a Great Household (*c*. 1500), Berkely Castle Muniments Select Book 89." In *Studies in Medieval and Renaissance History*. Edited by Cynthia Kosso and Anne Marie Scott, 87–251. 3rd ser. Vol. 12. AMS, 2016.

Walker Bynum, Caroline. "The Body of Christ in the Later Middle Ages: A Reply to Leo Steinberg." *Renaissance Quarterly* 39, no. 3 (Autumn 1986): 399–439.

——. *Jesus as Mother: Studies in the Spirituality of the High Middle Ages*. University of California Press, 1982.

Walsh, Christine. *The Cult of St. Katherine of Alexandria in Early Medieval Europe*. Ashgate, 2007.

——. "The Role of the Normans in the Development of the Cult of St. Katherine." In *St. Katherine of Alexandria: Texts and Contexts in Western Medieval Europe*. Edited by Katherine Lewis and Jacqueline Jenkins, 19–36. Brepols, 2013.

Ward, Emily. *Royal Childhood and Child Kingship: Boy Kings in England, Scotland, France and Germany, c. 1050–1262*. Cambridge University Press, 2022.

Warner, Kathryn. *Edward II: His Relationships and Sexuality*. Pen and Sword, 2024.

——. *Isabella of France: The Rebel Queen*. Amberley, 2016.

Watts, John. *Henry VI and the Politics of Kingship*. Cambridge University Press, 1996.

Webb, Diana. "Queen and Patron." In *Queens and Queenship in Medieval Europe: Proceedings of a Conference held at King's College London, April 1995*. Edited by Anne J. Duggan, 205–21. Boydell, 2008.

——. *Pilgrimage in Medieval England*. Bloomsbury, 2007.

Webster, Paul. "The Cult of St. Edmund, King and Martyr, and the Medieval Kings of England." *History* 105, no. 367 (2020): 636–51.

Weiler, Björn. "Matthew Paris and the Writing of History." *Journal of Medieval History* 35, no. 3 (September 2009): 254–78.

Weir, Alison. *Isabella, She-Wolf of France, Queen of England*. Random House, 2006.

Wickersheimer, Ernest. *Dictionnaire biographique des médecins en France au Moyen Âge*. 2 vols. Droz, 1936.

Williamson, Beth. "The Virgin *lactans* as Second Eve: Images of the *Salvatrix*." *Studies in Iconography* 10 (1998): 105–38.

Wogan-Browne, Jocelyn. "The Apple's Message: Some Post-Conquest Accounts of Hagiographic Textual Transmission." In *Late Medieval Religious Texts and Their Transmission*. Edited by Alastair Minnis, 39–51. Brewer, 1994.

——. *Saints' Lives and Women's Literary Culture, 1150–1300: Virginity and its Authorizations*. Oxford University Press, 2001.

——. "Women's Literary Culture in Twelfth- and Thirteenth-Century England." In *Saints' Lives and Women's Literary Culture, 1150–1300: Virginity and its Authorizations*. Edited by J. Wogan-Browne. Oxford University Press, 2001.

Woodacre, Elena. "Cousins & Queens: Family Ties, Political Ambition & Epistolary Diplomacy in Renaissance Europe." In *Women, Diplomacy and International Politics since 1500*. Edited by Glenda Sluga and Carolyn James, 30–45. Routledge, 2015.

——. "Ruling and Relationships: The Fundamental Basis of the Exercise of Power?" *Anuario de estudios medievales* 46, no. 1 (2016): 167–201.

Woolgar, Chris. *The Senses in Late Medieval England*. Yale University Press, 2006.

Youngs, Deborah. *The Life Cycle in Western Europe, c. 1300–c. 1500*. Manchester University Press, 2006.

INDEX

age, 1, 13, 20, 33, 35, 36, 41, 43, 44, 45, 51–59, 68, 72, 93, 97–98, 102, 120–29, 133–35, 153–55, 165–66, 174, 216, 218
  marriage, 8, 13, 51–52, 54–56, 58–59, 97, 112, 121–122, 125
  See also perfect age; consummation
Alexander II of Scotland, 57, 97, 102, 106–8, 112, 114–15, 116, 118–19, 127, 129, 208
  and Joan Plantagenet, 17, 54, 66, 68, 121–23, 150, 196, 204–5, 211
    See also Joan Plantagenet
  and Marie de Coucy, 1, 11, 66–71, 107, 208
    See also Marie de Coucy
  death of (1249), 12, 69
Alexander III of Scotland, 12, 30, 108, 166
  and Margaret of England, 9, 13, 20–21, 50, 55–57, 107, 125–26, 128, 133–34, 148, 207–9
    See also Margaret of England; *see also under* Matthew Paris
  and Yolande de Dreux, 9, 13–14, 83–84, 86, 92
    See also Yoland de Dreux
  death of (1286), 83–84, 86, 92
  minority of, 10
  See also succession, Scottish; Wars of Independence
Anglo-Scottish marriages, 11–14, 55–57, 68–69, 148, 208–9
Anglo-Scottish relations, 11, 194
  devotional unity through shared saints, 150, 207–9, 211
  political messaging through piety, 18, 103, 121, 186, 216–17
  Scottish royal interest in English saints and shrines, 18, 121, 196–97, 207–9, 211
apothecaries, 8, 146, 162
  John Adam, 162
  Odinet, 135–44, 147
    Odinet's medicines for Isabella of France, 131, 135–44
  Robert of Montpellier, 146
  See also physicians

Balmerino Abbey, Fife, 19, 106, 121–24, 204–5, 211
Battle of Neville's Cross (1346), 14, 103, 113, 160
Becket, Thomas, St., 77, 102–3, 106, 184, 193–97
  See also William of Canterbury
  See also under fertility: saints for
births, preparations for. *See* devotional practices for fertility and childbearing
Bower, Walter, 69, 74, 76–77, 79–80, 82–83, 104, 113, 163–64, 206
Bury St. Edmunds, 193, 198–200, 205, 207

childbearing, 49, 85, 89, 124–25, 132, 144, 153, 178–82, 198
  recorded vs. unrecorded pregnancies, 5–6, 72
  See also devotional practices for fertility and childbearing
childlessness, 28–31, 39
  historiographical focus on, 17–18
  vs. broader reproductive difficulties, 5, 18–22, 24, 37–38
  See also infertility; reproductive difficulties
children, sex of, 50, 57
  See also fertility

Chronicle of Bury St. Edmunds, 46, 49, 117–18, 200
Chronicle of Lanercost, 67–68, 83–86, 88, 92, 94, 113
Chronicle of Melrose, 50, 57, 66–68, 71, 194
chronicles, 46–50, 73–82
  emphasis on delayed conception in, 58–66
  recording practices, 46–49
  silences and omissions related to fertility, 49–50, 66–71
  See also individual chronicles and chroniclers
comparative methodology, 177
  eight royal couples, 8, 56, 124, 198
  English and Scottish patterns, 58, 97, 102, 106–7, 115
consummation, 13, 52–58, 107, 122, 125, 133–34, 148
  age at, 52–56, 58, 125

David II of Scotland, 14–17, 80–82, 112–14
  and Joan of the Tower, 14, 18, 54, 74–78, 102–3, 160, 191
    See also Joan of the Tower
  and Margaret Logie, 15, 78–79, 86–87, 90–91, 93–94, 103, 113, 162–63
    See also Margaret Logie
  capture and imprisonment, 15, 73–74, 80, 87, 102, 112, 160–61
  devotional practices, 102–6, 186, 191–92, 197–98
    See also devotional practices for fertility and childbearing
  relations with nephew, Robert the Steward, 15, 73–74, 106, 113, 163
De conferentibus et nocentibus, 155, 157–58
  See also Dietary of Queen Isabella
Despenser, Hugh. *See* Edward II
devotional practices for fertility and childbirth, 184–85, 211
  masses and prayers, 195
  offerings, votive, gold coins, and wax, 176, 184, 194–95
  visibility of, 181, 192, 195, 210
Dietary of Queen Isabella, 155, 157–58
  See also De conferentibus et nocentibus
dynastic connections. *See* Anglo-Scottish marriages

Edmund of Abingdon, St., 205–9
Edmund, king and martyr, St., 46, 99–100, 175, 184, 193, 198–201
Edward the Confessor, king, St., 19, 38, 97–102, 104, 126, 201–4, 211
  Scottish royal devotion to, 106, 121–23
  See also Balmerino Abbey
Edward I of England, 3, 9, 46, 48, 101, 108, 118–19
  and Eleanor of Castile, 4–5, 49–50, 54–55, 58, 115, 117, 134, 146
    See also Eleanor of Castile
  and Margaret of France, 4, 132–33, 148, 194, 201
    See also Margaret of France
  attitude toward replaceability of sons, 21
  fatherhood and historiography, 21
  minority of, 115–17, 128
Edward II of England, 5, 118
  and Isabella of France, 6–7, 58, 60–62, 64, 66, 72, 135–36, 146–47, 185, 195
    See also Isabella of France
  deposition, 7, 64–65
  relationship with Hugh Despenser, 6–7
  relationship with Piers Gaveston, 6, 62–63
Edward III of England, 7, 14–16, 34, 65, 74, 77, 160–62, 186, 197
Eleanor of Castile, 4, 16, 56, 72, 97, 128, 134–35, 147, 211, 216
  fecundity and historiographical emphasis, 20–21
  See also under Edward I
Eleanor of Provence, 16, 27, 56, 180–81, 192–93, 208–9, 211, 215–18
  accusations of sterility, 20
  suggestion of additional sons, 47–50
  See also under Henry III; Matthew Paris

fatherhood, 117–18, 177, 202–3
attitude of Edward I to, 21
neglect of, in historiography, 33–34
fertility, 43–44, 194
and kingship, 17–18, 25, 31–34, 110–15, 177, 216–17
as diplomacy, 56–57, 133, 148–50, 208–9
association with queens, 18, 27–31, 38–40, 66
See also individual queens
delayed conception. *See* reproductive difficulties
female reproductive body, 131–32, 135, 144, 173, 176–77, 179–80, 192, 212, 218
male reproductive body, 117, 155, 159, 174, 177, 212–13
prayers and masses for, 177, 195, 199, 201, 210–11
See also under devotional practices for fertility and childbearing
problems, in historiography, 35–38
See also historiography
saints for
demographic profiles of supplicants to, 191–92
Katherine of Alexandria, St., 188–91, 203
Margaret of Antioch, 177–82
Our Lady of Walsingham (shrine), 182–83
Thomas Becket, St., 193–94, 195, 201
See also individual saints
shared responsibility for, 66–67, 70–71, 173, 212–13, 216
visibility and public nature of, 46, 176
See also under devotional practices for fertility and childbearing
See also infertility; reproductive difficulties
Flores historiarum, 46–47, 49–50, 61, 63–66, 148
Fordun, John of, 68–69
Gesta annalia I, 68–69, 71
Gesta annalia II, 74–76, 78, 82

Gaveston, Piers. *See under* Edward II
gestation, length of, 92, 95, 216
Gray, Thomas, Sir, 80–82

heirs
birth of, 46, 57–58, 60–61, 66
female, 57–58
pressure to produce, 58–60, 194
significance of firstborn sons, 57, 117
Henry III of England, 11, 20–21, 27, 47, 55–57, 59, 66, 97–102, 106–8, 111–12, 117, 120, 126–28, 146, 172
and Eleanor of Provence, 2–4, 8, 11, 20, 46, 54, 66, 133, 145, 149–50, 152–55, 159, 165–68, 170, 173, 184, 187, 190, 194, 199, 201–2, 205
See also Eleanor of Provence
marriage of daughter Margaret to Alexander III, 11, 13, 55–56, 125
See also Alexander III of Scotland; Margaret of England
historiography
gender imbalance in analysis, 24–34
retrospective vs. contemporary perspectives, 16–21

illegitimate children, 63, 118–20
infant mortality. *See under* reproductive difficulties
infertility, 23–24, 44
definitions and terminology, 12, 23
perceptions of blame, 64–71, 76–82
secondary infertility, 23
subfertility, 24
visibility in sources, 43, 158
See also childlessness; reproductive difficulties: miscarriage; sterility
Isabella of France, 8, 16, 20, 56, 81, 97, 131, 135–44, 146, 155–58, 174, 211
deposition of Edward II, 7, 64–66, 216
reputation for successful fertility, 63–64, 71–72, 216
See also under Edward II

Joan of the Tower, 8, 74–78, 80–81, 124, 211
See also David II of Scotland
Joan Plantagenet, 18–19, 68–71, 107, 121–24, 150–51, 193, 197, 211
See also Alexander II of Scotland

Katherine of Alexandria, St., 126, 187, 191
devotional images, 190, 203
kingship. *See* masculinity; perfect age: of kings

Liber Pluscardensis, 74, 77–78, 80, 82–83, 86–88, 91, 93–94, 113

maidenhood. *See under* perfect age
Margaret Drummond. *See* Margaret Logie
Margaret Logie, 210, 215–16
divorce from David II, 162, 165
fake pregnancy claim, 86–95
marriage to David II. *See under* David II
Margaret of Antioch, St.,
devotional images, 180–82
protection in childbirth, 179–80, 182
Margaret of England, 3, 21, 46, 55–56, 133–34, 148, 173, 181–82, 211
and firstborn daughter, 10, 13–14, 50, 56–58
See also under Alexander III
Margaret of France, 4, 132–33, 148, 195, 200, 211
See also under Edward I
Marie de Coucy, 66–68
and Alexander II, 11, 69–70, 208
birth of Alexander III, 11
See also under Alexander II
marriage
separation of, 18, 75, 78, 80, 86–87, 90
See also age; consummation; Anglo-Scottish marriages
masculinity, 25–26, 31–34, 39–40, 65, 91, 98, 108–18, 120, 127, 159, 172–74, 203–4, 217–18
Matthew Paris, 46–48, 116–17, 150, 181–82, 194, 206–7
La estoire de Seint Aedward le rei, 100–101
on Eleanor of Provence, 3, 20, 58–60, 66, 97–98, 151, 192, 215–16
on Margaret of England and Alexander III's marriage, 55–56, 125
medical theory and practice, 32–33, 36–37, 44, 165–73
Aristotelian and Galenic models, 37, 43–44, 149
Ars medicinae, 44, 139, 143
colour
and fertility, 170–72
in humoral theory, 170–72
gardens and healthcare, 165–70
gender, theories of, 44–45, 124–25
humoral theory, 153–54, 165–67
See also under medical theory and practice: colour
Regimen sanitatis, 131, 144, 151–58, 172, 174
Trotula, 53, 138–44
two-seed model for conception, 43–44
See also fertility: female reproductive body; fertility: male reproductive body; menstruation; sterility. *See also under* apothecaries; physicians
menstruation, 44, 121, 141
miscarriage. *See under* reproductive difficulties
Monan, St., 104, 164
St. Monans (places), 104

Orygnale Cronykil. *See* Wyntoun, Andrew of
Our Lady of Walsingham (shrine), 182–85
fertility association with. *See under* fertility: saints for

patronage, religious, 7, 99
as political role, 175–77, 201
established patterns, 185, 192–96
new practices, 102, 107, 201–9
See also piety
perfect age, 53, 97, 107–17, 120–28, 159
of kings, 107–17
of maidenhood, 123–24

physicians (*individual physicians*)
Aldobrandino of Siena, 144, 151–55, 158, 174, 180
Arnald de Villanova, 155–58
Donald Bannerman, 162
Hector Beaton, 161–62
John of Fountains, 132, 148
John of Newcastle, 162
John of St. Giles, 150–51
Jordan of Canterbury, 162
Luke Matheu de Perrers, 148
Michael Scot, 149
Nicholas of Farnham, 133, 206
Nicholas of Menona, 147
Patrick of Carlisle, 150
Peter de Alpibus, 145
Ralph de Neketon, 146, 150
Raymond de Bariamondo, 145
Reginald of Bath, 133, 146, 148
Roger de Eyton, 160
Theobald de Troyes, 146–47
Thomas de Hall, 162
William of Bolton, 160
William of Provence, 145, 158
See also individual names under apothecaries
piety, 97–108, 175–77, 192–98, 200, 210, 216
See also individual saints; devotional practices for fertility and childbearing; pilgrimage
pilgrimage, 11, 66, 68–70, 77–78, 102, 104, 106, 151, 175–76, 182–90, 193, 197–99
See also David II: devotional practices; devotional practices for fertility and childbearing; fertility: prayers and masses for
pregnancy, 166–67
fake, 83–95
loss of. *See under* reproductive difficulties
prayers and masses for. *See under* devotional practices for fertility and childbearing; fertility; Margaret of Antioch, St.

queenship, 16–22, 24–31, 33, 40, 65, 94, 145–58, 173, 216
See fertility; historiography; individual queens

reproduction
anxieties about, 56–58, 66, 100, 217
contemporary vs. retrospective views, 1, 3–4, 20, 30
royal. *See under* fertility
reproductive bodies. *See* fertility
reproductive difficulties
birth intervals, 8
delayed conception, 8, 13–14, 20, 24, 51, 55, 64, 97–98
infant mortality, 5–6
miscarriage, 8, 136
stillbirth, 5, 54–55, 136
Robert the Steward, 16, 73–74, 87, 91, 114
See also David II

Scalacronica. See Gray, Thomas.
Scotichronicon. See Bower, Walter
sterility, 35, 125–26, 132, 141–42, 154, 171, 178, 188–92, 198
See also childlessness; infertility; medical theory; reproductive difficulties
succession, Scottish, 9–11
See also Alexander III; David II; heirs: birth of
succession-peace deals, 15–16, 77, 105, 162–63, 186

Wars of Independence, 4, 9–10
William of Canterbury, *Miracles of St. Thomas*, 198
Wyntoun, Andrew of, 69–70, 75–78, 113

Yolande de Dreux, 83–86
See also under Alexander III

Printed in the United States
by Baker & Taylor Publisher Services